ECG Strip Ease

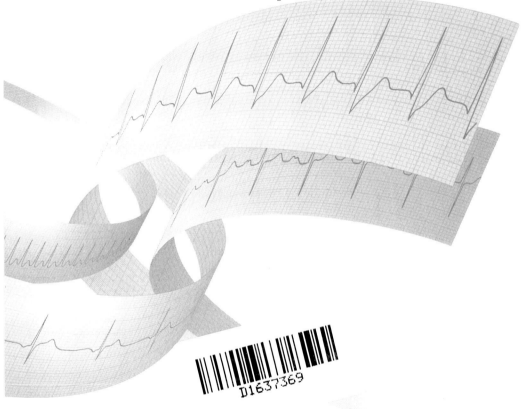

ECG Strip Ease

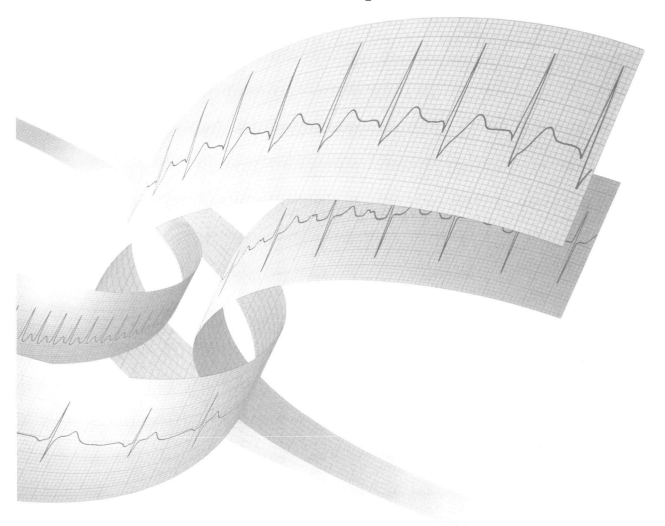

Wolters Kluwer | Lippincott Williams & Wilkins
Health

Philadelphia • Baltimore • New York • London
Buenos Aires • Hong Kong • Sydney • Tokyo

Staff

Executive Publisher
Judith A. Schilling McCann, RN, MSN

Editorial Director
David Moreau

Clinical Director
Joan M. Robinson, RN, MSN

Art Director
Mary Ludwicki

Senior Managing Editor
Jaime Stockslager Buss, MSPH, ELS

Clinical Manager
Collette Bishop Hendler, RN, BS, CCRN

Clinical Project Managers
Mary Perrong, RN, MSN, CRNP; Kate Stout, RN, MSN, CCRN

Editor
Beth Wegerbauer

Clinical Editor
Carol Knauff, RN, MSN, CCRN

Copy Editors
Kimberly Bilotta (supervisor), Amy Furman, Shana Harrington, Dorothy P. Terry, Pamela Wingrod

Designer
Lynn Foulk

Digital Composition Services
Diane Paluba (manager), Joyce Rossi Biletz, Donna S. Morris (project manager)

Associate Manufacturing Manager
Beth J. Welsh

Editorial Assistants
Megan L. Aldinger, Karen J. Kirk, Linda K. Ruhf

Design Assistant
Georg W. Purvis IV

Indexer
Barbara Hodgson

Library of Congress Cataloging-in-Publication Data

ECG strip ease.
    p. ; cm.
  Includes bibliographical references and index.
  1. Electrocardiography. 2. Cardiovascular diseases—Nursing. I. Lippincott Williams & Wilkins.
  [DNLM: 1. Electrocardiography—Nurses' Instruction. WG 140 E176 2007]
RC683.5.E5E2565 2007
616.1'207547—dc22
ISBN13: 978-1-58255-558-4 (alk. paper)
ISBN10: 1-58255-558-3 (alk. paper)   2006033579

■ CONTENTS

Helen C. Ballestas, RN, MSN, CRRN, PhD[C]
Nurse Educator
New York Institute of Technology
Old Westbury

Nancy J. Bekken, RN, MS, CCRN
Staff Educator, Adult Critical Care
Spectrum Health
Grand Rapids, Mich.

James S. Davis IV, RN, BSN
Clinical Leader, Medical Intensive Care
Abington (Pa.) Memorial Hospital

Kathleen M. Hill, RN, MSN, CCNS, CSC
Clinical Nurse Specialist
Cardiothoracic Intensive Care Units
The Cleveland Clinic Foundation

Cheryl Kline, RN, MSN, BC
Coordinator Education Services
St. Luke's Quakertown (Pa.) Hospital

Carol A. Knauff, RN, MSN, CCRN
Clinical Educator
Grand View Hospital
Sellersville, Pa.

Theresa M. Leonard, RN, BSN, CCRN
Unit Educator
Stony Brook (N.Y.) University Hospital

Deborah Murphy, RN, MSN, CRNP
Stroke Program Research Coordinator
Abington (Pa.) Memorial Hospital

Nancy M. Richards, RN, MSN, CCNS, CCRN
Cardiovascular Surgery Clinical Nurse Specialist
Mid America Heart Institute of Saint Luke's Hospital
Kansas City, Mo.

Cardiac anatomy and physiology

Correct electrocardiogram (ECG) interpretation provides an important challenge to any practitioner. With a good understanding of ECGs, you'll be better able to provide expert care to your patients. For example, when you're caring for a patient with an arrhythmia or a myocardial infarction, an ECG waveform can help you quickly assess his condition and, if necessary, begin lifesaving interventions.

To build ECG skills, begin with the basics covered in this chapter—an overview of the heart's anatomy and physiology and electrical conduction system.

Cardiac anatomy

The heart is a hollow, muscular organ that works like a mechanical pump. It delivers oxygenated blood to the body through the arteries. When blood returns through the veins, the heart pumps it to the lungs to be reoxygenated.

▨ Location and structure

The heart lies obliquely in the chest, behind the sternum in the mediastinal cavity, or mediastinum. It's located between the lungs, in front of the spine. The top of the heart, called the *base*, lies just below the second rib. The bottom of the heart, called the *apex*, tilts forward and down toward the left side of the body and rests on the diaphragm. (See *Location of the heart*, page 2.)

The heart varies in size, depending on the person's body size, but is roughly 5″ (12.5 cm) long and 3½″ (9 cm) wide, or about the size of the person's fist. The heart's weight, typically 9 to 12 oz (255 to 340 g), varies depending on the individual's size, age, gender, and athletic conditioning. An athlete's heart usually weighs more than average, whereas an elderly person's heart weighs less.

Life span considerations

An infant's heart is positioned more horizontally in the chest cavity than an adult's. As a result, the apex is positioned at the fourth left intercostal space. Until age 4, a child's apical impulse is left of the midclavicular line. By age 7, his heart is located in the same position as an adult's heart is.

As a person ages, his heart usually becomes slightly smaller and loses its contractile strength and efficiency. In people with hypertension, a moderate increase in left ventricular wall thickness may occur. As the myocardium of the aging heart becomes more irritable, extra systoles may occur, along with sinus arrhythmias and sinus bradycardia. In addition, increased fibrous tissue infiltrates the sinoatrial (SA) node and internodal atrial tracts, which may cause atrial fibrillation and flutter.

By age 70, cardiac output at rest has diminished by 30% to 35% in many people.

▨ Heart wall

The heart wall, which encases the heart, is made up of three layers: the epicardium, myocardium, and endocardium. The epicardium, the outermost layer, consists

Location of the heart

The heart lies within the mediastinum, a cavity that contains the tissues and organs separating the two pleural sacs. In most people, two-thirds of the heart extends to the left of the body's midline.

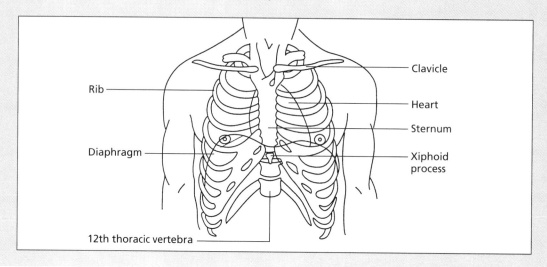

Rib

Diaphragm

12th thoracic vertebra

Clavicle

Heart

Sternum

Xiphoid process

of squamous epithelial cells overlying connective tissue. The myocardium, the middle and thickest layer, makes up the largest portion of the heart's wall. This layer of muscle tissue contracts with each heartbeat. The endocardium, the heart wall's innermost layer, consists of a thin layer of endothelial tissue that lines the heart valves and chambers. (See *Layers of the heart wall.*)

The pericardium is a fluid-filled sac that envelops the heart and acts as a tough, protective covering. It consists of the fibrous pericardium and the serous pericardium. The fibrous pericardium is composed of tough, white, fibrous tissue, which fits loosely around the heart and protects it. The serous pericardium, the thin, smooth, inner portion, has two layers:
- parietal layer, which lines the inside of the fibrous pericardium
- visceral layer, which adheres to the surface of the heart.

The pericardial space separates the visceral and parietal layers and contains 10 to 30 ml of thin, clear pericardial fluid, which lubricates the two surfaces and cushions the heart. Excess pericardial fluid, a condition called *pericardial effusion,* can compromise the heart's ability to pump blood.

Heart chambers

The heart contains four chambers—two atria and two ventricles. (See *Inside a normal heart,* page 4.) The right atrium lies in front of and to the right of the smaller but thicker-walled left atrium. An interatrial septum separates the two chambers and helps them contract. The right and left atria serve as volume reservoirs for blood being sent into the ventricles. The right atrium receives deoxygenated blood returning from the body through the inferior and superior venae cavae and from the heart through the coronary sinus. The left atrium receives oxygenated blood from the lungs through the four pulmonary veins.

The right and left ventricles serve as the pumping chambers of the heart. The right ventricle lies behind the sternum and forms the largest part of the heart's sternocostal surface and inferior border. The right ventricle receives deoxygenated blood from the right atrium and pumps it through the pulmonary arteries to the lungs, where it's reoxygenated. The left ventricle forms the heart's apex, most of its left border, and most of its posterior and diaphragmatic surfaces. The left ventricle receives oxygenated blood from the left atrium and pumps it through the aorta into the systemic circulation. The interventricular septum separates the ventricles and helps them pump.

The thickness of a chamber's walls is determined by the amount of pressure needed to eject its blood. Because the atria act as reservoirs for the ventricles and pump the blood a shorter distance, their walls are considerably thinner than the walls of the ventricles. Likewise, the left ventricle has a much thicker wall than the right ventricle because the left ventricle pumps blood against the higher

Layers of the heart wall

This cross section of the heart wall shows its various layers.

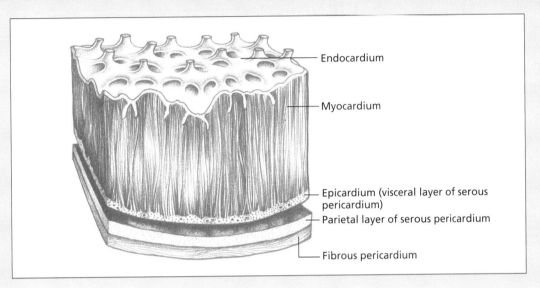

- Endocardium
- Myocardium
- Epicardium (visceral layer of serous pericardium)
- Parietal layer of serous pericardium
- Fibrous pericardium

pressures in the aorta. The right ventricle pumps blood against the lower pressures in the pulmonary circulation.

Heart valves

The heart contains four valves—two atrioventricular (AV) valves (tricuspid and mitral) and two semilunar valves (aortic and pulmonic). Each valve consists of cusps, or leaflets, that open and close in response to pressure changes within the chambers they connect. The primary function of the valves is to keep blood flowing forward through the heart. When the valves close, they prevent backflow, or regurgitation, of blood from one chamber to another. Closure of the valves is associated with heart sounds.

AV valves

The two AV valves are located between the atria and ventricles. The tricuspid valve, named for its three cusps, separates the right atrium from the right ventricle. The mitral valve, sometimes referred to as the bicuspid valve because of its two cusps, separates the left atrium from the left ventricle. Closure of the AV valves is associated with S_1, or the first heart sound.

The cusps of these valves are anchored to the papillary muscles of the ventricles by small tendinous cords called *chordae tendineae*. During ventricular contraction, the

papillary muscles and chordae tendineae work together to prevent the cusps from bulging backward into the atria. Disruption of either structure may prevent complete valve closure, allowing blood to flow backward into the atria. This backward blood flow may cause a heart murmur.

Semilunar valves

The semilunar valves are so called because their three cusps resemble half moons. The pulmonic valve, located where the pulmonary artery meets the right ventricle, permits blood to flow from the right ventricle to the pulmonary artery and prevents backflow into the right ventricle. The aortic valve, located where the left ventricle meets the aorta, allows blood to flow from the left ventricle to the aorta and prevents blood backflow into the left ventricle.

Increased pressure within the ventricles during ventricular systole causes the pulmonic and aortic valves to open, allowing ejection of blood into the pulmonary and systemic circulation. Loss of pressure as the ventricular chambers empty causes the valves to close. Closure of the semilunar valves is associated with S_2, or the second heart sound.

Inside a normal heart

This cross section shows the internal structure of a normal heart.

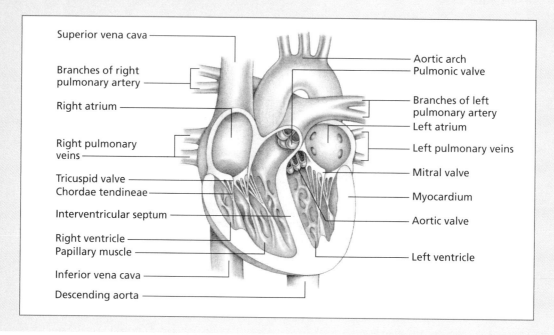

Superior vena cava

Branches of right pulmonary artery

Right atrium

Right pulmonary veins

Tricuspid valve
Chordae tendineae

Interventricular septum

Right ventricle
Papillary muscle

Inferior vena cava

Descending aorta

Aortic arch
Pulmonic valve

Branches of left pulmonary artery

Left atrium

Left pulmonary veins

Mitral valve

Myocardium

Aortic valve

Left ventricle

▉ Blood flow through the heart

Understanding the flow of blood through the heart is critical for understanding the overall functions of the heart and the way that changes in electrical activity affect peripheral blood flow. It's also important to remember that right- and left-sided heart events occur simultaneously.

Deoxygenated blood from the body returns to the heart through the inferior vena cava, superior vena cava, and coronary sinus and empties into the right atrium. The increasing volume of blood in the right atrium raises the pressure in that chamber above the pressure in the right ventricle. Then the tricuspid valve opens, allowing blood to flow into the right ventricle.

The right ventricle pumps blood through the pulmonic valve into the pulmonary arteries and lungs, where oxygen is picked up and excess carbon dioxide is released. From the lungs, the oxygenated blood flows through the pulmonary veins and into the left atrium. This completes a circuit called *pulmonic circulation.*

As the volume of blood in the left atrium increases, the pressure in the left atrium exceeds the pressure in the left ventricle. The mitral valve opens, allowing blood to flow into the left ventricle. The ventricle contracts and

ejects the blood through the aortic valve into the aorta. The blood is distributed throughout the body, releasing oxygen to the cells and picking up carbon dioxide. Blood then returns to the right atrium through the veins, completing a circuit called *systemic circulation.*

▉ Coronary blood supply

Like the brain and all other organs, the heart needs an adequate supply of oxygenated blood to survive. The main coronary arteries lie on the surface of the heart, with smaller arterial branches penetrating the surface into the cardiac muscle mass. The heart receives its blood supply almost entirely through these arteries. In fact, only a small percentage of the heart's endocardial surface can obtain sufficient amounts of nutrition directly from the blood in the cardiac chambers. (See *Vessels that supply the heart.*)

Understanding coronary blood flow can help you provide better care to a patient with coronary artery disease because you'll be able to predict which areas of the heart would be affected by a narrowing or occlusion of a particular coronary artery.

Vessels that supply the heart

The coronary circulation involves the arterial system of blood vessels, which supplies oxygenated blood to the heart, and the venous system, which removes oxygen-depleted blood from the heart.

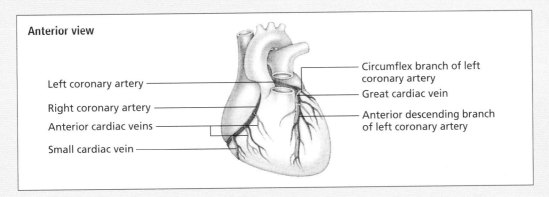

Anterior view

Left coronary artery

Right coronary artery

Anterior cardiac veins

Small cardiac vein

Circumflex branch of left coronary artery

Great cardiac vein

Anterior descending branch of left coronary artery

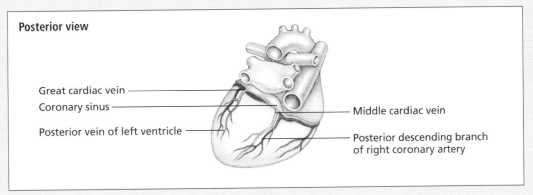

Posterior view

Great cardiac vein

Coronary sinus

Posterior vein of left ventricle

Middle cardiac vein

Posterior descending branch of right coronary artery

Coronary arteries

The left main and right coronary arteries arise from the coronary ostia, small orifices located just above the aortic valve cusps. The right coronary artery fills the groove between the atria and ventricles, giving rise to the acute marginal artery and ending as the posterior descending artery. The right coronary artery supplies blood to the right atrium, the right ventricle, and the inferior wall of the left ventricle. This artery also supplies blood to the SA node in about 50% of the population and to the AV node in 90% of the population. The posterior descending artery supplies the posterior wall of the left ventricle in 80% to 90% of the population.

The left main coronary artery varies in length from a few millimeters to a few centimeters. It splits into two major branches, the left anterior descending artery (also known as the *interventricular artery*) and the left circumflex artery. The left anterior descending artery runs down the anterior surface of the heart toward the apex. This ar-

tery and its branches—the diagonal arteries and the septal perforators—supply blood to the anterior wall of the left ventricle, the anterior interventricular septum, the bundle of His, the right bundle branch, and the anterior fasciculus of the left bundle branch.

The circumflex artery circles the left ventricle, ending on its posterior surface. The obtuse marginal artery arises from the circumflex artery. The circumflex artery provides oxygenated blood to the lateral wall of the left ventricle, the left atrium, the posterior wall of the left ventricle in 10% of the population, and the posterior fasciculus of the left bundle branch. In about 50% of the population, it supplies the SA node; in about 10% of the population, the AV node.

In most of the population, the right coronary artery is the dominant vessel, meaning that the right coronary artery supplies the posterior wall via the posterior descending artery. This system is described as *right coronary dominance* or a *dominant right coronary artery*. Likewise, patients in whom the left coronary artery supplies the posterior wall via the posterior descending artery, the terms *left coronary dominance* or *dominant left coronary artery* are used.

When two or more arteries supply the same region, they usually connect through anastomoses, junctions that provide alternative routes of blood flow. This network of smaller arteries, called *collateral circulation,* provides blood to capillaries that directly feed the heart muscle. Collateral circulation becomes so strong in many patients that even if major coronary arteries become narrowed with plaque, collateral circulation can continue to supply blood to the heart.

Coronary artery blood flow

In contrast to the other vascular beds in the body, the heart receives its blood supply primarily during ventricular relaxation, or diastole, when the left ventricle is filling with blood. This effect results because the coronary ostia lie near the aortic valve and become partially occluded when the aortic valve opens during ventricular contraction or systole. However, when the aortic valve closes, the ostia are unobstructed, allowing blood to fill the coronary arteries. Because diastole is the time when the coronary arteries receive their blood supply, anything that shortens diastole, such as periods of increased heart rate or tachycardia, also decreases coronary blood flow.

In addition, the left ventricular muscle compresses the intramuscular vessels during systole. During diastole, the cardiac muscle relaxes, and blood flow through the left ventricular capillaries is no longer obstructed.

Cardiac veins

Similar to other parts of the body, the heart has its own veins, which remove oxygen-depleted blood from the myocardium. About 75% of the total coronary venous blood flow leaves the left ventricle by way of the coronary sinus, an enlarged vessel that returns blood to the right atrium. Most of the venous blood from the right ventricle flows directly into the right atrium through the small anterior cardiac veins, not by way of the coronary sinus. A small amount of coronary blood flows back into the heart through the thebesian veins, minute veins that empty directly into all chambers of the heart.

Cardiac physiology

In this section, you'll find descriptions of the cardiac cycle, cardiac muscle innervation, depolarization and repolarization, and normal and abnormal impulse conduction.

Cardiac cycle

The cardiac cycle includes the cardiac events that occur from the beginning of one heartbeat to the beginning of the next. The cardiac cycle consists of ventricular diastole, or relaxation, and ventricular systole, or contraction. During ventricular diastole, blood flows from the atria through the open tricuspid and mitral valves into the relaxed ventricles. The aortic and pulmonic valves are closed during ventricular diastole. (See *Phases of the cardiac cycle.*)

During diastole, about 75% of the blood flows passively from the atria through the open tricuspid and mitral valves and into the ventricles even before the atria contract. Atrial contraction—or *atrial kick,* as it's sometimes called—contributes another 25% to ventricular filling. Loss of effective atrial contraction occurs with some arrhythmias such as atrial fibrillation. This loss results in a reduction in cardiac output.

During ventricular systole, the mitral and tricuspid valves are closed as the relaxed atria fill with blood. As ventricular pressure rises, the aortic and pulmonic valves open. The ventricles contract, and blood is ejected into the pulmonic and systemic circulation.

Cardiac output

Cardiac output is the amount of blood the left ventricle pumps into the aorta per minute. Cardiac output is measured by multiplying heart rate times stroke volume. Stroke volume refers to the amount of blood ejected with each ventricular contraction and is usually about 70 ml.

Normal cardiac output is 4 to 8 L/minute. The heart pumps only as much blood as the body requires, based on metabolic requirements. During exercise, for example, the heart increases cardiac output accordingly.

Three factors determine stroke volume: preload, afterload, and myocardial contractility. (See *Preload and afterload,* page 8.) Preload is the degree of stretch, or tension, on the muscle fibers when they begin to contract. It's usually considered to be the end-diastolic pressure when the ventricle has filled.

Afterload is the load (or amount of pressure) the left ventricle must work against to eject blood during systole and corresponds to the systolic pressure. The greater this resistance is, the greater the heart's workload. Afterload is also called *systemic vascular resistance.*

Myocardial contractility is the ventricle's ability to contract, which is determined by the degree of muscle fiber stretch at the end of diastole. The more the muscle fibers stretch during ventricular filling, up to an optimal length, the more forceful the contraction.

Phases of the cardiac cycle

The cardiac cycle consists of these phases:

1. Isovolumetric ventricular contraction—In response to ventricular depolarization, tension in the ventricles increases. The rise in pressure within the ventricles leads to closure of the mitral and tricuspid valves. The pulmonic and aortic valves stay closed during the entire phase.

2. Ventricular ejection—When ventricular pressure exceeds aortic and pulmonary artery pressures, the aortic and pulmonic valves open and the ventricles eject blood.

3. Isovolumetric relaxation—When ventricular pressure falls below the pressures in the aorta and pulmonary artery, the aortic and pulmonic valves close. All valves are closed during this phase. Atrial diastole occurs as blood fills the atria.

4. Ventricular filling—Atrial pressure exceeds ventricular pressure, which causes the mitral and tricuspid valves to open. Blood then flows passively into the ventricles. About 75% of ventricular filling takes place during this phase.

5. Atrial systole—Known as the *atrial kick,* atrial systole (coinciding with late ventricular diastole) supplies the ventricles with the remaining 25% of the blood for each heartbeat.

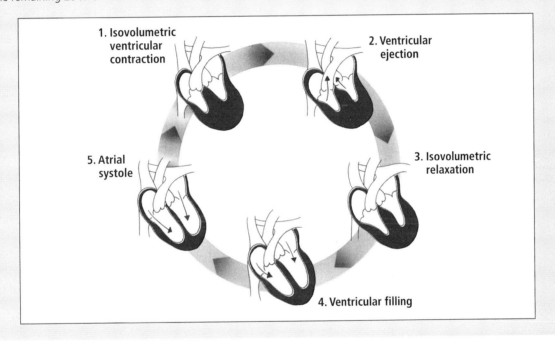

◼ Autonomic innervation of the heart

The two branches of the autonomic nervous system—the sympathetic (or adrenergic) nervous system and the parasympathetic (or cholinergic) nervous system—abundantly supply the heart. Sympathetic fibers innervate all the areas of the heart, whereas parasympathetic fibers primarily innervate the SA and AV nodes.

Sympathetic nerve stimulation causes the release of norepinephrine, which increases the heart rate by increasing SA node discharge, accelerates AV node conduction time, and increases the force of myocardial contraction and cardiac output.

Parasympathetic (vagal) stimulation causes the release of acetylcholine, which produces the opposite effects. The rate of SA node discharge is decreased, thus slowing heart rate and conduction through the AV node and reducing cardiac output.

◼ Transmission of electrical impulses

For the heart to contract and pump blood to the rest of the body, an electrical stimulus needs to occur first. Generation and transmission of electrical impulses depend on the four key characteristics of cardiac cells: automaticity, excitability, conductivity, and contractility.

Preload and afterload

Preload refers to a passive stretching that blood exerts on the ventricular muscle fibers at the end of diastole. According to Starling's law, the more the cardiac muscles are stretched in diastole, the more forcefully they contract in systole.

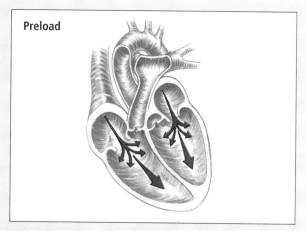

Preload

Afterload refers to the pressure that the ventricles need to generate to overcome higher pressure in the aorta to eject blood into the systemic circulation. This systemic vascular resistance corresponds to the systemic systolic pressure.

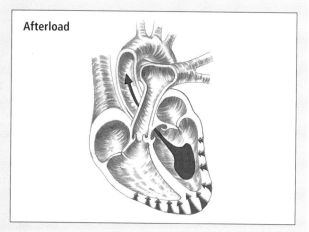

Afterload

Automaticity refers to a cell's ability to spontaneously initiate an electrical impulse. Pacemaker cells usually possess this ability. Excitability results from ion shifts across the cell membrane and refers to the cell's ability to respond to an electrical stimulus. Conductivity is the ability of a cell to transmit an electrical impulse from one cell to another. Contractility refers to the cell's ability to contract after receiving a stimulus by shortening and lengthening its muscle fibers.

It's important to remember that the first three characteristics are electrical properties of the cells, whereas contractility represents a mechanical response to the electrical activity. Of the four characteristics, automaticity has the greatest effect on the genesis of cardiac rhythms.

Depolarization and repolarization

As impulses are transmitted, cardiac cells undergo cycles of depolarization and repolarization. (See *Depolarization-repolarization cycle.*) Cardiac cells at rest are considered polarized, meaning that no electrical activity takes place. Cell membranes separate different concentrations of ions, such as sodium and potassium, and create a more negative charge inside the cell. This phenomenon is called the *resting potential.* After a stimulus occurs, ions cross the cell membrane and cause an action potential, or cell depolarization. When a cell is fully depolarized, it attempts to return to its resting state in a process called *repolarization.* Electrical charges in the cell reverse and return to normal.

A cycle of depolarization-repolarization consists of five phases—0 through 4. The action potential is represented by a curve that shows voltage changes during the five phases. (See *Action potential curves,* page 10.)

- During phase 0 (or rapid depolarization), the cell receives a stimulus, usually from a neighboring cell. The cell becomes more permeable to sodium, the inside of the cell becomes less negative, the cell is depolarized, and myocardial contraction occurs. In phase 1 (or early repolarization), sodium stops flowing into the cell, and the transmembrane potential falls slightly. Phase 2 (the plateau phase) is a prolonged period of slow repolarization, when little change occurs in the cell's transmembrane potential.
- During phases 1 and 2 and at the beginning of phase 3, the cardiac cell is said to be in its absolute refractory period. During that period, no stimulus—no matter how strong—can excite the cell.
- Phase 3 (or rapid repolarization) occurs as the cell returns to its original state. During the last half of this phase, when the cell is in its relative refractory period, a strong stimulus can depolarize it.
- Phase 4 is the resting phase of the action potential. By the end of phase 4, the cell is ready for another stimulus.

Electrical activity of the heart is represented on an ECG. Keep in mind that the ECG represents only electrical activity, not the mechanical activity or actual pumping of the heart.

Depolarization-repolarization cycle

The depolarization-repolarization cycle consists of these phases.

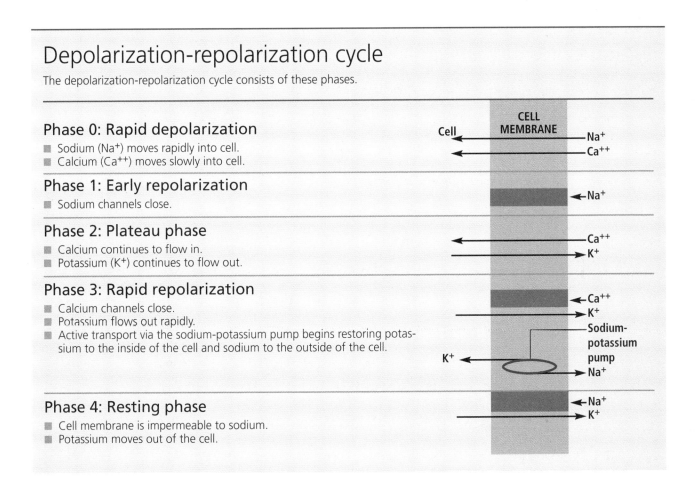

Phase 0: Rapid depolarization

- Sodium (Na^+) moves rapidly into cell.
- Calcium (Ca^{++}) moves slowly into cell.

Phase 1: Early repolarization

- Sodium channels close.

Phase 2: Plateau phase

- Calcium continues to flow in.
- Potassium (K^+) continues to flow out.

Phase 3: Rapid repolarization

- Calcium channels close.
- Potassium flows out rapidly.
- Active transport via the sodium-potassium pump begins restoring potassium to the inside of the cell and sodium to the outside of the cell.

Phase 4: Resting phase

- Cell membrane is impermeable to sodium.
- Potassium moves out of the cell.

■ Electrical conduction system of the heart

After depolarization and repolarization occur, the resulting electrical impulse travels through the heart along a pathway called the *conduction system*. (See *Cardiac conduction system*, page 11.)

Impulses travel out from the SA node and through the internodal tracts and the interatrial tract (Bachmann's bundle) to the AV node. From there, they travel through the bundle of His, the bundle branches, and finally to the Purkinje fibers.

The SA node, located in the right atrium where the superior vena cava joins the atrial tissue mass, is the heart's main pacemaker. Under resting conditions, the SA node generates impulses 60 to 100 beats/minute. When initiated, the impulses follow a specific path through the heart. Electrical impulses normally don't travel in a backward or retrograde direction because when the cells are activated they can't respond to another stimulus immediately after depolarization.

From the SA node, an impulse travels through the right and left atria. In the right atrium, the impulse is likely transmitted along three internodal tracts. These tracts include the anterior, the middle (or Wenckebach's), and the posterior (or Thorel's) internodal tracts. The impulse travels through the left atrium via Bachmann's bundle, the interatrial tract of tissue extending from the SA node to the left atrium. Impulse transmission through the right and left atria occurs so rapidly that the atria contract almost simultaneously

The AV node is located in the inferior right atrium, near the ostium of the coronary sinus. Although the AV node has no pacemaker cells, the tissue surrounding it, referred to as junctional tissue, contains pacemaker cells that can fire at a rate of 40 to 60 beats/minute. As the AV node conducts the atrial impulse to the ventricles, it causes a 0.04-second delay. This delay allows the ventricles to complete their filling phase as the atria contract.

Action potential curves

An action potential curve shows the changes in a cell's electrical charge during the five phases of the depolarization-repolarization cycle. These graphs show electrical changes for nonpacemaker and pacemaker cells. As the bottom graph shows, the action potential curve for pacemaker cells, such as those in the sinoatrial node, differs from that of other myocardial cells. Pacemaker cells have a resting membrane potential of –60 mV (instead of –90 mV), and they begin to depolarize spontaneously. Called *diastolic depolarization,* this effect results primarily from calcium and sodium leakage into the cell.

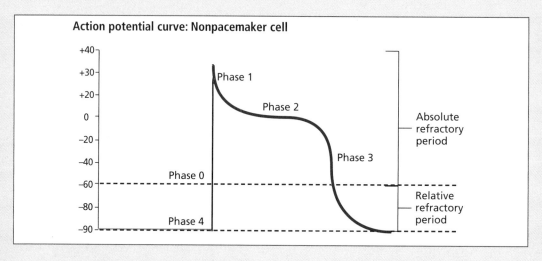

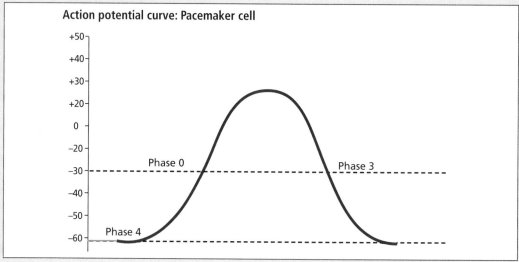

It also allows the cardiac muscle to stretch to its fullest for peak cardiac output.

Rapid conduction then resumes through the bundle of His, which divides into the right and left bundle branches and extends down either side of the interventricular septum. The right bundle branch extends down the right side of the interventricular septum and through the right ventricle. The left bundle branch extends down the left side of the interventricular septum and through the left ventricle. As a pacemaker site, the bundle of His has a firing rate between 40 and 60 beats/minute. The bundle of His usually fires when the SA node fails to generate an impulse at a normal rate or when the impulse fails to reach the AV junction.

Cardiac conduction system

The conduction system of the heart (shown below) begins with the heart's dominant pacemaker, the sinoatrial (SA) node. The intrinsic rate of the SA node is 60 to 100 beats/minute. When an impulse leaves the SA node, it travels through the atria along Bachmann's bundle and the internodal pathways, on its way to the atrioventricular (AV) node and ventricles.

After the impulse passes through the AV node, it travels to the ventricles, first down the bundle of His, then along the bundle branches, and finally down the Purkinje fibers. Pacemaker cells in the junctional tissue and Purkinje fibers of the ventricles normally remain dormant because they receive impulses from the SA node. They initiate an impulse only when they don't receive one from the SA node. The intrinsic rate of the AV junction is 40 to 60 beats/minute; the intrinsic rate of the ventricles, 20 to 40 beats/minute.

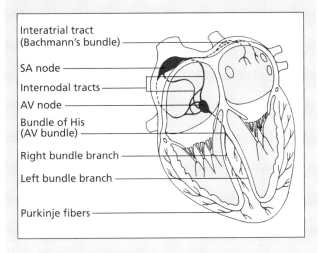

Interatrial tract
(Bachmann's bundle)

SA node

Internodal tracts

AV node

Bundle of His
(AV bundle)

Right bundle branch

Left bundle branch

Purkinje fibers

The left bundle branch then splits into two branches, or fasciculations. The left anterior fasciculus extends through the anterior portion of the left ventricle. The left posterior fasciculus extends through the lateral and posterior portions of the left ventricle. Impulses travel much faster down the left bundle branch, which feeds the larger, thicker-walled left ventricle, than they do down the right bundle branch, which feeds the smaller, thinner-walled right ventricle. The difference in the conduction speed allows both ventricles to contract simultaneously. The entire network of specialized nervous tissue that extends through the ventricles is known as the *His-Purkinje system.*

Purkinje fibers comprise a diffuse muscle fiber network beneath the endocardium that transmits impulses quicker than any other part of the conduction system does. This pacemaker site usually doesn't fire unless the SA and AV nodes fail to generate an impulse or the normal impulse is blocked in both bundle branches. The automatic firing rate of the Purkinje fibers ranges from 20 to 40 beats/minute. In children younger than age 3, the AV junction may discharge impulses at a rate of 50 to 80 times per minute; the Purkinje fibers may discharge at a rate of 40 to 50 times per minute.

◼ Abnormal impulse conduction

Causes of abnormal impulse conduction include altered automaticity, retrograde conduction of impulses, reentry abnormalities, and ectopy.

Automaticity, a special characteristic of pacemaker cells, allows them to generate electrical impulses spontaneously. If a cell's automaticity is increased or decreased, an arrhythmia—or abnormality in the cardiac rhythm—can occur. Tachycardia and premature beats are commonly caused by an increase in the automaticity of pacemaker cells below the SA node. Likewise, a decrease in automaticity of cells in the SA node can cause the development of bradycardia or escape rhythms generated by lower pacemaker sites.

When the electrical impulse is initiated at or below the AV node, it may be transmitted backward toward the atria. This backward, or retrograde, conduction usually takes longer than normal conduction and can cause the atria and ventricles to lose synchrony.

Reentry occurs when cardiac tissue is activated two or more times by the same impulse—for example, when conduction speed is slowed or when the refractory periods for neighboring cells occur at different times. Impulses are delayed long enough that cells have time to repolarize. In those cases, the active impulse reenters the same area and produces another impulse.

Injured pacemaker or nonpacemaker cells may partially depolarize, rather than fully depolarizing. Partial depolarization can lead to spontaneous or secondary depolarization, repetitive ectopic firings called *triggered activity.*

The resultant depolarization is called *afterdepolarization.* Early afterdepolarization occurs before the cell is fully repolarized and can be caused by hypokalemia, slow pacing rates, or drug toxicity. If it occurs after the cell has been fully repolarized, it's called *delayed afterdepolarization.* These problems can be caused by digoxin toxicity, hypercalcemia, or increased catecholamine release. Atrial or ventricular tachycardias may result.

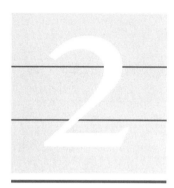

ECG basics

One of the most valuable diagnostic tools available, an electrocardiogram (ECG) records the heart's electrical activity as waveforms. By interpreting these waveforms accurately, you can identify rhythm disturbances, conduction abnormalities, and electrolyte imbalances. An ECG aids in diagnosing and monitoring such conditions as acute coronary syndromes and pericarditis.

To interpret an ECG correctly, you must first recognize its key components. Next, you need to analyze them separately. Then you can put your findings together to reach a conclusion about the heart's electrical activity. This chapter explains that analytic process, beginning with some fundamental information about electrocardiography.

The heart's electrical activity produces currents that radiate through the surrounding tissue to the skin. When electrodes are attached to the skin, they sense those electrical currents and transmit them to the electrocardiograph. This electrical activity is transformed into waveforms that represent the heart's depolarization-repolarization cycle.

Myocardial depolarization occurs when a wave of stimulation passes through the heart and causes the heart muscle to contract. Repolarization is the relaxation phase. An ECG shows the precise sequence of electrical events occurring in the cardiac cells throughout that process and identifies rhythm disturbances and conduction abnormalities.

Leads and planes

Because the electrical currents from the heart radiate to the skin in many directions, electrodes are placed at different locations to obtain a total picture of the heart's electrical activity. The ECG can then record information from different perspectives, which are called *leads* and *planes*.

Leads

A lead provides a view of the heart's electrical activity between two points, or poles. Each lead consists of one positive and one negative pole. Between the two poles lies an imaginary line representing the lead's axis, a term that refers to the direction of the current moving through the heart. Because each lead measures the heart's electrical potential from different directions, each generates its own characteristic tracing. (See *Current direction and waveform deflection.*)

The direction in which the electric current flows determines how the waveforms appear on the ECG tracing. When the current flows along the axis toward the positive pole of the electrode, the waveform deflects upward and is called a *positive deflection.* When the current flows away from the positive pole, the waveform deflects downward, below the baseline, and is called a *negative deflection.* When the current flows perpendicular to the axis, the wave may go in both directions or may be unusually small. When electrical activity is absent or too small to measure, the waveform is a straight line, also called an *isoelectric deflection.*

Planes

A plane is a cross section of the heart, which provides a different view of the heart's electrical activity. In the frontal plane—a vertical cut through the middle of the heart from top to bottom—electrical activity is viewed from right and left. The six limb leads are viewed from the frontal plane.

In the horizontal plane—a transverse cut through the middle of the heart dividing it into upper and lower por-

Current direction and waveform deflection

This illustration shows possible directions of electrical current and the corresponding waveform deflections. The direction of the electrical current through the heart determines the upward or downward deflection of an electrocardiogram waveform.

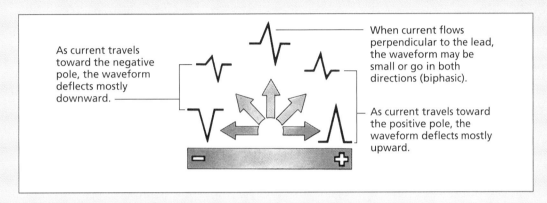

As current travels toward the negative pole, the waveform deflects mostly downward.

When current flows perpendicular to the lead, the waveform may be small or go in both directions (biphasic).

As current travels toward the positive pole, the waveform deflects mostly upward.

tions—electrical activity can be viewed moving anteriorly and posteriorly. The six precordial leads are viewed from the horizontal plane.

Types of ECG recordings

The two main types of ECG recordings are the 12-lead ECG and the rhythm strip. Both types give valuable information about the heart's electrical activity.

12-lead ECG

A 12-lead ECG records information from 12 different views of the heart and provides a complete picture of electrical activity. These 12 views are obtained by placing electrodes on the patient's limbs and chest. The limb leads and the chest, or precordial, leads reflect information from the different planes of the heart.

Different leads provide different information. The six limb leads—I, II, III, augmented vector right (aV_R), augmented vector left (aV_L), and augmented vector foot (aV_F)—provide information about the heart's frontal plane. Leads I, II, and III require a negative and positive electrode for monitoring, which makes these leads bipolar. The augmented leads—aV_R, aV_L, and aV_F—are unipolar, meaning they need only a positive electrode.

The six precordial, or V, leads—V_1, V_2, V_3, V_4, V_5, and V_6—provide information about the heart's horizontal plane. Like the augmented leads, the precordial leads are unipolar, requiring only a positive electrode. The negative pole of these leads, which is in the center of the heart, is calculated with the ECG.

Rhythm strip

A rhythm strip provides continuous information about the heart's electrical activity from one or more leads simultaneously. Commonly monitored leads include lead II, V_1, and V_6. A rhythm strip is used to monitor cardiac status. Chest electrodes pick up the heart's electrical activity for display on the monitor. The monitor also displays heart rate and other measurements and can print out strips of cardiac rhythms.

ECG monitoring systems

The type of ECG monitoring system used—hardwire monitoring or telemetry—depends on the patient's clinical status. With hardwire monitoring, the electrodes are connected directly to the cardiac monitor. Most hardwire monitors are mounted permanently on a shelf or wall near the patient's bed. Some monitors are mounted on an I.V. pole for portability, and some include a defibrillator.

The monitor provides a continuous cardiac rhythm display and transmits the ECG tracing to a console at the nurses' station. Both the monitor and the console have alarms and can print rhythm strips to show ectopic beats, for example, or other arrhythmias. Hardwire monitors also have the ability to track pulse oximetry, blood pressure, hemodynamic measurements, and other parameters through various attachments to the patient.

Hardwire monitoring is generally used in critical care units and emergency departments because it permits continuous observation of one or more patients from more than one area in the unit. However, this type of monitoring does have disadvantages, including limited mobility because the patient is tethered to a monitor.

With telemetry monitoring, the patient carries a small, battery-powered transmitter that sends electrical signals to another location, where the signals are displayed on a monitor screen. This type of ECG monitoring frees the patient from cumbersome wires and cables and protects him from the electrical leakage and accidental shock occasionally associated with hardwire monitoring.

Telemetry monitoring still requires skin electrodes to be placed on the patient's chest. Each electrode is connected by a thin wire to a small transmitter box carried in a pocket or pouch. Telemetry monitoring is especially useful for detecting arrhythmias that occur at rest or during sleep, exercise, or stressful situations. Most systems, however, can monitor only heart rate and rhythm.

Electrode placement

Electrode placement is different for each lead, and different leads provide different views of the heart. A lead may be chosen to highlight a particular part of the ECG complex or the electrical events of a specific area of the heart.

Although leads II, V_1, and V_6 are among the most commonly used leads for continuous monitoring, lead placement is varied according to the patient's clinical status. If your monitoring system has the capability, you may also monitor the patient in more than one lead. (See *Dual-lead monitoring.*)

Standard limb leads

All standard limb leads or bipolar limb leads have a third electrode, known as the *ground,* which is placed on the chest to prevent electrical interference from appearing on the ECG recording.

Lead I provides a view of the heart that shows current moving from right to left. Because current flows from negative to positive, the positive electrode for this lead is placed on the left arm or on the left side of the chest; the negative electrode is placed on the right arm. Lead I produces a positive deflection on ECG tracings.

Lead II is commonly used for routine monitoring. The positive electrode is placed on the patient's left leg and the negative electrode on the right arm. For continuous monitoring, place the electrodes on the patient's torso for convenience, with the positive electrode below the lowest palpable rib at the left midclavicular line and the negative electrode below the right clavicle. The current travels down and to the left in this lead. Lead II tends to produce a positive, high-voltage deflection, resulting in tall P, R, and T waves.

Lead III usually produces a positive deflection on the ECG. The positive electrode is placed on the left leg and the negative electrode on the left arm.

The axes of the three bipolar limb leads—I, II, and III—form a triangle around the heart and provide a frontal plane view of the heart. (See *Einthoven's triangle,* page 16.)

Augmented unipolar leads

Leads aV_R, aV_L, and aV_F are called *augmented leads* because the ECG enhances the small waveforms that would normally appear from these unipolar leads.

In lead aV_R, the positive electrode is placed on the right arm and produces a negative deflection on the ECG because the heart's electrical activity moves away from the lead. In lead aV_L, the positive electrode is on the left arm and usually produces a positive deflection on the ECG. In lead aV_F, the positive electrode is on the left leg and produces a positive deflection on the ECG. These three limb leads also provide a view of the heart's frontal plane.

Precordial unipolar leads

The six unipolar precordial leads are placed in sequence across the chest and provide a view of the heart's horizontal plane (see *Precordial views,* page 16):

- The precordial lead V_1 electrode is placed on the right side of the sternum at the fourth intercostal rib space.
- Lead V_2 is placed to the left of the sternum at the fourth intercostal space.
- Lead V_3 goes between V_2 and V_4 at the fifth intercostal space. Leads V_1, V_2, and V_3 are biphasic, with positive and negative deflections on the ECG.
- Lead V_4 is placed at the fifth intercostal space at the midclavicular line and produces a positive deflection on the ECG.
- Lead V_5 is placed at the fifth intercostal space at the anterior to the axillary line. Lead V_5 produces a positive deflection on the ECG.
- Lead V_6, the last of the precordial leads, is placed at the fifth intercostal space at the midaxillary line. Lead V_6 produces a positive deflection on the ECG.

Dual-lead monitoring

Monitoring in two leads provides a more complete picture than monitoring in one does. Therefore, if it's available, dual-lead monitoring should be used to detect ectopy or aberrant rhythms.

With simultaneous dual monitoring, the first lead—typically designated as the primary lead (lead II)—is usually reviewed for arrhythmias. The second lead (lead V_1) helps detect ectopic beats or aberrant rhythms. Leads II and V_1 are the leads most commonly monitored simultaneously.

Lead II

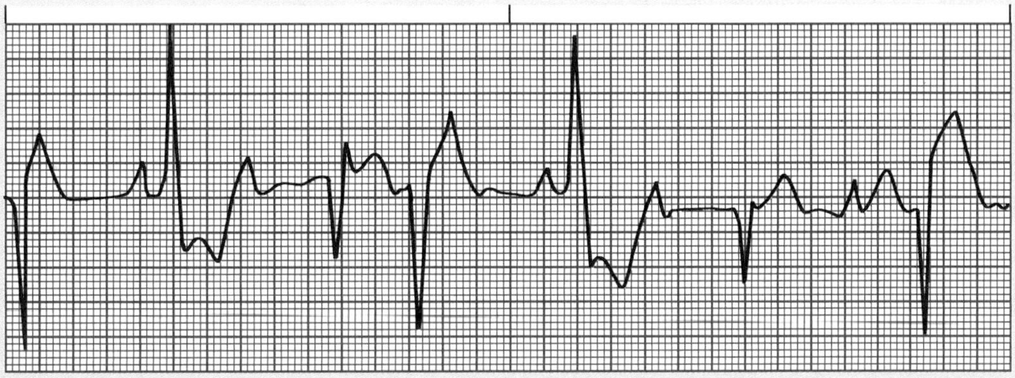

Lead V_1

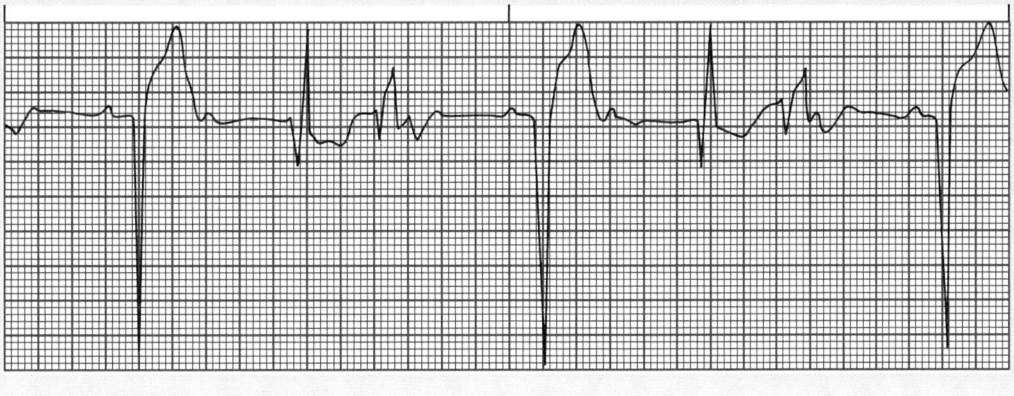

These precordial leads are useful in monitoring ventricular arrhythmias, ST-segment changes, and bundle-branch blocks.

Modified chest leads

The modification of the chest lead occurs because a negative electrode is placed on the left side of the chest, rather than having the center of the heart function as the negative lead. MCL_1 is created by placing the negative electrode on the left upper chest, the positive electrode on the right side of the heart, and the ground electrode usually on the right upper chest. The MCL_1 lead most closely approximates the ECG pattern produced by the chest lead V_1.

When the positive electrode is on the right side of the heart and the electrical current travels toward the left ventricle, the waveform has a negative deflection. As a result, ectopic, or abnormal, beats deflect in a positive direction.

Choose MCL_1 to assess QRS-complex arrhythmias as a bipolar substitute for V_1. You can use this lead to monitor premature ventricular beats and to distinguish different types of tachycardia, such as ventricular and supraventricular tachycardia. MCL_1 can also be used to assess bundle-branch defects and P-wave changes.

Einthoven's triangle

The axes of the three bipolar limb leads (I, II, and III) form a triangle, known as *Einthoven's triangle*. Because the electrodes for these leads are about equidistant from the heart, the triangle is equilateral.

The axis of lead I extends from shoulder to shoulder, with the right arm lead being the negative electrode and the left arm lead being the positive electrode. The axis of lead II runs from the negative right arm lead electrode to the positive left leg lead electrode. The axis of lead III extends from the negative left arm lead electrode to the positive left leg lead electrode.

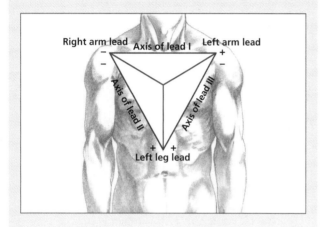

MCL$_6$ is an alternative to MCL$_1$ and most closely approximates the ECG pattern produced by the chest lead V$_6$. Like MCL$_1$, it monitors ventricular conduction

changes. The positive lead in MCL$_6$ is placed at the midaxillary line of the left fifth intercostal space, the negative electrode below the left shoulder, and the ground below the right shoulder.

Application of electrodes

Before attaching electrodes to your patient, make sure he knows you're monitoring his heart rate and rhythm, not controlling them. Tell him not to become upset if he hears an alarm during the procedure; it probably just means a leadwire has come loose.

Explain the electrode placement procedure to the patient, provide privacy, and wash your hands. Expose the patient's chest, and select electrode sites for the chosen lead. Choose sites over soft tissues or close to bone, not over bony prominences, thick muscles, or skin folds. Those areas can produce ECG artifact—waveforms not produced by the heart's electrical activity.

▇ Skin preparation

Wash the patient's chest with soap and water, and then dry it thoroughly. Use a special rough patch on the back of the electrode, a dry washcloth, or a gauze pad to briskly rub each site until the skin reddens. Be sure not to damage or break the skin. Brisk scrubbing helps to remove dead skin cells and improves electrical contact.

Hair may interfere with electrical contact; therefore, it may be necessary to clip areas with dense hair. Dry the areas if you moistened them. If the patient has oily skin,

Precordial views

These illustrations show the different views of the heart obtained from each precordial (chest) lead.

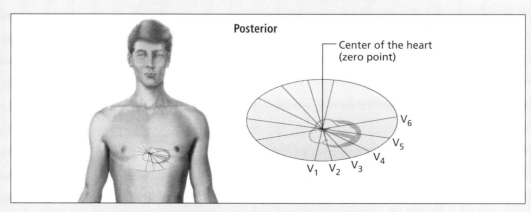

clean each site with an alcohol pad and allow it to air-dry. This process ensures proper adhesion and prevents alcohol from becoming trapped beneath the electrode, which can irritate the skin and cause skin breakdown.

Application of electrode pads

To apply the electrodes, remove the backing and make sure each pregelled electrode is still moist. If an electrode has become dry, discard it and select another. A dry electrode decreases electrical contact and interferes with waveforms.

Apply one electrode to each prepared site using this method:

- Press one side of the electrode against the patient's skin, pull gently, and then press the opposite side of the electrode against the skin.
- Using two fingers, press the adhesive edge around the outside of the electrode to the patient's chest. This fixes the gel and stabilizes the electrode.
- Repeat this procedure for each electrode.
- Every 24 hours or according to your facility's policy and procedure, remove the electrodes, assess the patient's skin, and replace the old electrodes with new ones.

Attaching leadwires

A three- or five-leadwire system may be used for bedside monitoring. (See *Leadwire systems,* page 18.) You'll need to attach leadwires and the cable connections to the monitor. Then attach leadwires to the electrodes. Leadwires may clip on or, more commonly, snap on. If you're using the snap-on type, attach the electrode to the leadwire before applying it to the patient's chest. You can even do this step ahead of time if you know when the patient will arrive, to prevent patient discomfort and disturbances of the contact between the electrode and the skin. When you use a clip-on leadwire, apply it after the electrode has been secured to the patient's skin. That way, applying the clip won't interfere with the electrode's contact with the skin.

Cardiac monitoring

After the electrodes are properly positioned, the monitor is on, and the necessary cables are attached, observe the screen. You should see the patient's ECG waveform. Although most monitoring systems allow you to make adjustments by touching the screen, some require you to manipulate knobs and buttons. If the waveform appears too large or too small, change the size by adjusting the gain control. If the waveform appears too high or too low on the screen, adjust the position dial.

Verify that the monitor detects each heartbeat by comparing the patient's apical rate with the rate displayed on the monitor. Set the upper and lower limits of the heart rate according to your facility's policy and the patient's condition. Heart rate alarms are generally set 10 to 20 beats/minute higher or lower than the patient's heart rate.

Monitors with arrhythmia detection generate a rhythm strip automatically whenever the alarm goes off. You can obtain other views of your patient's cardiac rhythm by selecting different leads. You can select leads with the lead selector button or switch.

To get a printout of the patient's cardiac rhythm, press the record control on the monitor on the control console. The ECG strip will be printed at the central console. Some systems print the rhythm from a recorder box on the monitor itself.

Most monitors can input the patient's name, date, and time as a permanent record; however, if the monitor you're using can't do this, label the rhythm strip with the patient's name, date, time, and rhythm interpretation. Add appropriate clinical information to the ECG strip, such as any medication administered, presence of chest pain, or patient activity at the time of the recording. Be sure to place the rhythm strip in the appropriate section of the patient's medical record.

▨ Troubleshooting monitor problems

For optimal cardiac monitoring, you need to recognize problems that can interfere with obtaining a reliable ECG recording and performing an accurate rhythm strip interpretation. (See *Common monitor problems,* pages 19 and 20.) Causes of interference include artifact from patient movement and poorly placed or poorly functioning equipment.

Artifact, also called *waveform interference,* may be seen with excessive movement (somatic tremor). It causes the baseline of the ECG to appear wavy, bumpy, or tremulous. Dry electrodes may also cause this problem because of poor contact.

Electrical interference, also called *AC interference* or *60-cycle interference,* is caused by electrical power leakage. It may also result from interference from other room equipment or improperly grounded equipment. As a result, the lost current pulses at a rate of 60 cycles/second. This interference appears on the ECG as a baseline that's thick and unreadable.

A wandering baseline undulates, meaning that all waveforms are present but the baseline isn't stationary.

Leadwire systems

The illustrations below show the correct electrode positions for some of the leads you'll use most often—the five-leadwire, three-leadwire, and telemetry systems. The abbreviations used are RA for the right arm, LA for the left arm, RL for the right leg, LL for the left leg, C for the chest, and G for the ground.

Electrode positions

In the three- and five-leadwire systems, electrode positions for one lead may be identical to those for another lead. When that happens, change the lead selector switch to the setting that corresponds to the lead you want. In some cases, you'll need to reposition the electrodes.

Telemetry

In a telemetry monitoring system, you can create the same leads as the other systems with just two electrodes and a ground wire.

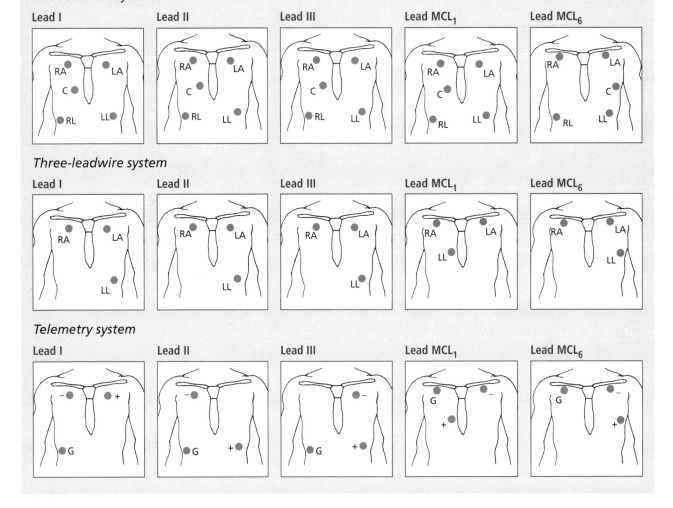

Five-leadwire system

Lead I   Lead II   Lead III   Lead MCL₁   Lead MCL₆

Three-leadwire system

Lead I   Lead II   Lead III   Lead MCL₁   Lead MCL₆

Telemetry system

Lead I   Lead II   Lead III   Lead MCL₁   Lead MCL₆

Movement of the chest wall during respiration, poor electrode placement, or poor electrode contact usually causes this problem.

Faulty equipment, such as broken leadwires and cables, can also cause monitoring problems. Excessively

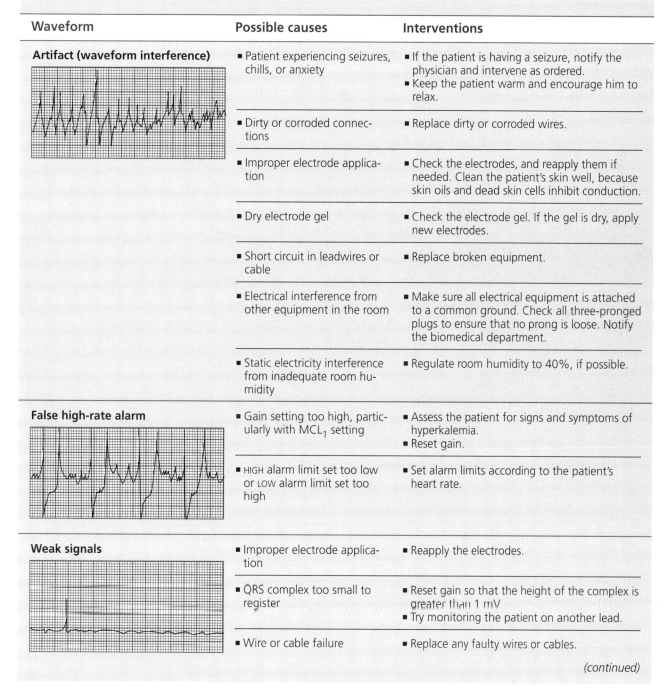

Common monitor problems

These illustrations present the most commonly encountered monitor problems, including the way to identify them, their possible causes, and interventions.

Waveform	Possible causes	Interventions
Artifact (waveform interference)	▪ Patient experiencing seizures, chills, or anxiety	▪ If the patient is having a seizure, notify the physician and intervene as ordered. ▪ Keep the patient warm and encourage him to relax.
	▪ Dirty or corroded connections	▪ Replace dirty or corroded wires.
	▪ Improper electrode application	▪ Check the electrodes, and reapply them if needed. Clean the patient's skin well, because skin oils and dead skin cells inhibit conduction.
	▪ Dry electrode gel	▪ Check the electrode gel. If the gel is dry, apply new electrodes.
	▪ Short circuit in leadwires or cable	▪ Replace broken equipment.
	▪ Electrical interference from other equipment in the room	▪ Make sure all electrical equipment is attached to a common ground. Check all three-pronged plugs to ensure that no prong is loose. Notify the biomedical department.
	▪ Static electricity interference from inadequate room humidity	▪ Regulate room humidity to 40%, if possible.
False high-rate alarm	▪ Gain setting too high, particularly with MCL$_1$ setting	▪ Assess the patient for signs and symptoms of hyperkalemia. ▪ Reset gain.
	▪ HIGH alarm limit set too low or LOW alarm limit set too high	▪ Set alarm limits according to the patient's heart rate.
Weak signals	▪ Improper electrode application	▪ Reapply the electrodes.
	▪ QRS complex too small to register	▪ Reset gain so that the height of the complex is greater than 1 mV ▪ Try monitoring the patient on another lead.
	▪ Wire or cable failure	▪ Replace any faulty wires or cables.

(continued)

Common monitor problems *(continued)*

Waveform	Possible causes	Interventions
Wandering baseline ![wandering baseline waveform]	▪ Patient restlessness	▪ Encourage the patient to relax.
	▪ Chest wall movement during respiration	▪ Make sure that tension on the cable isn't pulling the electrode away from the patient's body.
	▪ Improper electrode application; electrode positioned over bone	▪ Reposition improperly placed electrodes.
Fuzzy baseline (electrical interference) ![fuzzy baseline waveform]	▪ Electrical interference from other equipment in the room	▪ Make sure that all electrical equipment being used, such as an I.V. pump, is attached to a common ground. ▪ Check all three-pronged plugs to make sure no prong is loose. Notify the biomedical department.
	▪ Improper grounding of the patient's bed	▪ Make sure that the bed ground is attached to the room's common ground.
	▪ Electrode malfunction	▪ Replace the electrodes.
Baseline (no waveform) ![baseline no waveform]	▪ Improper electrode placement (perpendicular to axis of heart) ▪ Electrode disconnection ▪ Dry electrode gel ▪ Wire or cable failure	▪ Reposition improperly placed electrodes. ▪ Check for disconnected electrodes. ▪ Check the electrode gel. If the gel is dry, apply new electrodes. ▪ Replace any faulty wires or cables.

worn equipment can cause improper grounding, putting the patient at risk for accidental shock.

Be aware that some types of artifact resemble arrhythmias and that the monitor will interpret them as such. For example, the monitor may sense a small movement, such as the patient brushing his teeth, as a potentially lethal ventricular tachycardia. So, remember to treat the patient, not the monitor. The more familiar you become with your unit's monitoring system—and with your patient—the more quickly you can recognize and interpret monitor problems and act appropriately.

The ECG grid

Waveforms produced by the heart's electrical current are recorded on graphed ECG paper by a heated stylus. ECG paper consists of horizontal and vertical lines forming a grid. A piece of ECG paper is called an *ECG strip* or *tracing*. (See *Understanding the ECG grid.*)

The horizontal axis of the ECG strip represents time. Each small block equals 0.04 second, and five small blocks form a large block, which equals 0.2 second. This time increment is determined by multiplying 0.04 second (for one small block) by five, the number of small blocks that make up a large block. Five large blocks equal 1 second (5 × 0.2). When measuring or calculating a patient's heart rate, a 6-second strip consisting of 30 large blocks is usually used.

The ECG strip's vertical axis measures amplitude in millimeters (mm) or electrical voltage in millivolts (mV). Each small block represents 1 mm or 0.1 mV; each large block, 5 mm or 0.5 mV. To determine the amplitude of a wave, segment, or interval, count the number of small

Understanding the ECG grid

This electrocardiogram (ECG) grid shows the horizontal axis and vertical axis and their respective measurement values.

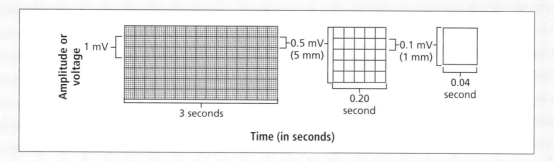

blocks from the baseline to the highest or lowest point of the wave, segment, or interval.

ECG waveform components

An ECG complex represents the heart's electrical activity (depolarization-repolarization cycle) occurring in one cardiac cycle. The ECG tracing consists of three basic waveforms: the P wave, the QRS complex, and the T wave. These units of electrical activity can be further broken down into these segments and intervals: the PR interval, the ST segment, and the QT interval.

In addition, a U wave may sometimes be present. The J point marks the end of the QRS complex and the beginning of the ST segment. (See *Identifying ECG waveform components.*)

The upward and downward movement of the ECG machine's stylus, which forms the various waves, reflects the directional flow of the heart's electrical impulse. When the electrodes are placed correctly, an upward deflection is positive and a downward deflection is negative. Between each cardiac cycle, when the heart's electrical activity is absent, the stylus on the ECG recorder re-

Identifying ECG waveform components

This illustration shows the components of a normal electrocardiogram (ECG) waveform.

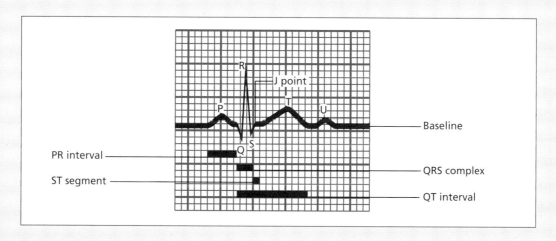

turns to the baseline or isoelectric line and records a straight line.

P wave

The P wave is the first component of a normal ECG waveform. It represents atrial depolarization or conduction of an electrical impulse through the atria. When evaluating a P wave, look closely at its characteristics, especially its location, configuration, and deflection. A normal P wave has the following characteristics:

- Location: precedes the QRS complex
- Amplitude: 2 to 3 mm high
- Duration: 0.06 to 0.12 second
- Configuration: usually rounded and smooth

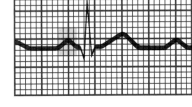

- Deflection: positive or upright in leads I, II, aV_F, and V_2 to V_6; usually positive but may vary in leads III and aV_L; negative or inverted in lead aV_R; biphasic or variable in lead V_1

If the deflection and configuration of a P wave are normal—for example, if the P wave is upright in lead II and is rounded and smooth—and if the P wave precedes each QRS complex, you can assume that this electrical impulse originated in the sinoatrial (SA) node. The atria start to contract partway through the P wave, but you won't see this on the ECG. Remember, the ECG records only electrical activity, not mechanical activity or contraction.

Peaked, notched, or enlarged P waves may represent atrial hypertrophy or enlargement associated with chronic obstructive pulmonary disease, pulmonary emboli, valvular disease, or heart failure. Inverted P waves may signify retrograde or reverse conduction from the atrioventricular (AV) junction toward the atria. Whenever an upright sinus P wave becomes inverted, consider retrograde conduction and reverse conduction as possible conditions.

Varying P waves indicate that the impulse may be coming from different sites, as with a wandering pacemaker rhythm, irritable atrial tissue, or damage near the SA node. Absent P waves may signify impulse initiation by tissue other than the SA node, as with a junctional or atrial fibrillation rhythm. When a P wave doesn't precede the QRS complex, heart block may be present.

PR interval

The PR interval tracks the atrial impulse from the atria through the AV node, bundle of His, and right and left bundle branches. When evaluating a PR interval, look

particularly at its duration. Changes in the PR interval indicate an altered impulse formation or a conduction delay, as seen in AV block. A normal PR interval has the following characteristics (amplitude, configuration, and deflection aren't measured):

- Location: from the beginning of the P wave to the beginning of the QRS complex
- Duration: 0.12 to 0.20 second

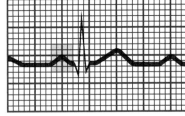

Short PR intervals (less than 0.12 second) indicate that the impulse originated somewhere other than the SA node. This variation is associated with junctional arrhythmias and preexcitation syndromes. Prolonged PR intervals (greater than 0.20 second) may represent a conduction delay through the atria or AV junction resulting from digoxin toxicity or heart block—slowing related to ischemia or conduction tissue disease.

QRS complex

The QRS complex follows the P wave and represents depolarization of the ventricles, or impulse conduction. Immediately after the ventricles depolarize, as represented by the QRS complex, they contract. That contraction ejects blood from the ventricles and pumps it through the arteries, creating a pulse.

Whenever you're monitoring cardiac rhythm, remember that the waveform you see represents only the heart's electrical activity. It doesn't guarantee a mechanical contraction of the heart and a subsequent pulse. The contraction could be weak, as happens with premature ventricular contractions, or absent, as happens with pulseless electrical activity. So, before you treat what the rhythm strip shows, check the patient.

Pay special attention to the duration and configuration when evaluating a QRS complex. A normal complex has the following characteristics:

- Location: follows the PR interval
- Amplitude: 5 to 30 mm high, but differs for each lead used
- Duration: 0.06 to 0.10 second or half of the PR interval (Duration is measured from the beginning of the Q wave to the end of the S wave or from the beginning of the R wave if the Q wave is absent.)

QRS waveform variety

These illustrations show the various configurations of QRS complexes. When documenting the QRS complex, use uppercase letters to indicate a wave with a normal or high amplitude (greater than 5 mm) and lowercase letters to indicate one with a low amplitude (less than 5 mm).

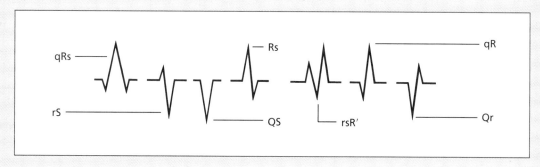

- Configuration: consists of the Q wave (the first negative deflection, or deflection below the baseline, after the P wave), the R wave (the first positive deflection after the Q wave), and the S wave (the first negative deflection after the R wave) (You may not always see all three waves. It may also look different in each lead.) (See *QRS waveform variety.*)
- Deflection: positive (with most of the complex above the baseline) in leads I, II, III, aV_L, aV_F, and V_4 to V_6; negative in leads aV_R and V_1 to V_2; biphasic in lead V_3

Remember that the QRS complex represents intraventricular conduction time. That's why identifying and correctly interpreting it is so crucial. If no P wave appears before the QRS complex, then the impulse may have originated in the ventricles, indicating a ventricular arrhythmia.

Deep, wide Q waves may represent a myocardial infarction. In this case, the Q wave amplitude (depth) is greater than or equal to 25% of the height of the succeeding R wave, or the duration of the Q wave is 0.04 second or more. A notched R wave may signify a bundle-branch block. A widened QRS complex (greater than 0.12 second) may signify a ventricular conduction delay. A missing QRS complex may indicate AV block or ventricular standstill.

ST segment

The ST segment represents the end of ventricular conduction or depolarization and the beginning of ventricular recovery or repolarization. The point that marks the end of the QRS complex and the beginning of the ST segment is known as the *J point.*

Pay special attention to the deflection of an ST segment. A normal ST segment has the following characteristics (amplitude, duration, and configuration aren't observed):

- Location: extends from the S wave to the beginning of the T wave
- Deflection: usually isoelectric or on the baseline (neither positive nor negative); may vary from –0.5 to +1 mm in some precordial leads

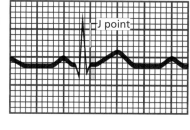

A change in the ST segment may indicate myocardial injury or ischemia. An ST segment may become either elevated or depressed. (See *Changes in the ST segment,* page 24.)

T wave

The peak of the T wave represents the relative refractory period of repolarization or ventricular recovery. When evaluating a T wave, look at the amplitude, configuration, and deflection.

Normal T waves have the following characteristics (duration isn't measured):

- Location: follows the ST segment
- Amplitude: 0.5 mm in leads I, II, and III and up to 10 mm in the precordial leads
- Configuration: typically rounded and smooth

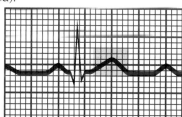

Changes in the ST segment

Closely monitoring the ST segment on a patient's electrocardiogram can help you detect myocardial ischemia or injury before infarction develops.

ST-segment depression
An ST segment is considered depressed when it's 0.5 mm or more below the baseline. A depressed ST segment may indicate myocardial ischemia or digoxin toxicity.

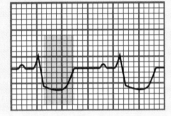

ST-segment elevation
An ST segment is considered elevated when it's 1 mm or more above the baseline. An elevated ST segment may indicate myocardial injury.

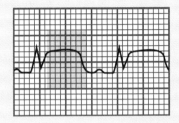

■ Deflection: usually positive or upright in leads I, II, and V_2 to V_6; inverted in lead aV_R; variable in leads III and V_1

The T wave's peak represents the relative refractory period of ventricular repolarization, a period during which cells are especially vulnerable to extra stimuli. Bumps in a T wave may indicate that a P wave is hidden in it. If a P wave is hidden, atrial depolarization has occurred, the impulse having originated at a site above the ventricles.

Tall, peaked, or "tented" T waves may indicate myocardial injury or electrolyte imbalances such as hyperkalemia. Inverted T waves in leads I, II, aV_L, aV_F, or V_2 through V_6 may represent myocardial ischemia. Heavily notched or pointed T waves in an adult may indicate pericarditis.

■ QT interval

The QT interval measures the time needed for ventricular depolarization and repolarization. The length of the QT interval varies according to heart rate. The faster the heart rate, the shorter the QT interval. When checking the QT interval, look closely at the duration.

A normal QT interval has the following characteristics (amplitude, configuration, and deflection aren't observed):
■ Location: extends from the beginning of the QRS complex to the end of the T wave
■ Duration: varies according to age, gender, and heart rate; usually lasts

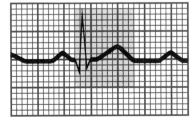

from 0.36 to 0.44 second; shouldn't be greater than half the distance between the two consecutive R waves (called the *R-R interval*) when the rhythm is regular

The QT interval measures the time needed for ventricular depolarization and repolarization. Prolonged QT intervals indicate that ventricular repolarization time is slowed, meaning that the relative refractory, or vulnerable, period of the cardiac cycle is longer.

This variation is also associated with certain medications, such as class I antiarrhythmics. Prolonged QT syndrome is a congenital conduction-system defect present in certain families. Short QT intervals may result from digoxin toxicity or electrolyte imbalances such as hypercalcemia.

■ U wave

The U wave represents repolarization of the His-Purkinje system or ventricular conduction fibers. It usually isn't present on a rhythm strip. The configuration is the most important characteristic of the U wave.

When present, a U wave has the following characteristics (amplitude and duration aren't measured):
■ Location: follows the T wave
■ Configuration: typically rounded
■ Deflection: upright

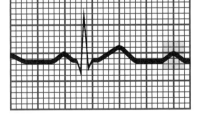

The U wave may not appear on an ECG. A prominent U wave may result from hypercalcemia, hypokalemia, or digoxin toxicity.

The 8-step method

Analyzing a rhythm strip is a skill developed through practice. You can use several methods, as long as you're consistent. Rhythm strip analysis requires a sequential and systematic approach such as the eight steps outlined here.

▉ Step 1: Determine rhythm

To evaluate the heart's atrial and ventricular rhythms, use either the paper-and-pencil method or the caliper method. (See *Methods of measuring rhythm.*)

For atrial rhythm, measure the P-P intervals—that is, the intervals between consecutive P waves. These intervals should occur regularly, with only small variations associated with respirations. Then compare the P-P intervals in several cycles. Consistently similar P-P intervals indicate regular atrial rhythm; dissimilar P-P intervals indicate irregular atrial rhythm.

To determine the ventricular rhythm, measure the intervals between two consecutive R waves in the QRS complexes. If an R wave isn't present, use either the Q wave or the S wave of consecutive QRS complexes. The R-R intervals should occur regularly. Then compare R-R intervals in several cycles. As with atrial rhythms, consistently similar R-R intervals mean a regular ventric-

---

Methods of measuring rhythm

You can use either of the following methods to determine atrial or ventricular rhythm.

Paper-and-pencil method

- ▉ Place the electrocardiogram (ECG) strip on a flat surface.
- ▉ Position the straight edge of a piece of paper along the strip's baseline.
- ▉ Move the paper up slightly so the straight edge is near the peak of the R wave.
- ▉ With a pencil, mark the paper at the R waves of two consecutive QRS complexes, as shown below. This distance is the R-R interval.
- ▉ Move the paper across the strip lining up the two marks with succeeding R-R intervals. If the distance for each R-R interval is the same, the ventricular rhythm is regular. If the distance varies, the rhythm is irregular.
- ▉ Using the same method, measure the distance between P waves (the P-P interval) to determine whether the atrial rhythm is regular or irregular.

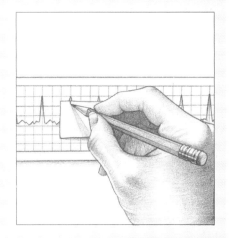

Caliper method

- ▉ With the ECG on a flat surface, place one point of the calipers on the peak of the first R wave of two consecutive QRS complexes.
- ▉ Adjust the caliper legs so the other point is on the peak of the next R wave, as shown below. This distance is the R-R interval.
- ▉ Pivot the first point of the calipers toward the third R wave, and note whether it falls on the peak of that wave.
- ▉ Check succeeding R-R intervals in the same way. If they're all the same, the ventricular rhythm is regular. If they vary, the rhythm is irregular.
- ▉ Using the same method, measure the P-P intervals to determine whether the atrial rhythm is regular or irregular.

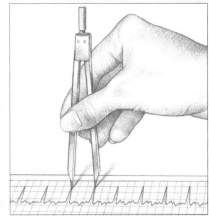

ular rhythm; dissimilar R-R intervals point to an irregular ventricular rhythm.

After completing your measurements, ask yourself:
■ Is the rhythm regular or irregular? Consider a rhythm with only slight variations, up to 0.04 second, to be regular.
■ If the rhythm is irregular, is it slightly irregular or markedly so? Does the irregularity occur in a pattern (a regularly irregular pattern)?

■ Step 2: Calculate rate

You can use one of three methods to determine atrial and ventricular heart rates from an ECG waveform. Although these methods can provide accurate information, you shouldn't rely solely on them when assessing your patient. Keep in mind that the ECG waveform represents electrical, not mechanical, activity. Therefore, although an ECG can show you that ventricular depolarization has occurred, it doesn't mean that ventricular contraction has occurred. To determine this, you must assess the patient's pulse. So remember, always check a pulse to correlate it with the heart rate on the ECG.

■ Times-10 method: The first method that's the simplest, quickest, and most common way to calculate rate is the times-10 method, especially if the rhythm is irregular. ECG paper is marked in increments of 3 seconds, or 15 large boxes. To calculate the atrial rate, obtain a 6-second strip, count the number of P waves on it, and multiply by 10. Ten 6-second strips equal 1 minute. Calculate ventricular rate the same way, using the R waves.

■ 1,500 method: If the heart rhythm is regular, use the second method—the 1,500 method, so named because 1,500 small squares equal 1 minute. Count the number of small squares between identical points on two consecutive P waves, and then divide 1,500 by that number to get the atrial rate. To obtain the ventricular rate, use the same method with two consecutive R waves.

■ Sequence method: The third method of estimating heart rate is the sequence method, which requires memorizing a sequence of numbers. For atrial rate, find a P wave that peaks on a heavy black line and assign the following numbers to the next six heavy black lines: 300, 150, 100, 75, 60, and 50. Then find the next P wave peak and estimate the atrial rate, based on the number assigned to the nearest heavy black line. Estimate the ventricular rate the same way, using the R wave. (See *Calculating heart rate*.)

Calculating heart rate

This table can help make the sequencing method of determining heart rate more precise. After counting the number of boxes between the R waves, use this table to find the rate.

For example, if you count 20 small blocks, or 4 large blocks, the rate would be 75 beats/minute. To calculate the atrial rate, use the same method with P waves instead of R waves.

Rapid estimation

This rapid-rate calculation is also called the countdown method. Using the number of large boxes between R waves or P waves as a guide, you can rapidly estimate ventricular or atrial rates by memorizing the sequence "300, 150, 100, 75, 60, 50."

Number of small blocks	Heart rate
5 (1 large block)	300
6	250
7	214
8	188
9	167
10 (2 large blocks)	150
11	136
12	125
13	115
14	107
15 (3 large blocks)	100
16	94
17	88
18	83
19	79
20 (4 large blocks)	75
21	71
22	68
23	65
24	63
25 (5 large blocks)	60
26	58
27	56
28	54
29	52
30 (6 large blocks)	50
31	48
32	47
33	45
34	44
35 (7 large blocks)	43
36	42
37	41
38	39
39	38
40 (8 large blocks)	37

Step 3: Evaluate the P wave

When examining a rhythm strip for P waves, ask yourself:
■ Are P waves present?
■ Do the P waves have a normal configuration?
■ Do all the P waves have a similar size and shape?
■ Is there one P wave for every QRS complex?

Step 4: Calculate the PR interval

To measure the PR interval, count the small squares between the start of the P wave and the start of the QRS complex; then multiply the number of squares by 0.04 second. After performing this calculation, ask yourself:
■ Does the duration of the PR interval fall within normal limits, 0.12 to 0.20 second (or 3 to 5 small squares)?
■ Is the PR interval constant?

Step 5: Evaluate the QRS complex

When determining QRS-complex duration, make sure you measure straight across from the end of the PR interval to the end of the S wave, not just to the peak. Remember, the QRS complex has no horizontal components. To calculate duration, count the number of small squares between the beginning and end of the QRS complex and multiply this number by 0.04 second. Then ask yourself:
■ Does the duration of the QRS complex fall within normal limits, 0.06 to 0.10 second?
■ Are all QRS complexes the same size and shape? (If not, measure each one and describe them individually.)
■ Does a QRS complex appear after every P wave?

Step 6: Evaluate the T wave

Examine the T waves on the ECG strip. Then ask yourself:
■ Are T waves present?
■ Do all of the T waves have a normal shape?
■ Could a P wave be hidden in a T wave?
■ Do all T waves have a normal amplitude?
■ Do the T waves have the same deflection as the QRS complexes?

Step 7: Calculate the duration of the QT interval

To determine the duration of the QT interval, count the number of small squares between the beginning of the QRS complex and the end of the T wave, where the T wave returns to the baseline. Multiply this number by 0.04 second. Ask yourself:
■ Does the duration of the QT interval fall within normal limits, 0.36 to 0.44 second?

Step 8: Evaluate other components

Note the presence of ectopic beats or other abnormalities such as aberrant conduction. Also, check the ST segment for abnormalities, and look for the presence of a U wave.

Now, interpret your findings by classifying the rhythm strip according to one or all of the following.
■ Origin of the rhythm: for example, sinus node, atria, AV node, or ventricles
■ Rate: normal (60 to 100 beats/minute), bradycardia (fewer than 60 beats/minute), or tachycardia (greater than 100 beats/minute)
■ Rhythm interpretation: normal or abnormal—for example, flutter, fibrillation, heart block, escape rhythm, or other arrhythmias

Normal sinus rhythm

Before you can recognize an arrhythmia, you first need to be able to recognize a normal cardiac rhythm. The term *arrhythmia* literally means an absence of rhythm. The more accurate term *dysrhythmia* means an abnormality in rhythm. These terms, however, are typically used interchangeably.

Normal sinus rhythm (NSR) occurs when an impulse starts in the sinus node and progresses to the ventricles through a normal conduction pathway—from the sinus node to the atria and AV node, through the bundle of His, to the bundle branches, and on to the Purkinje fibers. No premature or aberrant contractions are present. NSR is the standard against which all other rhythms are compared. (See *Identifying normal sinus rhythm.*)

The ECG characteristics of NSR include:

- Rhythm—atrial and ventricular rhythms regular
- Rate—atrial and ventricular rates 60 to 100 beats/minute, the SA node's normal firing rate
- P wave—normally shaped (round and smooth) and upright in lead II; all P waves similar in size and shape; one P wave for every QRS complex
- PR interval—within normal limits (0.12 to 0.20 second)
- QRS complex—within normal limits (0.06 to 0.10 second)
- T wave—normally shaped; upright and rounded in lead II
- QT interval—within normal limits (0.36 to 0.44 second)
- Other—no ectopic or aberrant beats.

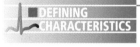

Identifying normal sinus rhythm

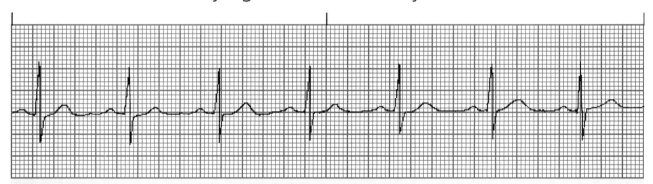

Rhythm
- Atrial regular
- Ventricular regular

Rate
- 60 to 100 beats/minute (sinoatrial node's normal firing rate)

P wave
- Normal shape (round and smooth)
- Upright in lead II
- One for every QRS complex
- All similar in size and shape

PR interval
- Within normal limits (0.12 to 0.20 second)

QRS complex
- Within normal limits (0.06 to 0.10 second)

T wave
- Normal shape
- Upright and rounded in lead II

QT interval
- Within normal limits (0.36 to 0.44 second)

Other
- No ectopic or aberrant beats

PRACTICE # Normal sinus rhythm

Use the 8-step method to interpret the following rhythm strip. Place your answers on the blank lines. See the answer key below.

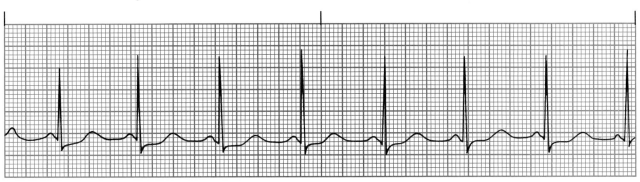

Rhythm: _____

Rate: _____

P wave: _____

PR interval: _____

QRS complex: _____

T wave: _____

QT interval: _____

Other: _____

■ **ANSWER KEY**

Rhythm: Atrial and ventricular rhythms regular

Rate: Atrial and ventricular rates normal; 78 beats/ minute

P wave: Normal; precedes each QRS complex; all P waves similar in size and shape

PR interval: Normal; 0.12 second

QRS complex: 0.08 second

T wave: Upright

QT interval: Normal; 0.44 second

Other: No ectopic or aberrantly conducted impulses

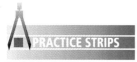

PRACTICE STRIPS

■ PRACTICE 2-1

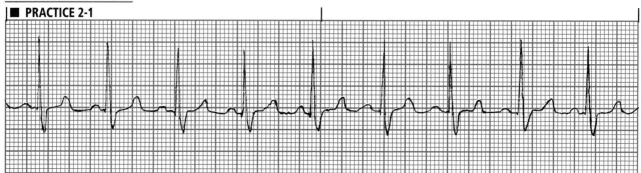

Rhythm: _____

PR interval: _____

QT interval: _____

Rate: _____

QRS complex: _____

Other: _____

P wave: _____

T wave: _____

Interpretation: _____

■ PRACTICE 2-2

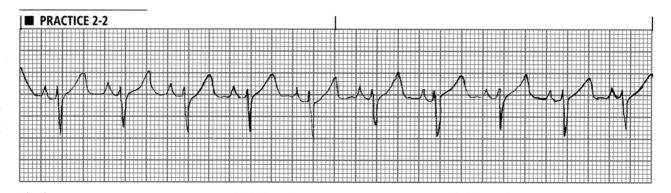

Rhythm: _____

PR interval: _____

QT interval: _____

Rate: _____

QRS complex: _____

Other: _____

P wave: _____

T wave: _____

Interpretation: _____

■ PRACTICE 2-3

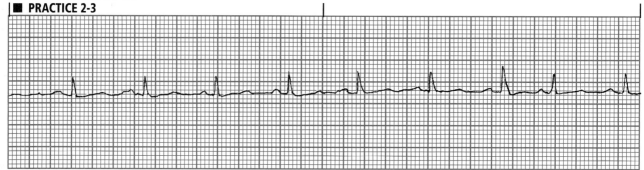

Rhythm: _____

PR interval: _____

QT interval: _____

Rate: _____

QRS complex: _____

Other: _____

P wave: _____

T wave: _____

Interpretation: _____

■ PRACTICE STRIP ANSWERS

PRACTICE 2-1
- Rhythm: Regular
- Rate: 94 beats/minute
- P wave: Normal
- PR interval: 0.16 second
- QRS complex: 0.12 second
- T wave: Normal
- QT interval: 0.34 second
- Other: None
- Interpretation: NSR

PRACTICE 2-2
- Rhythm: Regular
- Rate: 100 beats/minute
- P wave: Normal
- PR interval: 0.16 second
- QRS complex: 0.12 second
- T wave: Normal
- QT interval: 0.34 second
- Other: None
- Interpretation: NSR

PRACTICE 2-3
- Rhythm: Regular
- Rate: 88 beats/minute
- P wave: Normal
- PR interval: 0.18 second
- QRS complex: 0.08 second
- T wave: Normal
- QT interval: 0.36 second
- Other: None
- Interpretation: NSR

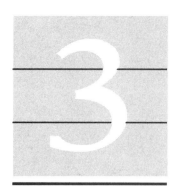

Sinus node arrhythmias

When the heart functions normally, the sinoatrial (SA) node, also called the *sinus node,* acts as the primary pacemaker. The sinus node assumes this role because its automatic firing rate exceeds that of the heart's other pacemakers. In an adult at rest, the sinus node has an inherent firing rate of 60 to 100 times per minute.

Changes in the automaticity of the sinus node, alterations in its blood supply, and autonomic nervous system (ANS) influences may all lead to sinus node arrhythmias. (See *SA node arrhythmias.*)

Sinus node arrhythmias include:
- sinus arrhythmia
- sinus bradycardia
- sinus tachycardia
- sinus arrest
- sinoatrial exit block
- sick sinus syndrome.

SA node arrhythmias

Impulses originate in the sinus node, the normal pacemaker of the heart, but changes in automaticity, blood supply, and autonomic nervous system influences lead to the development of sinoatrial (SA) node arrhythmias.

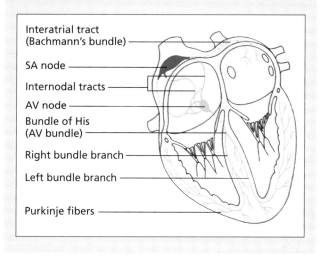

Interatrial tract (Bachmann's bundle)
SA node
Internodal tracts
AV node
Bundle of His (AV bundle)
Right bundle branch
Left bundle branch
Purkinje fibers

Sinus arrhythmia

In sinus arrhythmia, the rate stays within normal limits but the rhythm is irregular and corresponds to the respiratory cycle. Sinus arrhythmia can occur normally in athletes, children, and older adults, but it rarely occurs in infants. (See *Identifying sinus arrhythmia*.)

■ DEFINING
CHARACTERISTICS

Identifying sinus arrhythmia

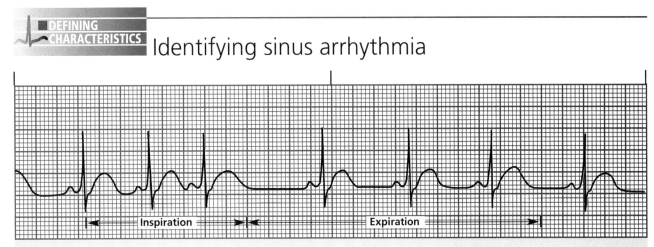

Inspiration ◄ ► ◄ Expiration ►

Rhythm
- Irregular
- Corresponds to the respiratory cycle
- P-P interval and R-R interval shorter during inspiration; longer during expiration
- Difference between the longest and the shortest P-P interval exceeds 0.12 second

Rate
- Usually within normal limits (60 to 100 beats/minute); rate may be less than 60 beats/minute
- Varies with respiration
- Increases during inspiration
- Decreases during expiration

P wave
- Normal size
- Normal configuration

PR interval
- May vary slightly
- Within normal limits

QRS complex
- Preceded by P wave
- Normal configuration

T wave
- Normal size
- Normal configuration

QT interval
- May vary slightly
- Usually within normal limits

Other
- Phasic slowing and quickening

Sinus arrhythmia

Use the 8-step method to interpret the following rhythm strip. Place your answers on the blank lines. See the answer key below.

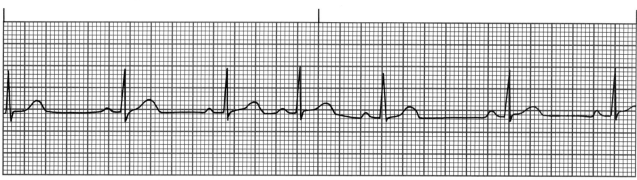

Rhythm:

Rate:

P wave:

PR interval:

QRS complex:

T wave:

QT interval:

Other:

■ **ANSWER KEY**

Rhythm: **Irregular**

Rate: **60 beats/minute**

P wave: **Normal**

PR interval: **0.18 second**

QRS complex: **0.08 second**

T wave: **Normal**

QT interval: **0.36 second**

Other: **Phasic slowing and quickening**

Sinus bradycardia

Sinus bradycardia is characterized by a sinus rate below 60 beats/minute and a regular rhythm. All impulses originate in the SA node. This arrhythmia's significance depends on the patient's symptoms and the underlying cause. (See *Identifying sinus bradycardia.*)

■ DEFINING CHARACTERISTICS

Identifying sinus bradycardia

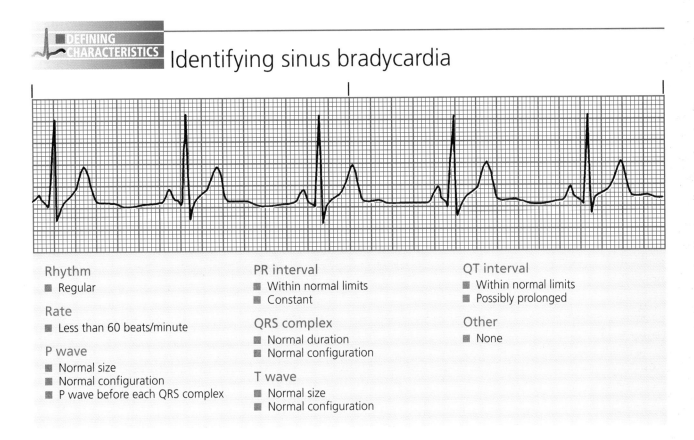

Rhythm
- Regular

Rate
- Less than 60 beats/minute

P wave
- Normal size
- Normal configuration
- P wave before each QRS complex

PR interval
- Within normal limits
- Constant

QRS complex
- Normal duration
- Normal configuration

T wave
- Normal size
- Normal configuration

QT interval
- Within normal limits
- Possibly prolonged

Other
- None

■ PRACTICE **Sinus bradycardia**

Use the 8-step method to interpret the following rhythm strip. Place your answers on the blank lines. See the answer key below.

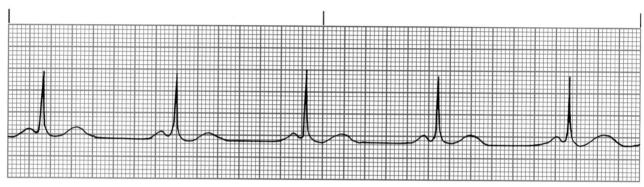

Rhythm: _____

Rate: _____

P wave: _____

PR interval: _____

QRS complex: _____

T wave: _____

QT interval: _____

Other: _____

■ **ANSWER KEY**

Rhythm: **Regular**

Rate: **48 beats/minute**

P wave: **Normal; precedes each QRS complex**

PR interval: **0.16 second**

QRS complex: **0.08 second**

T wave: **Normal**

QT interval: **0.50 second**

Other: **None**

Sinus tachycardia

Sinus tachycardia is an acceleration of the firing of the SA node beyond its normal discharge rate. Sinus tachycardia in an adult is characterized by a sinus rate of more than 100 beats/minute. The rate rarely exceeds 160 beats/minute, except during strenuous exercise; the maximum rate achievable with exercise decreases with age. (See *Identifying sinus tachycardia*.)

DEFINING CHARACTERISTICS

Identifying sinus tachycardia

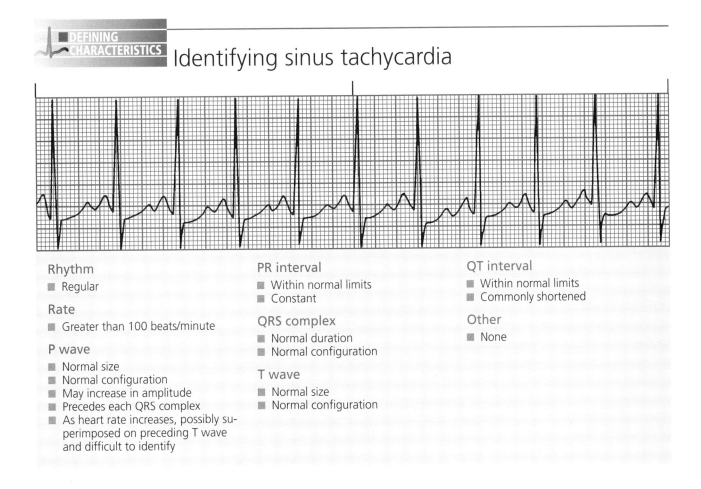

Rhythm
■ Regular

Rate
■ Greater than 100 beats/minute

P wave
■ Normal size
■ Normal configuration
■ May increase in amplitude
■ Precedes each QRS complex
■ As heart rate increases, possibly superimposed on preceding T wave and difficult to identify

PR interval
■ Within normal limits
■ Constant

QRS complex
■ Normal duration
■ Normal configuration

T wave
■ Normal size
■ Normal configuration

QT interval
■ Within normal limits
■ Commonly shortened

Other
■ None

PRACTICE # Sinus tachycardia

Use the 8-step method to interpret the following rhythm strip. Place your answers on the blank lines. See the answer key below.

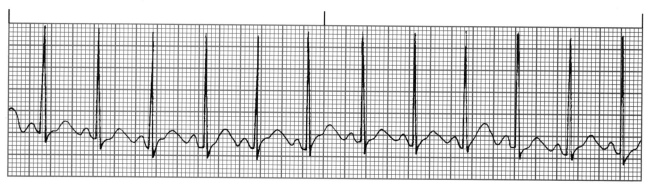

Rhythm:

Rate:

P wave:

PR interval:

QRS complex:

T wave:

QT interval:

Other:

Sinus arrest

In sinus arrest, the normal sinus rhythm is interrupted by an occasional, prolonged failure of the SA node to initiate an impulse. Therefore, sinus arrest is caused by episodes of failure in the automaticity or impulse forma- tion of the SA node. The atria aren't stimulated, and an entire PQRST complex is missing from the ECG strip. Except for this missing complex, or pause, the ECG usually remains normal. (See *Identifying sinus arrest*.)

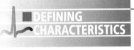

Identifying sinus arrest

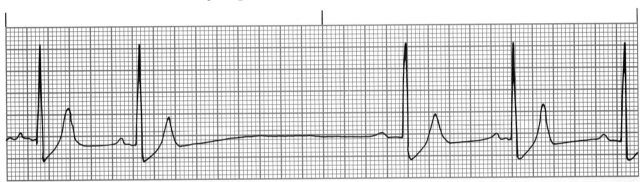

Rhythm
- Regular except during arrest (irregular as a result of missing complexes)

Rate
- Usually within normal limits (60 to 100 beats/minute) before arrest
- Length or frequency of pause may result in bradycardia

P wave
- Periodically absent, with entire PQRST complexes missing
- When present, normal size and configuration
- Precedes each QRS complex

PR interval
- Within normal limits when a P wave is present
- Constant when a P wave is present

QRS complex
- Normal duration
- Normal configuration
- Absent during arrest

T wave
- Normal size
- Normal configuration
- Absent during arrest

QT interval
- Within normal limits
- Absent during arrest

Other
- The pause isn't a multiple of the underlying P-P intervals

Sinus arrest

Use the 8-step method to interpret the following rhythm strip. Place your answers on the blank lines. See the answer key below.

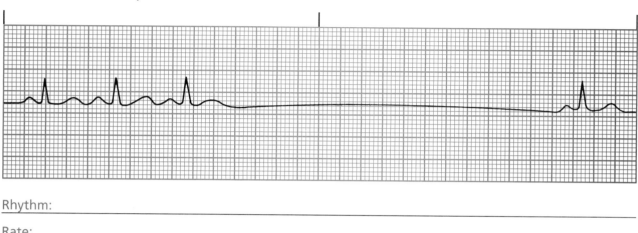

Rhythm:

Rate:

P wave:

PR interval:

QRS complex:

T wave:

QT interval:

Other:

■ **ANSWER KEY**

Rhythm: **Regular, except for missing PQRST complexes**

Rate: **Underlying rhythm, 88 beats/minute**

P wave: **Normal; missing during pause**

PR interval: **0.20 second**

QRS complex: **0.08 second; missing during pause**

T wave: **Normal; missing during pause**

QT interval: **0.40 second; missing during pause**

Other: **None**

Sinoatrial exit block

In sinoatrial exit block, the SA node discharges at regular intervals, but some impulses are delayed or blocked from reaching the atria, resulting in long sinus pauses. SA block results from failure to conduct impulses, whereas sinus arrest results from failure to form impulses in the SA node. In sinoatrial exit block, the pause occurs for an indefinite period and ends with a sinus rhythm. (See *Identifying sinoatrial exit block.*)

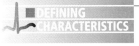 **DEFINING CHARACTERISTICS**

Identifying sinoatrial exit block

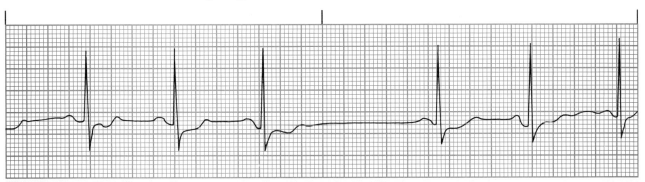

Rhythm
- Regular except during pause (irregular as result of pause)

Rate
- Usually within normal limits (60 to 100 beats/minute) before pause
- Length or frequency of pause may result in bradycardia

P wave
- Periodically absent, with entire PQRST complexes missing
- When present, normal size and configuration and precedes each QRS complex

PR interval
- Within normal limits
- Constant when a P wave is present

QRS complex
- Normal duration
- Normal configuration
- Absent during a pause

T wave
- Normal size
- Normal configuration
- Absent during a pause

QT interval
- Within normal limits
- Absent during a pause

Other
- The pause is a multiple of the underlying P-P interval

PRACTICE # Sinoatrial exit block

Use the 8-step method to interpret the following rhythm strip. Place your answers on the blank lines. See the answer key below.

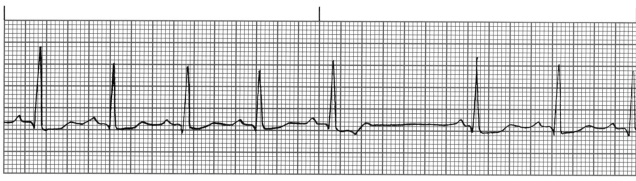

Rhythm: _____

Rate: _____

P wave: _____

PR interval: _____

QRS complex: _____

T wave: _____

QT interval: _____

Other: _____

■ **ANSWER KEY**

Rhythm: **Regular, except for pauses**

Rate: **Underlying rhythm, 83 beats/minute before sinoatrial block; length or frequency of the pause may result in bradycardia**

P wave: **Periodically absent**

PR interval: **0.18 second**

QRS complex: **0.10 second; missing during pause**

T wave: **Normal; missing during pause**

QT interval: **0.42 second; missing during pause**

Other: **Entire PQRST complex missing; pause ends with sinus rhythm**

Sick sinus syndrome

Also known as *SA syndrome, sinus nodal dysfunction,* and *Stokes-Adams syndrome,* sick sinus syndrome (SSS) refers to a wide spectrum of SA node arrhythmias. SSS is caused by disturbances in the way impulses are generated or in the ability to conduct impulses to the atria. These disturbances may be either intrinsic or mediated by the ANS.

SSS usually shows up as bradycardia, with episodes of sinus arrest and SA block interspersed with sudden, brief periods of rapid atrial fibrillation. Patients are also prone to paroxysms of other atrial tachyarrhythmias, such as atrial flutter and ectopic atrial tachycardia, a condition sometimes referred to as bradycardia-tachycardia (or "brady-tachy") syndrome.

Most patients with SSS are older than age 60, but anyone can develop the arrhythmia. It's rare in children, except after open-heart surgery that results in SA node damage. The arrhythmia affects men and women equally. The onset is progressive, insidious, and chronic. (See *Identifying sick sinus syndrome.*)

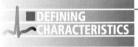

Identifying sick sinus syndrome

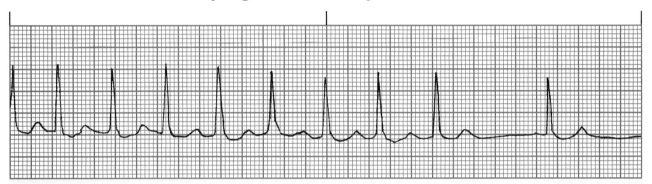

Rhythm
■ Irregular with sinus pauses

Rate
■ Fast, slow, or alternating
■ Abrupt rate changes
■ Interrupted by a long sinus pause

P wave
■ Varies with rhythm changes
■ May be normal size and configuration
■ May be absent
■ Usually precedes each QRS complex

PR interval
■ Usually within normal limits
■ Varies with rhythm changes

QRS complex
■ Duration within normal limits
■ Varies with rhythm changes
■ Normal configuration

T wave
■ Normal size
■ Normal configuration

QT interval
■ Usually within normal limits
■ Varies with rhythm changes

Other
■ Usually more than one arrhythmia on a 6-second strip

PRACTICE # Sick sinus syndrome

Use the 8-step method to interpret the following rhythm strip. Place your answers on the blank lines. See the answer key below.

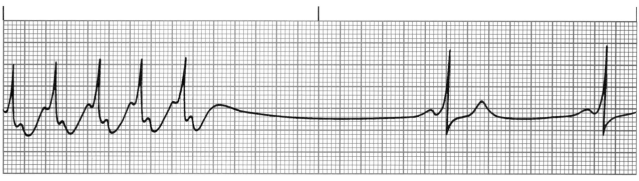

Rhythm:

Rate:

P wave:

PR interval:

QRS complex:

T wave:

QT interval:

Other:

■ **ANSWER KEY**

Rhythm: **Irregular**

Rate: **Atrial and ventricular rates fast (150 beats/minute) or slow (41 beats/minute) or alternate between fast and slow; interrupted by a long sinus pause**

P wave: **Varies with prevailing rhythm**

PR interval: **Varies with rhythm**

QRS complex: **0.12 second; may vary with rhythm**

T wave: **Configuration varies**

QT interval: **Varies with rhythm changes**

Other: **Sinus pause due to nonfiring sinus node**

■ PRACTICE 3-1

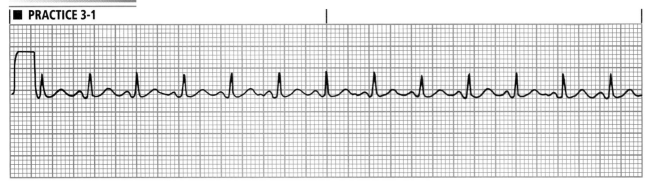

Rhythm: _____

Rate: _____

P wave: _____

PR interval: _____

QRS complex: _____

T wave: _____

QT interval: _____

Other: _____

Interpretation: _____

■ PRACTICE 3-2

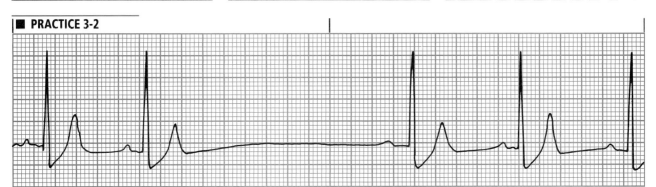

Rhythm: _____

Rate: _____

P wave: _____

PR interval: _____

QRS complex: _____

T wave: _____

QT interval: _____

Other: _____

Interpretation: _____

■ PRACTICE 3-3

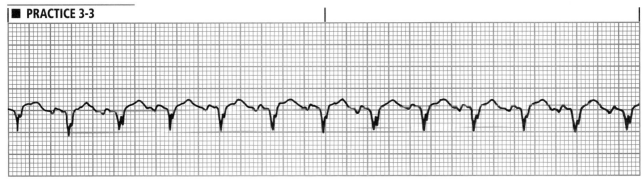

Rhythm: _____

Rate: _____

P wave: _____

PR interval: _____

QRS complex: _____

T wave: _____

QT interval: _____

Other: _____

Interpretation: _____

■ PRACTICE 3-4

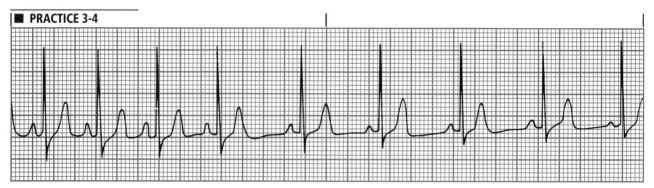

Rhythm: _____   PR interval: _____   QT interval: _____

Rate: _____   QRS complex: _____   Other: _____

P wave: _____   T wave: _____   Interpretation: _____

■ PRACTICE 3-5

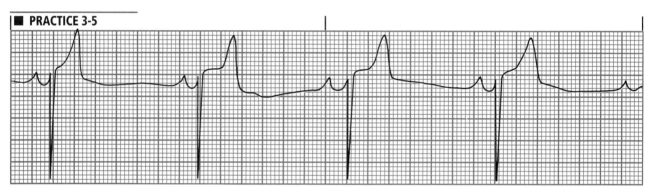

Rhythm: _____   PR interval: _____   QT interval: _____

Rate: _____   QRS complex: _____   Other: _____

P wave: _____   T wave: _____   Interpretation: _____

■ PRACTICE 3-6

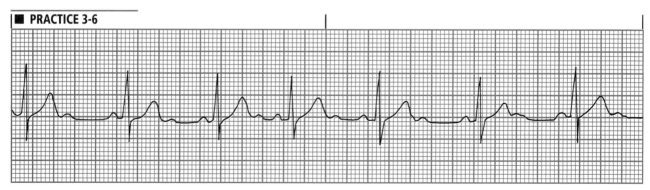

Rhythm: _____   PR interval: _____   QT interval: _____

Rate: _____   QRS complex: _____   Other: _____

P wave: _____   T wave: _____   Interpretation: _____

■ PRACTICE 3-7

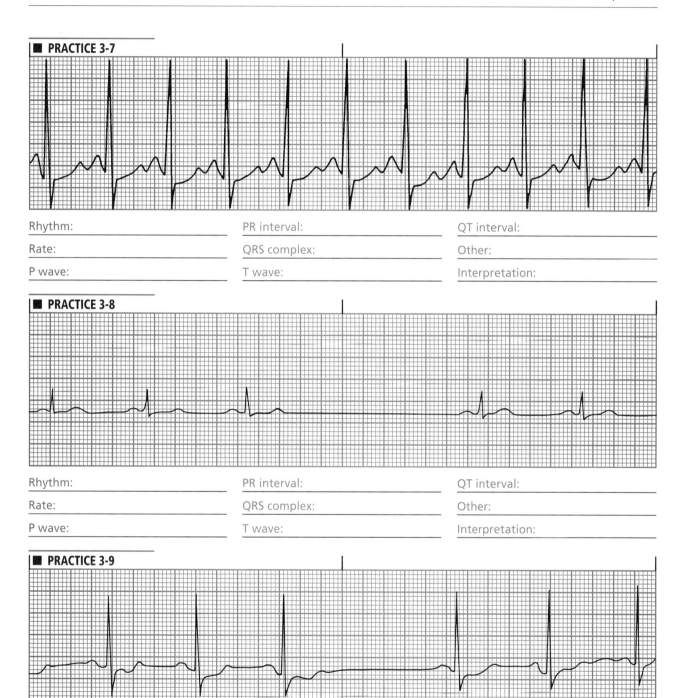

Rhythm: _____ PR interval: _____ QT interval: _____

Rate: _____ QRS complex: _____ Other: _____

P wave: _____ T wave: _____ Interpretation: _____

■ PRACTICE 3-8

Rhythm: _____ PR interval: _____ QT interval: _____

Rate: _____ QRS complex: _____ Other: _____

P wave: _____ T wave: _____ Interpretation: _____

■ PRACTICE 3-9

Rhythm: _____ PR interval: _____ QT interval: _____

Rate: _____ QRS complex: _____ Other: _____

P wave: _____ T wave: _____ Interpretation: _____

■ **PRACTICE 3-10**

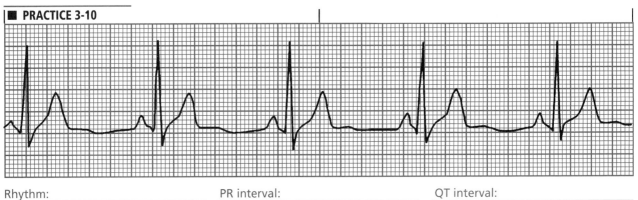

Rhythm: _____ PR interval: _____ QT interval: _____

Rate: _____ QRS complex: _____ Other: _____

P wave: _____ T wave: _____ Interpretation: _____

■ **PRACTICE 3-11**

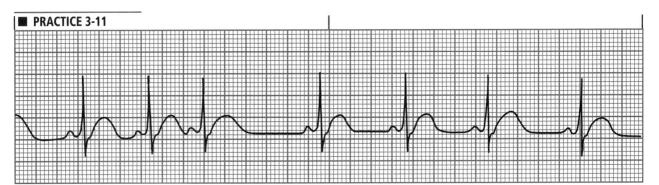

Rhythm: _____ PR interval: _____ QT interval: _____

Rate: _____ QRS complex: _____ Other: _____

P wave: _____ T wave: _____ Interpretation: _____

■ **PRACTICE 3-12**

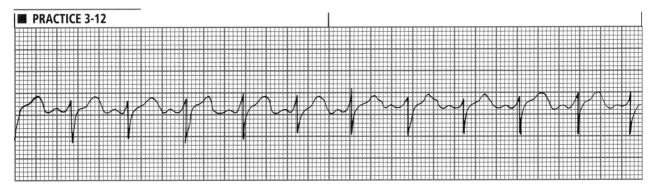

Rhythm: _____ PR interval: _____ QT interval: _____

Rate: _____ QRS complex: _____ Other: _____

P wave: _____ T wave: _____ Interpretation: _____

■ PRACTICE 3-13

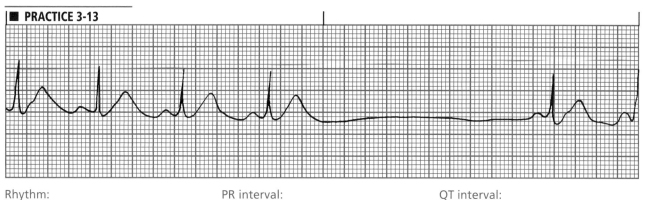

Rhythm: _____

Rate: _____

P wave: _____

PR interval: _____

QRS complex: _____

T wave: _____

QT interval: _____

Other: _____

Interpretation: _____

■ PRACTICE 3-14

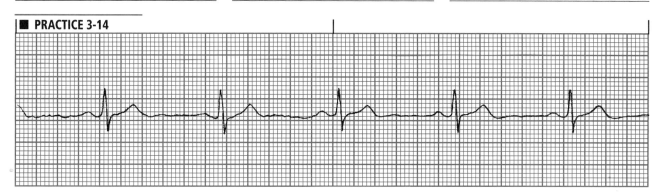

Rhythm: _____

Rate: _____

P wave: _____

PR interval: _____

QRS complex: _____

T wave: _____

QT interval: _____

Other: _____

Interpretation: _____

■ PRACTICE 3-15

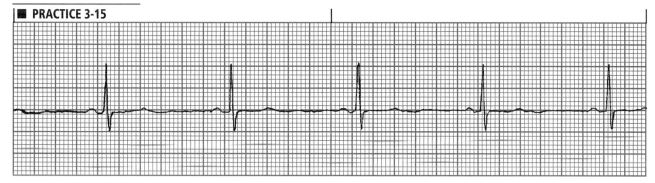

Rhythm: _____

Rate: _____

P wave: _____

PR interval: _____

QRS complex: _____

T wave: _____

QT interval: _____

Other: _____

Interpretation: _____

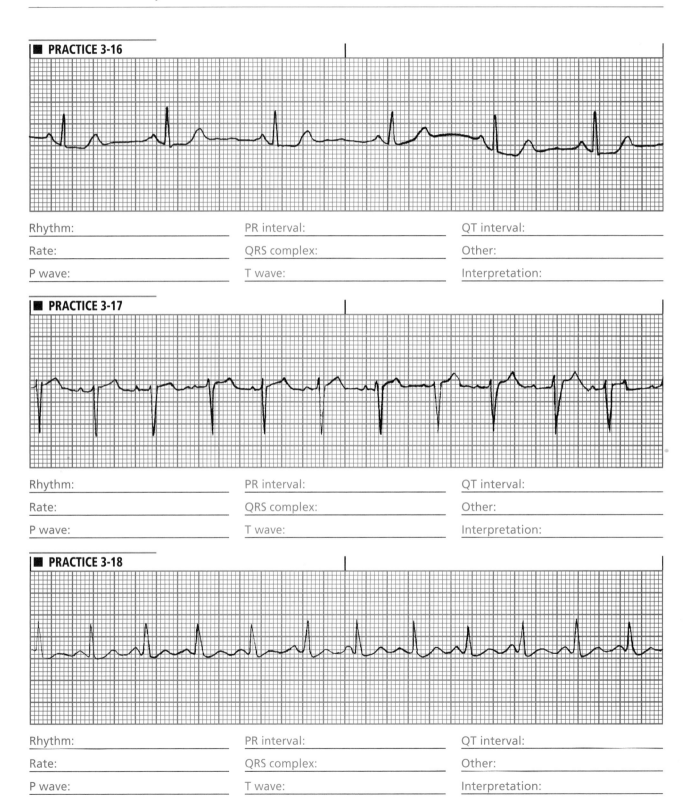

■ **PRACTICE 3-16**

Rhythm: _____ PR interval: _____ QT interval: _____

Rate: _____ QRS complex: _____ Other: _____

P wave: _____ T wave: _____ Interpretation: _____

■ **PRACTICE 3-17**

Rhythm: _____ PR interval: _____ QT interval: _____

Rate: _____ QRS complex: _____ Other: _____

P wave: _____ T wave: _____ Interpretation: _____

■ **PRACTICE 3-18**

Rhythm: _____ PR interval: _____ QT interval: _____

Rate: _____ QRS complex: _____ Other: _____

P wave: _____ T wave: _____ Interpretation: _____

■ PRACTICE 3-19

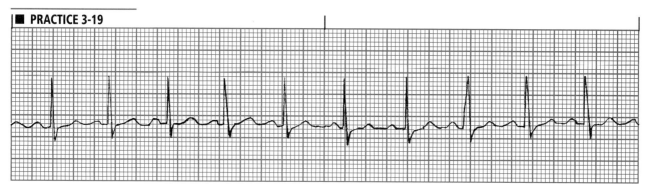

Rhythm: _____

Rate: _____

P wave: _____

PR interval: _____

QRS complex: _____

T wave: _____

QT interval: _____

Other: _____

Interpretation: _____

■ PRACTICE 3-20

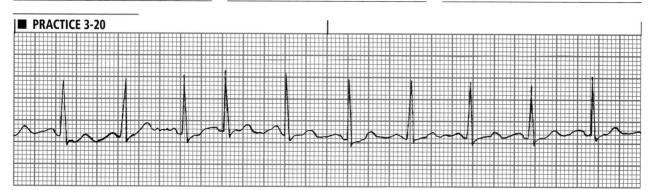

Rhythm: _____

Rate: _____

P wave: _____

PR interval: _____

QRS complex: _____

T wave: _____

QT interval: _____

Other: _____

Interpretation: _____

■ PRACTICE 3-21

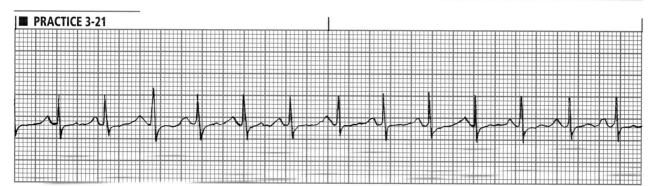

Rhythm: _____

Rate: _____

P wave: _____

PR interval: _____

QRS complex: _____

T wave: _____

QT interval: _____

Other: _____

Interpretation: _____

■ PRACTICE 3-22

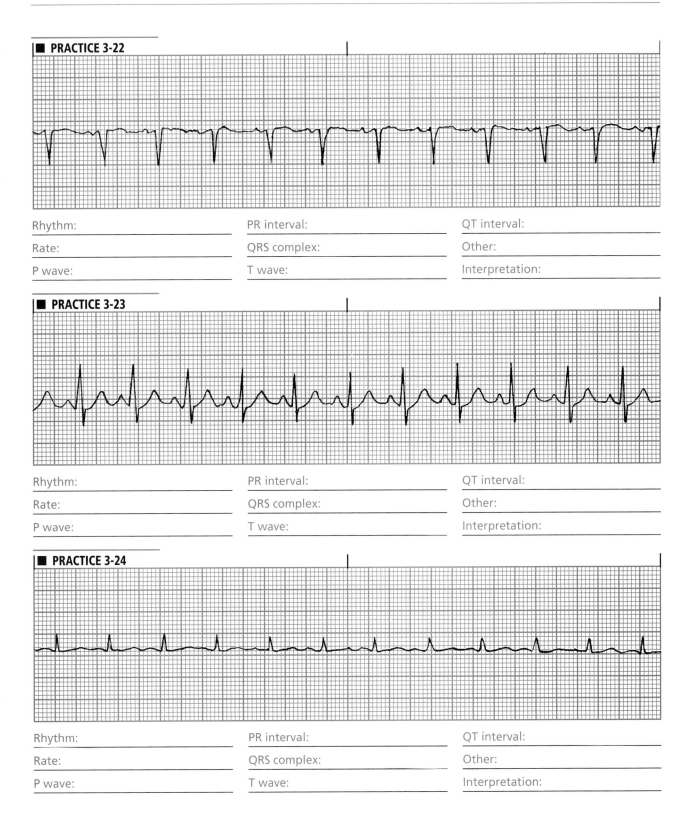

Rhythm: _____

Rate: _____

P wave: _____

PR interval: _____

QRS complex: _____

T wave: _____

QT interval: _____

Other: _____

Interpretation: _____

■ PRACTICE 3-23

Rhythm: _____

Rate: _____

P wave: _____

PR interval: _____

QRS complex: _____

T wave: _____

QT interval: _____

Other: _____

Interpretation: _____

■ PRACTICE 3-24

Rhythm: _____

Rate: _____

P wave: _____

PR interval: _____

QRS complex: _____

T wave: _____

QT interval: _____

Other: _____

Interpretation: _____

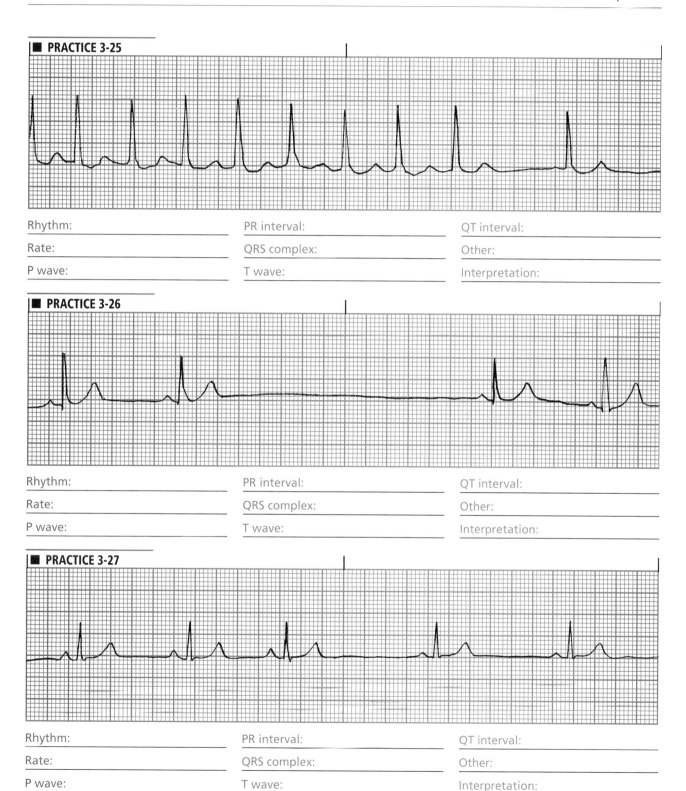

■ PRACTICE 3-25

Rhythm: _____   PR interval: _____   QT interval: _____

Rate: _____   QRS complex: _____   Other: _____

P wave: _____   T wave: _____   Interpretation: _____

■ PRACTICE 3-26

Rhythm: _____   PR interval: _____   QT interval: _____

Rate: _____   QRS complex: _____   Other: _____

P wave: _____   T wave: _____   Interpretation: _____

■ PRACTICE 3-27

Rhythm: _____   PR interval: _____   QT interval: _____

Rate: _____   QRS complex: _____   Other: _____

P wave: _____   T wave: _____   Interpretation: _____

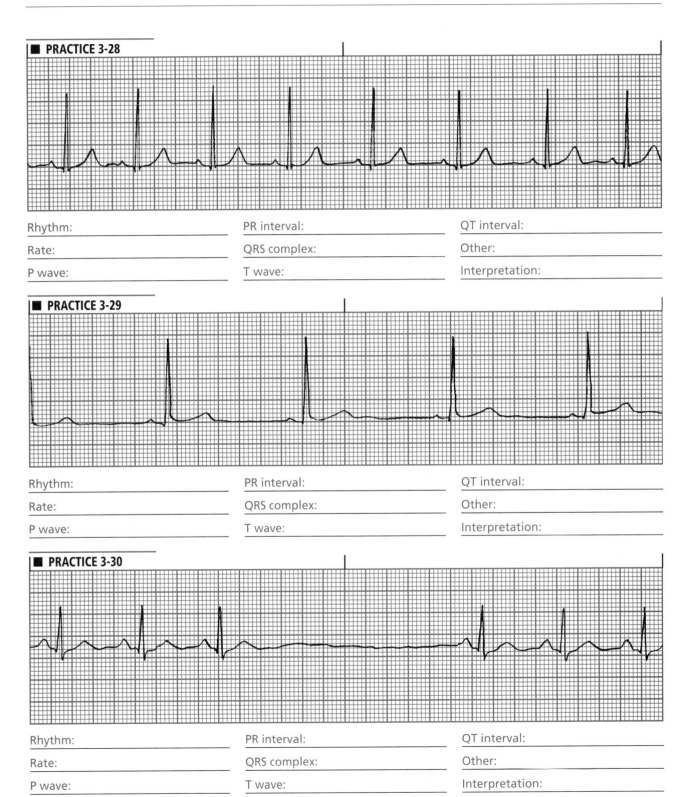

PRACTICE 3-28

Rhythm: _____   PR interval: _____   QT interval: _____

Rate: _____   QRS complex: _____   Other: _____

P wave: _____   T wave: _____   Interpretation: _____

PRACTICE 3-29

Rhythm: _____   PR interval: _____   QT interval: _____

Rate: _____   QRS complex: _____   Other: _____

P wave: _____   T wave: _____   Interpretation: _____

PRACTICE 3-30

Rhythm: _____   PR interval: _____   QT interval: _____

Rate: _____   QRS complex: _____   Other: _____

P wave: _____   T wave: _____   Interpretation: _____

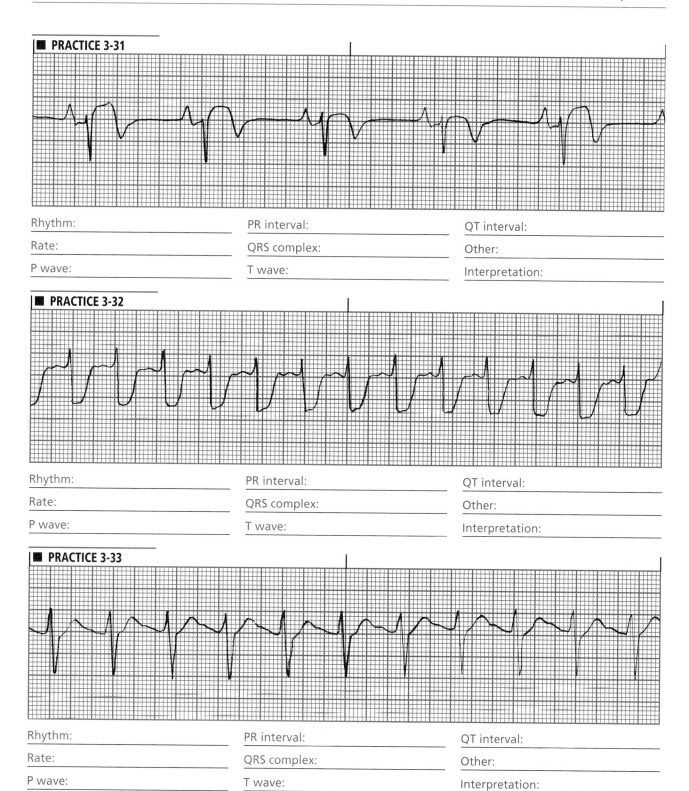

■ **PRACTICE 3-31**

Rhythm: _____

Rate: _____

P wave: _____

PR interval: _____

QRS complex: _____

T wave: _____

QT interval: _____

Other: _____

Interpretation: _____

■ **PRACTICE 3-32**

Rhythm: _____

Rate: _____

P wave: _____

PR interval: _____

QRS complex: _____

T wave: _____

QT interval: _____

Other: _____

Interpretation: _____

■ **PRACTICE 3-33**

Rhythm: _____

Rate: _____

P wave: _____

PR interval: _____

QRS complex: _____

T wave: _____

QT interval: _____

Other: _____

Interpretation: _____

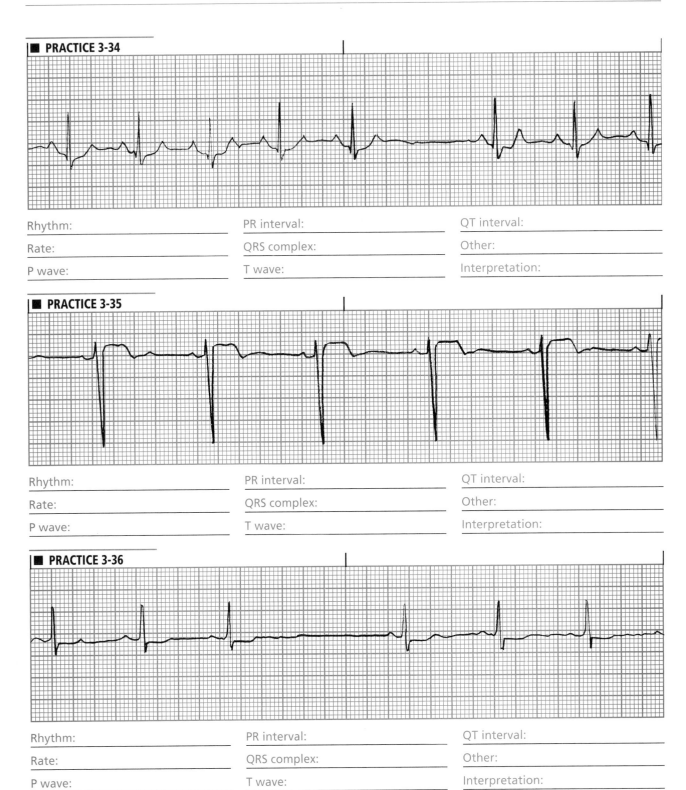

■ PRACTICE 3-34

Rhythm: _____ PR interval: _____ QT interval: _____

Rate: _____ QRS complex: _____ Other: _____

P wave: _____ T wave: _____ Interpretation: _____

■ PRACTICE 3-35

Rhythm: _____ PR interval: _____ QT interval: _____

Rate: _____ QRS complex: _____ Other: _____

P wave: _____ T wave: _____ Interpretation: _____

■ PRACTICE 3-36

Rhythm: _____ PR interval: _____ QT interval: _____

Rate: _____ QRS complex: _____ Other: _____

P wave: _____ T wave: _____ Interpretation: _____

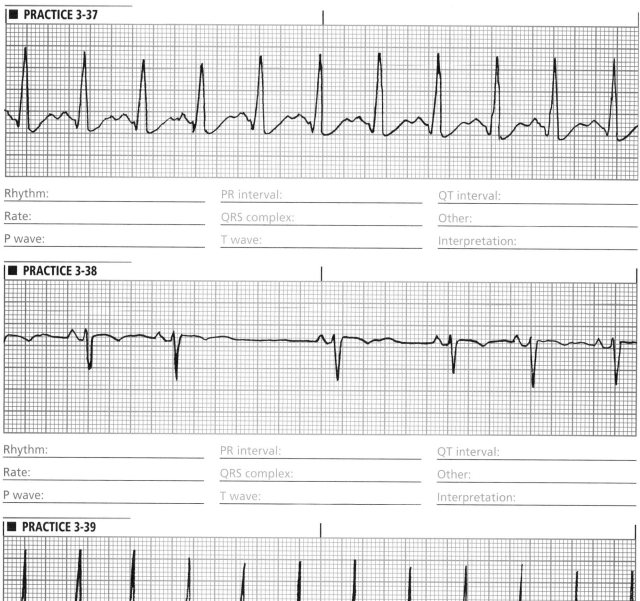

■ **PRACTICE 3-37**

Rhythm: _____

Rate: _____

P wave: _____

PR interval: _____

QRS complex: _____

T wave: _____

QT interval: _____

Other: _____

Interpretation: _____

■ **PRACTICE 3-38**

Rhythm: _____

Rate: _____

P wave: _____

PR interval: _____

QRS complex: _____

T wave: _____

QT interval: _____

Other: _____

Interpretation: _____

■ **PRACTICE 3-39**

Rhythm: _____

Rate: _____

P wave: _____

PR interval: _____

QRS complex: _____

T wave: _____

QT interval: _____

Other: _____

Interpretation: _____

■ **PRACTICE 3-40**

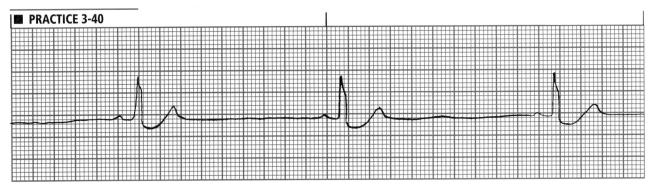

Rhythm: _____   PR interval: _____   QT interval: _____

Rate: _____   QRS complex: _____   Other: _____

P wave: _____   T wave: _____   Interpretation: _____

■ **PRACTICE 3-41**

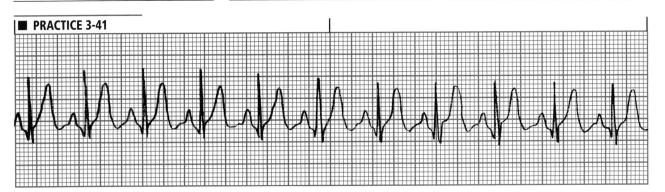

Rhythm: _____   PR interval: _____   QT interval: _____

Rate: _____   QRS complex: _____   Other: _____

P wave: _____   T wave: _____   Interpretation: _____

■ **PRACTICE 3-42**

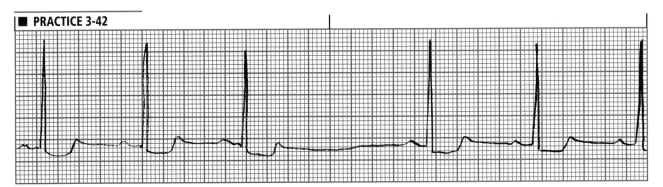

Rhythm: _____   PR interval: _____   QT interval: _____

Rate: _____   QRS complex: _____   Other: _____

P wave: _____   T wave: _____   Interpretation: _____

■ **PRACTICE 3-43**

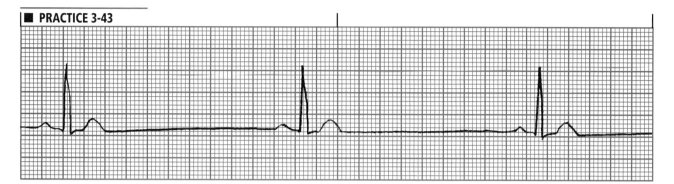

Rhythm: _____   PR interval: _____   QT interval: _____

Rate: _____   QRS complex: _____   Other: _____

P wave: _____   T wave: _____   Interpretation: _____

■ **PRACTICE 3-44**

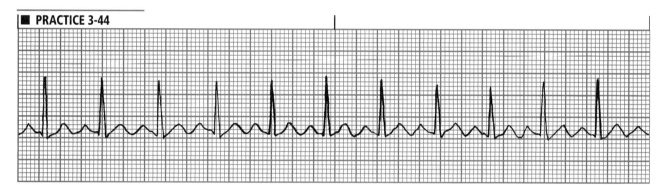

Rhythm: _____   PR interval: _____   QT interval: _____

Rate: _____   QRS complex: _____   Other: _____

P wave: _____   T wave: _____   Interpretation: _____

■ **PRACTICE 3-45**

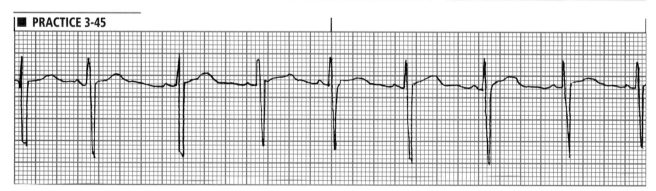

Rhythm: _____   PR interval: _____   QT interval: _____

Rate: _____   QRS complex: _____   Other: _____

P wave: _____   T wave: _____   Interpretation: _____

■ **PRACTICE 3-46**

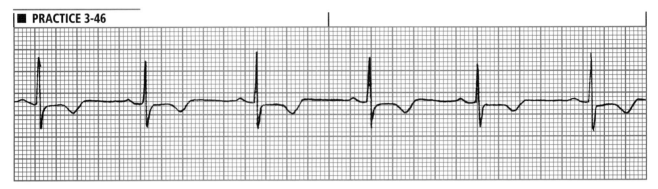

Rhythm: _____   PR interval: _____   QT interval: _____

Rate: _____   QRS complex: _____   Other: _____

P wave: _____   T wave: _____   Interpretation: _____

■ **PRACTICE 3-47**

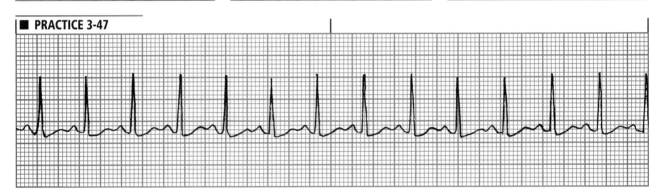

Rhythm: _____   PR interval: _____   QT interval: _____

Rate: _____   QRS complex: _____   Other: _____

P wave: _____   T wave: _____   Interpretation: _____

■ **PRACTICE 3-48**

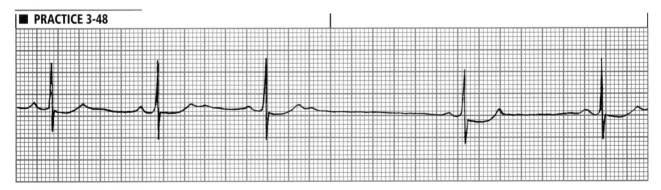

Rhythm: _____   PR interval: _____   QT interval: _____

Rate: _____   QRS complex: _____   Other: _____

P wave: _____   T wave: _____   Interpretation: _____

■ PRACTICE 3-49

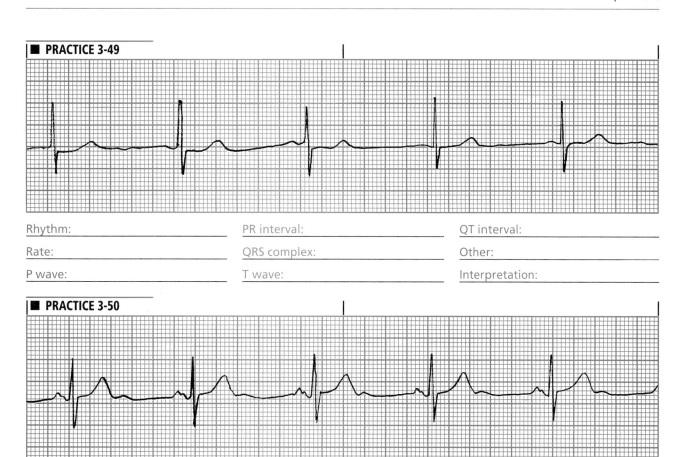

Rhythm: _____ PR interval: _____ QT interval: _____

Rate: _____ QRS complex: _____ Other: _____

P wave: _____ T wave: _____ Interpretation: _____

■ PRACTICE 3-50

Rhythm: _____ PR interval: _____ QT interval: _____

Rate: _____ QRS complex: _____ Other: _____

P wave: _____ T wave: _____ Interpretation: _____

■ PRACTICE 3-51

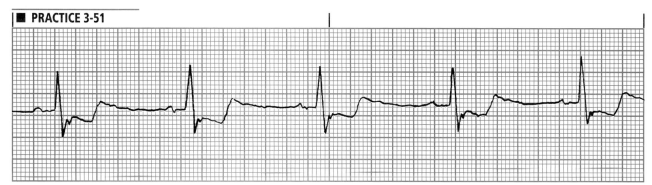

Rhythm: _____ PR interval: _____ QT interval: _____

Rate: _____ QRS complex: _____ Other: _____

P wave: _____ T wave: _____ Interpretation: _____

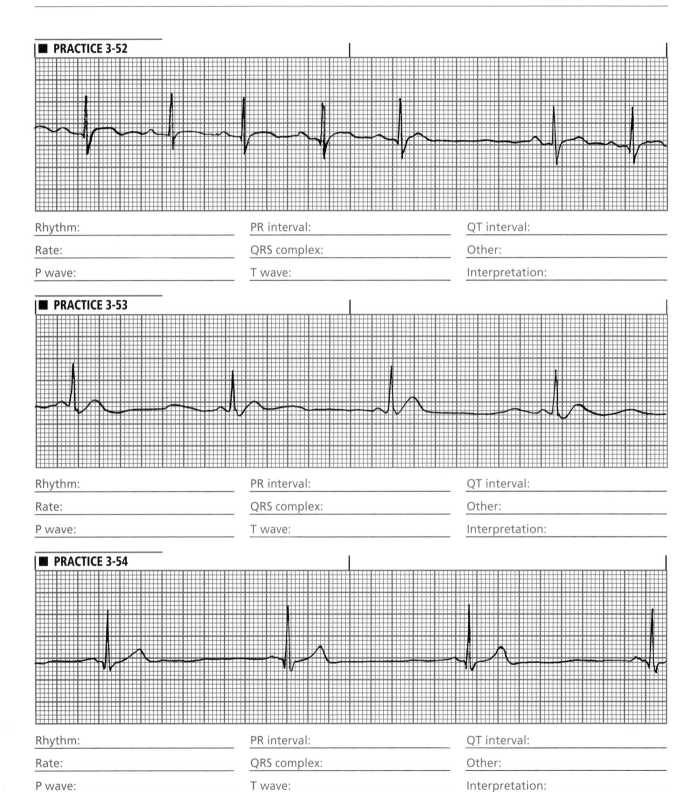

■ **PRACTICE 3-52**

Rhythm: _____ PR interval: _____ QT interval: _____

Rate: _____ QRS complex: _____ Other: _____

P wave: _____ T wave: _____ Interpretation: _____

■ **PRACTICE 3-53**

Rhythm: _____ PR interval: _____ QT interval: _____

Rate: _____ QRS complex: _____ Other: _____

P wave: _____ T wave: _____ Interpretation: _____

■ **PRACTICE 3-54**

Rhythm: _____ PR interval: _____ QT interval: _____

Rate: _____ QRS complex: _____ Other: _____

P wave: _____ T wave: _____ Interpretation: _____

■ PRACTICE 3-55

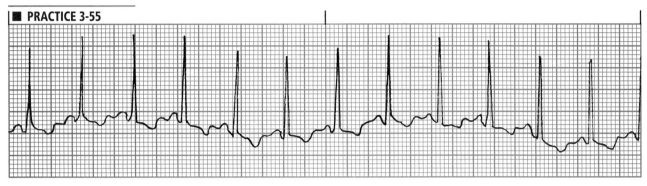

Rhythm: _____   PR interval: _____   QT interval: _____

Rate: _____   QRS complex: _____   Other: _____

P wave: _____   T wave: _____   Interpretation: _____

■ PRACTICE 3-56

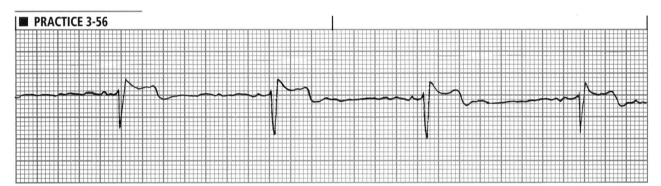

Rhythm: _____   PR interval: _____   QT interval: _____

Rate: _____   QRS complex: _____   Other: _____

P wave: _____   T wave: _____   Interpretation: _____

■ PRACTICE 3-57

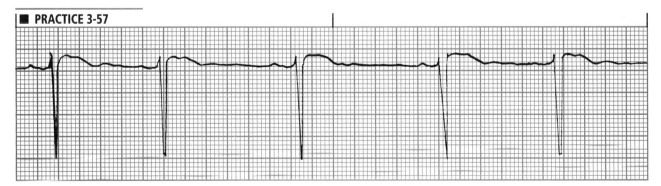

Rhythm: _____   PR interval: _____   QT interval: _____

Rate: _____   QRS complex: _____   Other: _____

P wave: _____   T wave: _____   Interpretation: _____

■ PRACTICE 3-58

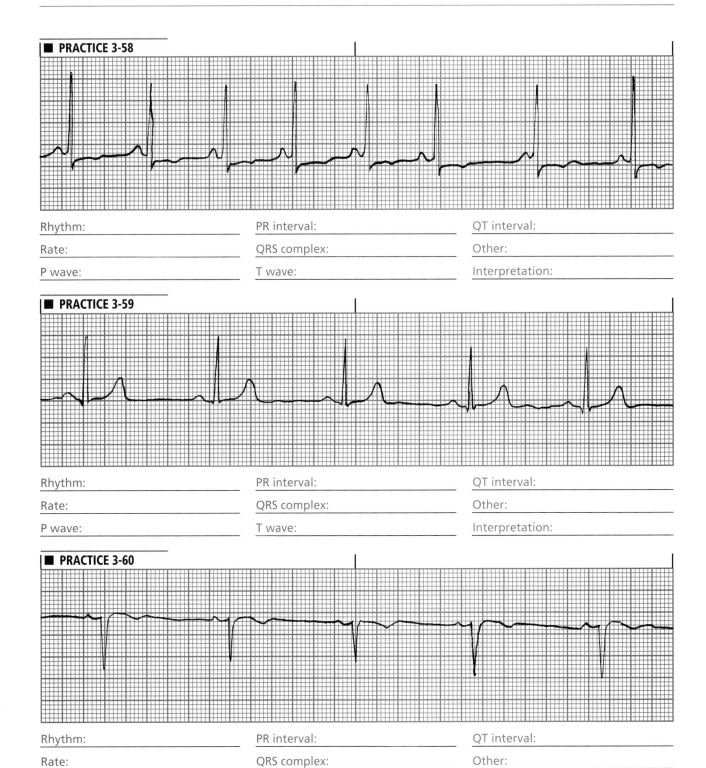

Rhythm: _____   PR interval: _____   QT interval: _____

Rate: _____   QRS complex: _____   Other: _____

P wave: _____   T wave: _____   Interpretation: _____

■ PRACTICE 3-59

Rhythm: _____   PR interval: _____   QT interval: _____

Rate: _____   QRS complex: _____   Other: _____

P wave: _____   T wave: _____   Interpretation: _____

■ PRACTICE 3-60

Rhythm: _____   PR interval: _____   QT interval: _____

Rate: _____   QRS complex: _____   Other: _____

P wave: _____   T wave: _____   Interpretation: _____

■ PRACTICE STRIP ANSWERS

PRACTICE 3-1
Rhythm: Regular
Rate: 136 beats/minute
P wave: Normal
PR interval: 0.12 second
QRS complex: 0.08 second
T wave: Normal
QT interval: 0.28 second
Other: None
Interpretation: Sinus tachycardia

PRACTICE 3-2
Rhythm: Irregular
Rate: 50 beats/minute
P wave: Normal
PR interval: 0.20 second
QRS complex: 0.08 second
T wave: Normal
QT interval: 0.40 second
Other: Pause present
Interpretation: Sinus bradycardia with premature atrial contraction (PAC)

PRACTICE 3-3
Rhythm: Regular
Rate: 125 beats/minute
P wave: Slightly peaked
PR interval: 0.12 second
QRS complex: 0.10 second
T wave: Normal
QT interval: 0.28 second
Other: None
Interpretation: Sinus tachycardia

PRACTICE 3-4
Rhythm: Irregular
Rate: 90 beats/minute
P wave: Normal
PR interval: 0.12 second
QRS complex: 0.10 second
T wave: Normal
QT interval: 0.30 second
Other: Phasic slowing and quickening
Interpretation: Sinus arrhythmia

PRACTICE 3-5
Rhythm: Regular
Rate: 40 beats/minute
P wave: Normal
PR interval: 0.20 second
QRS complex: 0.08 second
T wave: Normal
QT interval: 0.44 second
Other: None
Interpretation: Sinus bradycardia

PRACTICE 3-6
Rhythm: Irregular
Rate: 70 beats/minute
P wave: Normal
PR interval: 0.16 second
QRS complex: 0.10 second
T wave: Biphasic
QT interval: 0.38 second
Other: None
Interpretation: Sinus arrhythmia

PRACTICE 3-7
Rhythm: Regular
Rate: 110 beats/minute
P wave: Normal
PR interval: 0.16 second
QRS complex: 0.10 second
T wave: Normal
QT interval: 0.38 second
Other: None
Interpretation: Sinus tachycardia

PRACTICE 3-8
Rhythm: Regular except for pause
Rate: Underlying, 68 beats/minute
P wave: Normal
PR interval: 0.18 second
QRS complex: 0.08 second
T wave: Normal
QT interval: 0.38 second
Other: None
Interpretation: Sinus arrest

PRACTICE 3-9
Rhythm: Regular except for pause
Rate: Underlying, 60 beats/minute
P wave: Normal
PR interval: 0.20 second
QRS complex: 0.10 second
T wave: Inverted
QT interval: 0.38 second
Other: None
Interpretation: Sinoatrial exit block

PRACTICE 3-10
Rhythm: Regular
Rate: 50 beats/minute
P wave: Normal
PR interval: 0.16 second
QRS complex: 0.12 second
T wave: Normal
QT interval: 0.44 second
Other: None
Interpretation: Sinus bradycardia

PRACTICE 3-11
Rhythm: Irregular
Rate: 70 beats/minute
P wave: Normal
PR interval: 0.14 second
QRS complex: 0.12 second
T wave: Normal
QT interval: 0.36 second
Other: None
Interpretation: Sinus arrhythmia

PRACTICE 3-12
Rhythm: Regular
Rate: 110 beats/minute
P wave: Normal
PR interval: 0.16 second
QRS complex: 0.12 second
T wave: Slightly elevated
QT interval: 0.34 second
Other: None
Interpretation: Sinus tachycardia

PRACTICE 3-13
Rhythm: Regular except for pause
Rate: Underlying, 75 beats/minute
P wave: Normal
PR interval: 0.20 second
QRS complex: 0.12 second
T wave: Normal
QT interval: 0.42 second
Other: None
Interpretation: Sinus arrest

PRACTICE 3-14
Rhythm: Regular
Rate: 56 beats/minute
P wave: Normal
PR interval: 0.20 second
QRS complex: 0.12 second
T wave: Normal
QT interval: 0.40 second
Other: None
Interpretation: Sinus bradycardia

PRACTICE 3-15
Rhythm: Regular
Rate: 50 beats/minute
P wave: Normal
PR interval: 0.16 second
QRS complex: 0.08 second
T wave: Flattened
QT interval: 0.44 second
Other: None
Interpretation: Sinus bradycardia

PRACTICE 3-16
Rhythm: Irregular
Rate: 60 beats/minute
P wave: Normal
PR interval: 0.16 second
QRS complex: 0.08 second
T wave: Normal
QT interval: 0.40 second
Other: None
Interpretation: Sinus arrhythmia

PRACTICE 3-17
Rhythm: Regular
Rate: 110 beats/minute
P wave: Normal
PR interval: 0.12 second
QRS complex: 0.10 second
T wave: Normal
QT interval: 0.28 second
Other: None
Interpretation: Sinus tachycardia

PRACTICE 3-18
Rhythm: Regular
Rate: 115 beats/minute
P wave: Normal
PR interval: 0.16 second
QRS complex: 0.08 second
T wave: Normal
QT interval: 0.32 second
Other: None
Interpretation: Sinus tachycardia

PRACTICE 3-19
Rhythm: Regular
Rate: 107 beats/minute
P wave: Normal
PR interval: 0.18 second
QRS complex: 0.10 second
T wave: Normal
QT interval: 0.32 second
Other: None
Interpretation: Sinus tachycardia

PRACTICE 3-20
Rhythm: Irregular
Rate: 100 beats/minute
P wave: Normal
PR interval: 0.18 second
QRS complex: 0.12 second
T wave: Normal
QT interval: 0.32 second
Other: None
Interpretation: Sinus tachycardia with one PAC (beat #4)

PRACTICE 3-21
Rhythm: Regular
Rate: 136 beats/minute
P wave: Normal
PR interval: 0.16 second
QRS complex: 0.08 second
T wave: Flattened
QT interval: Unmeasurable
Other: None
Interpretation: Sinus tachycardia

PRACTICE 3-22
Rhythm: Regular
Rate: 115 beats/minute
P wave: Normal
PR interval: 0.14 second
QRS complex: 0.10 second
T wave: Normal
QT interval: 0.28 second
Other: None
Interpretation: Sinus tachycardia

PRACTICE 3-23
Rhythm: Regular
Rate: 115 beats/minute
P wave: Normal
PR interval: 0.16 second
QRS complex: 0.08 second
T wave: Normal
QT interval: 0.30 second
Other: None
Interpretation: Sinus tachycardia

PRACTICE 3-24
Rhythm: Regular
Rate: 120 beats/minute
P wave: Normal
PR interval: 0.16 second
QRS complex: 0.08 second
T wave: Normal
QT interval: 0.30 second
Other: None
Interpretation: Sinus tachycardia

RACTICE 3-25
Rhythm: Irregular
Rate: 100 beats/minute
P wave: Normal
PR interval: Varies
QRS complex: 0.08 second
T wave: Normal
QT interval: 0.40 second
Other: None
Interpretation: Sick sinus syndrome

PRACTICE 3-26
Rhythm: Regular except for pause
Rate: Underlying, 40 beats/minute
P wave: Normal
PR interval: 0.16 second
QRS complex: 0.10 second
T wave: Normal
QT interval: 0.40 second
Other: None
Interpretation: Sinus arrest

PRACTICE 3-27
Rhythm: Irregular
Rate: 50 beats/minute
P wave: Normal
PR interval: 0.16 second
QRS complex: 0.06 second
T wave: Normal
QT interval: 0.38 second
Other: None
Interpretation: Sinus bradyarrhythmia

PRACTICE 3-28
Rhythm: Irregular
Rate: 80 beats/minute
P wave: Normal
PR interval: 0.14 second
QRS complex: 0.06 second
T wave: Normal
QT interval: 0.36 second
Other: None
Interpretation: Sinus arrhythmia

PRACTICE 3-29
Rhythm: Irregular
Rate: 40 to 50 beats/minute
P wave: Normal
PR interval: 0.16 second
QRS complex: 0.08 second
T wave: Normal
QT interval: 0.48 second
Other: None
Interpretation: Sinus bradyarrhythmia

PRACTICE 3-30
Rhythm: Regular except for pause
Rate: Underlying, 79 beats/minute
P wave: Normal
PR interval: 0.18 second
QRS complex: 0.08 second
T wave: Normal
QT interval: 0.38 second
Other: None
Interpretation: Sinus arrest

PRACTICE 3-31
- Rhythm: Regular
- Rate: 54 beats/minute
- P wave: Peaked
- PR interval: 0.20 second
- QRS complex: 0.08 second
- T wave: Inverted
- QT interval: 0.44 second
- Other: None
- Interpretation: Sinus bradycardia

PRACTICE 3-32
- Rhythm: Regular
- Rate: 136 beats/minute
- P wave: Normal
- PR interval: 0.12 second
- QRS complex: 0.04 second
- T wave: Inverted
- QT interval: 0.26 second
- Other: None
- Interpretation: Sinus tachycardia

PRACTICE 3-33
- Rhythm: Regular
- Rate: 107 beats/minute
- P wave: Flattened
- PR interval: 0.20 second
- QRS complex: 0.12 second
- T wave: Normal
- QT interval: 0.34 second
- Other: None
- Interpretation: Sinus tachycardia

PRACTICE 3-34
- Rhythm: Regular except for pause
- Rate: Underlying, 80 beats/minute
- P wave: Normal
- PR interval: 0.18 second
- QRS complex: 0.10 second
- T wave: Normal
- QT interval: 0.30 second
- Other: None
- Interpretation: Sinoatrial exit block

PRACTICE 3-35
- Rhythm: Regular
- Rate: 58 beats/minute
- P wave: Normal
- PR interval: 0.16 second
- QRS complex: 0.08 second
- T wave: Normal
- QT interval: 0.38 second
- Other: None
- Interpretation: Sinus bradycardia

PRACTICE 3-36
- Rhythm: Regular except missed beat
- Rate: Underlying, 72 beats/minute
- P wave: Normal
- PR interval: 0.16 second
- QRS complex: 0.08 second
- T wave: Normal
- QT interval: 0.32 second
- Other: Slight ST segment depression
- Other: None
- Interpretation: Sinoatrial exit block

PRACTICE 3-37
- Rhythm: Regular
- Rate: 107 beats/minute
- P wave: Normal
- PR interval: 0.16 second
- QRS complex: 0.12 second
- T wave: Normal
- QT interval: 0.40 second
- Other: None
- Interpretation: Sinus tachycardia

PRACTICE 3-38
- Rhythm: Irregular
- Rate: 60 beats/minute
- P wave: Normal
- PR interval: 0.16 second
- QRS complex: 0.10 second
- T wave: Inverted
- QT interval: 0.40 second
- Other: None
- Interpretation: Sinus arrhythmia

PRACTICE 3-39
- Rhythm: Regular
- Rate: 115 beats/minute
- P wave: Normal
- PR interval: 0.18 second
- QRS complex: 0.08 second
- T wave: Inverted
- QT interval: 0.28 second
- Other: None
- Interpretation: Sinus tachycardia

PRACTICE 3-40
- Rhythm: Irregular
- Rate: 30 beats/minute
- P wave: Normal
- PR interval: 0.20 second
- QRS complex: 0.10 second
- T wave: Normal
- QT interval: 0.44 second
- Other: None
- Interpretation: Sinus bradyarrhythmia

PRACTICE 3-41
- Rhythm: Regular
- Rate: 107 beats/minute
- P wave: Peaked
- PR interval: 0.16 second
- QRS complex: 0.08 second
- T wave: Peaked
- QT interval: 0.28 second
- Other: None
- Interpretation: Sinus tachycardia

PRACTICE 3-42
- Rhythm: Regular except for pause
- Rate: Underlying, 60 beats/minute
- P wave: Normal
- PR interval: 0.20 second
- QRS complex: 0.04 second
- T wave: Normal
- QT interval: 0.40 second
- Other: Depressed ST segment
- Interpretation: Sinus arrest

PRACTICE 3-43
- Rhythm: Regular
- Rate: 27 beats/minute
- P wave: Normal
- PR interval: 0.20 second
- QRS complex: 0.08 second
- T wave: Normal
- QT interval: 0.40 second
- Other: None
- Interpretation: Sinus bradycardia

PRACTICE 3-44
- Rhythm: Regular
- Rate: 115 beats/minute
- P wave: Normal
- PR interval: 0.20 second
- QRS complex: 0.08 second
- T wave: Normal
- QT interval: 0.28 second
- Other: None
- Interpretation: Sinus tachycardia

PRACTICE 3-45
- Rhythm: Irregular
- Rate: 90 beats/minute
- P wave: Normal
- PR interval: 0.12 second
- QRS complex: 0.08 second
- T wave: Normal
- QT interval: 0.38 second
- Other: None
- Interpretation: Sinus arrhythmia

PRACTICE 3-46
- Rhythm: Regular
- Rate: 56 beats/minute
- P wave: Normal
- PR interval: 0.18 second
- QRS complex: 0.08 second
- T wave: Inverted
- QT interval: 0.44 second
- Other: None
- Interpretation: Sinus bradycardia

PRACTICE 3-47
- Rhythm: Regular
- Rate: 136 beats/minute
- P wave: Normal
- PR interval: 0.16 second
- QRS complex: 0.06 second
- T wave: Normal
- QT interval: 0.28 second
- Other: None
- Interpretation: Sinus bradycardia

PRACTICE 3-48
- Rhythm: Irregular
- Rate: 50 beats/minute
- P wave: Normal
- PR interval: 0.16 second
- QRS complex: 0.08 second
- T wave: Normal
- QT interval: 0.44 second
- Other: None
- Interpretation: Sinus arrest

PRACTICE 3-49
- Rhythm: Regular
- Rate: 48 beats/minute
- P wave: Normal
- PR interval: 0.18 second
- QRS complex: 0.08 second
- T wave: Normal
- QT interval: 0.46 second
- Other: None
- Interpretation: Sinus bradycardia

PRACTICE 3-50
- Rhythm: Regular
- Rate: 54 beats/minute
- P wave: Notched
- PR interval: 0.16 second
- QRS complex: 0.10 second
- T wave: Peaked
- QT interval: 0.44 second
- Other: None
- Interpretation: Sinus bradycardia

PRACTICE 3-51
- Rhythm: Regular
- Rate: 48 beats/minute
- P wave: Normal
- PR interval: 0.20 second
- QRS complex: 0.12 second
- T wave: Biphasic
- QT interval: 0.52 second
- Other: None
- Interpretation: Sinus bradycardia

PRACTICE 3-52
- Rhythm: Irregular
- Rate: 70 beats/minute
- P wave: Normal
- PR interval: 0.20 second
- QRS complex: 0.08 second
- T wave: Normal
- QT interval: 0.34 second
- Other: None
- Interpretation: Sinoatrial exit block

PRACTICE 3-53
- Rhythm: Regular
- Rate: 40 beats/minute
- P wave: Normal
- PR interval: 0.16 second
- QRS complex: 0.08 second
- T wave: Normal
- QT interval: 0.36 second
- Other: None
- Interpretation: Sinus bradycardia

PRACTICE 3-54
- Rhythm: Regular
- Rate: 35 beats/minute
- P wave: Normal
- PR interval: 0.18 second
- QRS complex: 0.12 second
- T wave: Normal
- QT interval: 0.44 second
- Other: None
- Interpretation: Sinus bradycardia

PRACTICE 3-55
- Rhythm: Regular
- Rate: 130 beats/minute
- P wave: Normal
- PR interval: 0.12 second
- QRS complex: 0.08 second
- T wave: Inverted
- QT interval: 0.28 second
- Other: None
- Interpretation: Sinus tachycardia

PRACTICE 3-56
- Rhythm: Regular
- Rate: 42 beats/minute
- P wave: Normal
- PR interval: 0.16 second
- QRS complex: 0.08 second
- T wave: Normal
- QT interval: 0.42 second
- Other: ST segment elevation
- Interpretation: Sinus bradycardia

PRACTICE 3-57
- Rhythm: Irregular
- Rate: 50 beats/minute
- P wave: Normal
- PR interval: 0.20 second
- QRS complex: 0.08 second
- T wave: Normal
- QT interval: 0.40 second
- Other: Slight ST segment elevation
- Interpretation: Sinus bradyarrhythmia

PRACTICE 3-58
- Rhythm: Irregular
- Rate: 80 beats/minute
- P wave: Normal
- PR interval: 0.16 second
- QRS complex: 0.08 second
- T wave: Inverted
- QT interval: 0.34 second
- Other: None
- Interpretation: Sinus arrhythmia

PRACTICE 3-59
- Rhythm: Irregular
- Rate: 50 beats/minute
- P wave: Normal
- PR interval: 0.20 second
- QRS complex: 0.08 second
- T wave: Normal
- QT interval: 0.40 second
- Other: None
- Interpretation: Sinus bradyarrhythmia

PRACTICE 3-60
- Rhythm: Regular
- Rate: 50 beats/minute
- P wave: Normal
- PR interval: 0.20 second
- QRS complex: 0.08 second
- T wave: Inverted
- QT interval: 0.44 second
- Other: None
- Interpretation: Sinus bradycardia

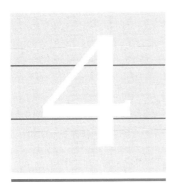

Atrial arrhythmias

Atrial arrhythmias, the most common cardiac rhythm disturbances, result from impulses originating in the atrial tissue in areas outside the sinoatrial (SA) node. These arrhythmias can affect ventricular filling time and diminish atrial kick. The term *atrial kick* refers to the complete filling of the ventricles during atrial systole and normally contributes about 25% to ventricular end-diastolic volume.

Atrial arrhythmias are thought to result from three mechanisms: altered automaticity, reentry, and afterdepolarization:

- Altered automaticity—The term *automaticity* refers to the ability of cardiac cells to initiate electrical impulses spontaneously. An increase in the automaticity of the atrial fibers can trigger abnormal impulses. Causes of increased automaticity include extracellular factors, such as hypoxia, hypocalcemia, and digoxin toxicity, as well as conditions in which the function of the heart's normal pacemaker, the SA node, is diminished. For example, increased vagal tone or hypokalemia can increase the refractory period of the SA node and allow atrial fibers to initiate impulses.
- Reentry—In reentry, an impulse is delayed along a slow conduction pathway. Despite the delay, the impulse remains active enough to produce another impulse during myocardial repolarization. Reentry may occur with coronary artery disease, cardiomyopathy, or myocardial infarction.
- Afterdepolarization—Afterdepolarization can occur as a result of cell injury, digoxin toxicity, and other conditions. An injured cell sometimes only partially repolarizes. Partial repolarization can lead to repetitive ectopic firing called *triggered activity*. The depolarization produced by triggered activity, known as *afterdepolarization,* can lead to atrial or ventricular tachycardia.

Atrial arrhythmias

Impulses originate in atrial tissue in areas outside the sinoatrial (SA) node.

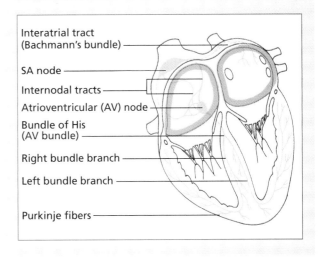

Interatrial tract (Bachmann's bundle)

SA node

Internodal tracts

Atrioventricular (AV) node

Bundle of His (AV bundle)

Right bundle branch

Left bundle branch

Purkinje fibers

This chapter will help you identify atrial arrhythmias, including premature atrial contractions (PACs), atrial tachycardia, atrial flutter, atrial fibrillation, Ashman's phenomenon, and wandering pacemaker. The chapter reviews causes and electrocardiogram (ECG) characteristics of each arrhythmia.

Premature atrial contractions

PACs originate in the atria, outside the SA node. They arise from either a single ectopic focus or from multiple atrial foci that supersede the SA node as pacemaker for one or more beats. PACs are generally caused by enhanced automaticity in the atrial tissue.

PACs may be conducted or nonconducted (blocked) through the atrioventricular (AV) node and the rest of the heart, depending on the status of the AV and intraventricular conduction system. If the atrial ectopic pacemaker discharges too soon after the preceding QRS complex, the AV junction or bundle branches may still be refractory from conducting the previous electrical impulse. If they're still refractory, they may not be sufficiently repolarized to conduct the premature electrical impulse into the ventricles normally. (See *Identifying premature atrial contractions.*)

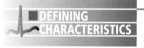

Identifying premature atrial contractions

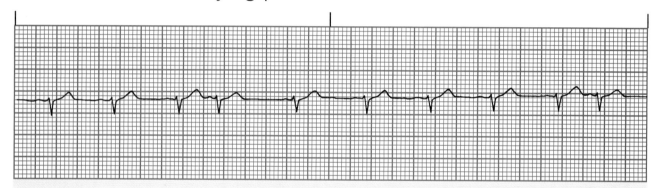

Rhythm

- Atrial: Irregular
- Ventricular: Irregular
- Underlying: Possibly regular

Rate

- Atrial and ventricular: Vary with underlying rhythm

P wave

- Premature
- Abnormal configuration compared to a sinus P wave
- If varying configurations, multiple ectopic sites
- May be hidden in preceding T wave

PR interval

- Usually within normal limits
- May be shortened or slightly prolonged for the ectopic beat, depending on the origin of ectopic focus

QRS complex

- Conducted: Duration and configuration usually normal
- Nonconducted: No QRS complex follows PAC

T wave

- Usually normal
- May be distorted if P wave is hidden in T wave

QT interval

- Usually within normal limits

Other

- May be a single beat
- May be bigeminal (every other beat premature)
- May be trigeminal (every third beat premature)
- May be quadrigeminal (every fourth beat premature)
- May occur in couplets (pairs)
- Three or more PACs in a row indicate atrial tachycardia

Distinguishing nonconducted PACs from SA block

To differentiate nonconducted premature atrial contractions (PACs) from sinoatrial (SA) block:

▪ Whenever you see a pause in a rhythm, look carefully for a nonconducted P wave, which may occur before, during, or just after the T wave preceding the pause.

▪ Compare T waves that precede a pause with the other T waves in the rhythm strip, and look for a distortion of the slope of the T wave or a difference in its height or shape. These are clues showing you where the nonconducted P wave may be hidden.

▪ If you find a P wave in the pause, check to see whether it's premature or if it occurs earlier than subsequent sinus P waves. If it's premature (see shaded area below, top), you can be certain it's a nonconducted PAC.

▪ If there's no P wave in the pause or T wave (see shaded area below, bottom), the rhythm is SA block.

Nonconducted PAC

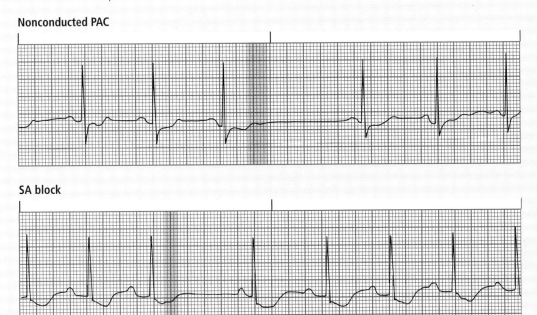

SA block

When a PAC is conducted, ventricular conduction is usually normal. Nonconducted, or blocked, PACs aren't followed by a QRS complex. At times, it may be difficult to distinguish nonconducted PACs from SA block. (See *Distinguishing nonconducted PACs from SA block.*)

PRACTICE   # Premature atrial contractions

Use the 8-step method to interpret the following rhythm strip. Place your answers on the blank lines. See the answer key below.

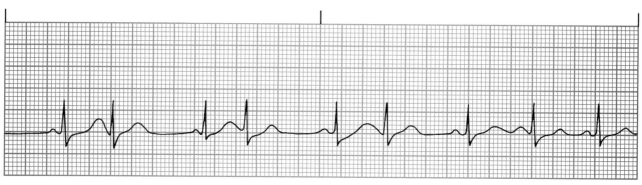

Rhythm:
_____

Rate:
_____

P wave:
_____

PR interval:
_____

QRS complex:
_____

T wave:
_____

QT interval:
_____

Other:
_____

■ **ANSWER KEY**

Rhythm: **Irregular**

Rate: **90 beats/minute**

P wave: **Premature and abnormally shaped with PACs**

PR interval: **0.16 second for the underlying rhythm; unmeasurable for the PAC**

QRS complex: **0.08 second**

T wave: **Abnormal with embedded P waves of PACs**

QT interval: **0.36 second**

Other: **Noncompensatory pause**

Atrial tachycardia

Atrial tachycardia is characterized by an atrial rate of 150 to 250 beats/minute. It's a supraventricular tachycardia, which means that the impulses driving the rapid rhythm originate above the ventricles. The rapid rate shortens diastole, resulting in a loss of atrial kick, reduced cardiac output, reduced coronary perfusion, and the potential for myocardial ischemia.

Leads II, V_1, V_6, MCL_1, and MCL_6 are the best choices for monitoring patients with atrial tachycardia. (See *Identifying atrial tachycardia.*)

Three forms of atrial tachycardia are discussed here: atrial tachycardia with block; multifocal atrial tachycardia (MAT), or chaotic atrial rhythm; and paroxysmal atrial tachycardia (PAT). In MAT, the tachycardia originates from multiple foci. PAT is generally a transient event in which the tachycardia starts and stops suddenly. (See *Distinguishing types of atrial tachycardia*, page 74.)

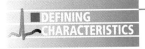

Identifying atrial tachycardia

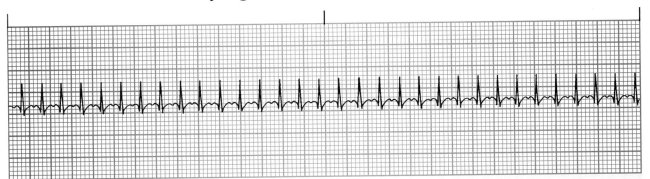

Rhythm

- Atrial: Usually regular
- Ventricular: Regular or irregular depending on AV conduction ratio and type of atrial tachycardia

Rate

- Atrial: Three or more consecutive ectopic atrial beats at 150 to 250 beats/minute; rarely exceeds 250 beats/minute
- Ventricular: Varies, depending on AV conduction ratio

P wave

- Deviates from normal appearance
- May be hidden in preceding T wave
- If visible, usually upright and preceding each QRS complex

PR interval

- Within normal limits or may be difficult to measure if P wave can't be distinguished from preceding T wave

QRS complex

- Usually normal duration and configuration
- May be abnormal if impulses conducted abnormally through ventricles

T wave

- Usually visible
- May be distorted by P wave
- May be inverted if ischemia is present

QT interval

- Usually within normal limits
- May be shorter because of rapid rate

Other

- None

Distinguishing types of atrial tachycardia
Characteristics of atrial tachycardia with block

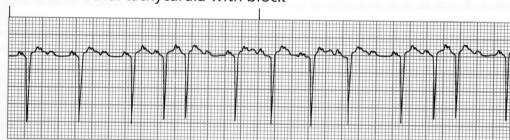

- Rhythm: Atrial—regular; ventricular—regular if block is constant, irregular if block is variable
- Rate: Atrial—150 to 250 beats/minute and a multiple of ventricular rate; ventricular—varies with block
- P wave: Abnormal
- PR interval: Can vary but is usually constant for conducted P waves

- QRS complex: Usually normal
- T wave: Usually distorted
- QT interval: May be indiscernible
- Other: More than one P wave for each QRS complex

Characteristics of multifocal atrial tachycardia

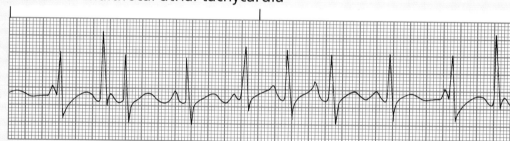

- Rhythm: Both irregular
- Rate: Atrial—100 to 250 beats/minute; ventricular—100 to 250 beats/minute
- P wave: Configuration varies; usually at least three different P-wave shapes must appear

- PR interval: Varies
- QRS complex: Usually normal; may become aberrant if arrhythmia persists
- T wave: Usually distorted
- QT interval: May be indiscernible

Characteristics of paroxysmal atrial tachycardia

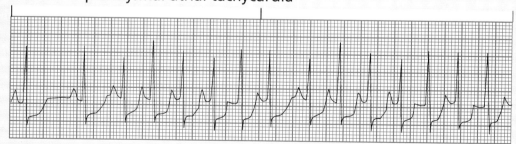

- Rhythm: Both regular in underlying rhythm; both irregular with PAC
- Rate: 150 to 250 beats/minute
- P wave: Abnormal; may not be visible or may be difficult to distinguish from the preceding T wave
- PR interval: Usually within normal limits but may be unmeasurable if the P wave can't be distinguished from the preceding T wave

- QRS complex: Usually normal but can be aberrantly conducted
- T wave: Usually distorted
- QT interval: May be indistinguishable
- Other: Sudden onset, typically initiated by a premature atrial contraction

PRACTICE # Atrial tachycardia

Use the 8-step method to interpret the following rhythm strip. Place your answers on the blank lines. See the answer key below.

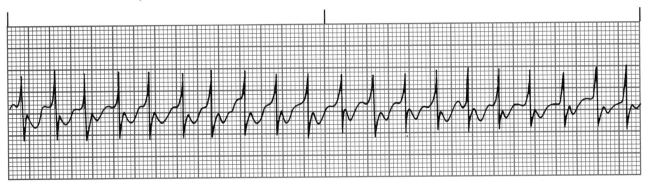

Rhythm: _____

Rate: _____

P wave: _____

PR interval: _____

QRS complex: _____

T wave: _____

QT interval: _____

Other: _____

■ **ANSWER KEY**

Rhythm: **Regular**

Rate: **214 beats/minute**

P wave: **Hidden in the preceding T wave**

PR interval: **Not visible**

QRS complex: **0.10 second**

T wave: **Inverted**

QT interval: **0.20 second**

Other: **T-wave changes (inversion may indicate ischemia)**

Atrial flutter

Atrial flutter, a supraventricular tachycardia, is characterized by a rapid atrial rate of 250 to 400 beats/minute (usually around 300 beats/minute). Originating in a single atrial focus, this rhythm results from a reentry mechanism and, possibly, increased automaticity.

On an ECG, the P waves lose their normal appearance because of the rapid atrial rate. The waves blend together in a sawtoothed configuration called *flutter waves,* or F waves. These waves are the hallmark of atrial flutter. (See *Identifying atrial flutter.*)

Leads II and III are the best leads for monitoring the patient with atrial flutter.

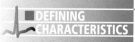

DEFINING CHARACTERISTICS

Identifying atrial flutter

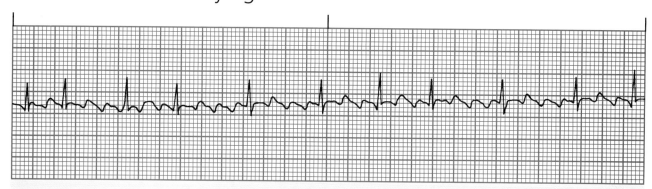

Rhythm

- Atrial: Regular
- Ventricular: Typically regular; may be irregular because cycles may alternate (depends on AV conduction pattern)

Rate

- Atrial: 250 to 400 beats/minute
- Ventricular: Usually 60 to 150 beats/minute (one-half to one-fourth of atrial rate) but varies depending on degree of AV block
- Usually expressed as a ratio (2:1 or 4:1, for example)
- Commonly 300 beats/minute atrial and 150 beats/minute ventricular (known as *2:1 block*)

- Only every second, third, or fourth impulse is conducted to ventricles because the AV node usually won't accept more than 180 impulses/minute
- When atrial flutter is first recognized, ventricular rate typically exceeds 100 beats/minute

P wave

- Abnormal
- Sawtoothed appearance known as *flutter waves* or *F waves*

PR interval

- Unmeasurable

QRS complex

- Duration: Usually within normal limits
- May be widened if flutter waves are buried within the complex

T wave

- Not identifiable

QT interval

- Unmeasurable because T wave isn't identifiable

Other

- Atrial rhythm may vary between a fibrillatory line and flutter waves (called *atrial fib-flutter*), with an irregular ventricular response
- May be difficult to differentiate atrial flutter from atrial fibrillation

■ PRACTICE Atrial flutter

Use the 8-step method to interpret the following rhythm strip. Place your answers on the blank lines. See the answer key below.

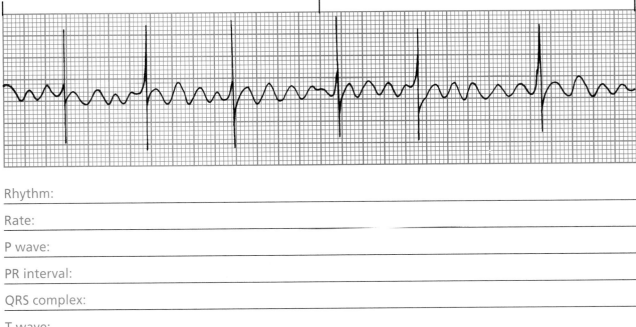

Rhythm: _____

Rate: _____

P wave: _____

PR interval: _____

QRS complex: _____

T wave: _____

QT interval: _____

Other: _____

■ **ANSWER KEY**

Rhythm: **Atrial—regular; ventricular—irregular**

Rate: **Atrial—280 beats/minute; ventricular—60 beats/minute, but depends on degree of AV block**

P wave: **Sawtoothed appearance**

PR interval: **Unmeasurable**

QRS complex: **0.08 second**

T wave: **Unidentifiable**

QT interval: **Unmeasurable**

Other: **Atrial rate greater than ventricular rate**

Atrial fibrillation

Atrial fibrillation, sometimes called *AFib,* is defined as chaotic, asynchronous, electrical activity in atrial tissue. It results from the firing of multiple impulses from numerous ectopic pacemakers in the atria. Atrial fibrillation is characterized by the absence of P waves and an irregularly irregular ventricular response.

When a number of ectopic sites in the atria initiate impulses, depolarization can't spread in an organized manner. Small sections of the atria are depolarized individually, resulting in the atrial muscle quivering instead of contracting. Uneven baseline fibrillatory waves—rather than clearly distinguishable P waves—appear on the ECG.

The AV node protects the ventricles from the 400 to 600 erratic atrial impulses that occur each minute by acting as a filter and blocking some of the impulses. The ventricles respond only to impulses conducted through the AV node—hence the characteristic wide variation in R-R intervals. When the ventricular response rate drops below 100, atrial fibrillation is considered controlled. When the ventricular rate exceeds 100, atrial fibrillation is considered uncontrolled.

Lead II is the best choice for monitoring a patient with atrial fibrillation; however, you should be able to identify fibrillatory waves and the irregular R-R intervals in most leads.

Patients may develop an atrial rhythm that varies between a fibrillatory line and flutter waves. This variation is referred to as *atrial fib-flutter,* but the rhythm is interpreted as atrial fibrillation. The ventricular response is irregular. (See *Identifying atrial fibrillation.*)

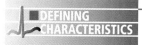
DEFINING CHARACTERISTICS

Identifying atrial fibrillation

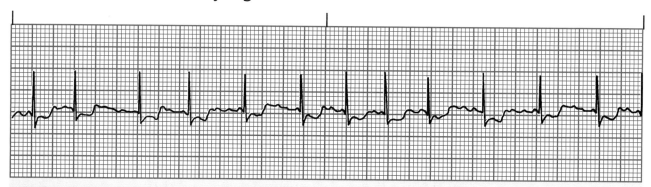

Rhythm

- Atrial: Irregularly irregular
- Ventricular: Irregularly irregular

Rate

- Atrial: Almost indiscernible, usually above 400 beats/minute; far exceeds ventricular rate because most impulses aren't conducted through the atrioventricular junction
- Ventricular: Usually 100 to 150 beats/minute but can be below 100 beats/minute

P wave

- Absent
- Replaced by baseline fibrillatory waves that represent atrial tetanization from rapid atrial depolarizations

PR interval

- Indiscernible

QRS complex

- Duration and configuration usually normal

T wave

- May be indiscernible

QT interval

- May be unmeasurable

Other

- Atrial rhythm may vary between fibrillatory line and flutter waves (called *atrial fib-flutter*)
- May be difficult to differentiate atrial fibrillation from atrial flutter and multifocal atrial tachycardia

Distinguishing atrial flutter from atrial fibrillation

It's common to see atrial flutter that has an irregular pattern of impulse conduction to the ventricles. In some leads, this may be confused with atrial fibrillation. Here's how to tell the two arrhythmias apart.

Atrial flutter

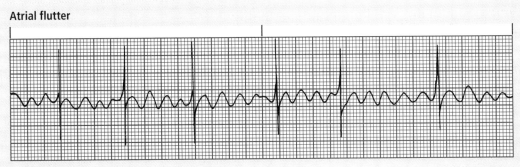

- Look for characteristic abnormal P waves that produce a sawtoothed appearance, referred to as *flutter waves* or *F waves*. These can best be identified in leads II, III, and V₁ on the 12-lead electrocardiogram.

- Remember that the atrial rhythm is regular. You should be able to map the flutter waves across the rhythm strip. Although some flutter waves may occur within the QRS or T waves, subsequent flutter waves will be visible and will occur on time.

Atrial fibrillation

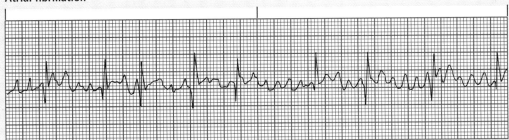

- Fibrillatory waves, or f waves, occur in an irregular pattern, making the atrial rhythm irregular.
- If you identify atrial activity that at times looks like flutter waves and seems to be regular for a short time, and in other places the rhythm strip contains fibrillatory waves, interpret the rhythm as atrial fibrillation. Coarse fibrillatory waves may intermittently look similar to the characteristic sawtoothed appearance of flutter waves.

At times, it may be difficult to distinguish atrial flutter from atrial fibrillation. (See *Distinguishing atrial flutter from atrial fibrillation.*)

PRACTICE ## Atrial fibrillation

Use the 8-step method to interpret the following rhythm strip. Place your answers on the blank lines. See the answer key below.

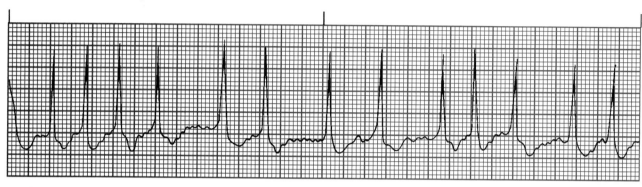

Rhythm:

Rate:

P wave:

PR interval:

QRS complex:

T wave:

QT interval:

Other:

■ **ANSWER KEY**

Rhythm: Irregularly irregular

Rate: Atrial—indiscernible; ventricular—130 beats/minute

P wave: Absent; replaced by fine fibrillatory waves

PR interval: Indiscernible

QRS complex: 0.08 second

T wave: Indiscernible

QT interval: Unmeasurable

Other: None

Ashman's phenomenon

Ashman's phenomenon refers to the aberrant conduction of premature supraventricular beats to the ventricles. This benign phenomenon is commonly associated with atrial fibrillation but can occur with any arrhythmia that affects the R-R interval. (See *Identifying Ashman's phenomenon.*)

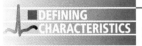 **DEFINING CHARACTERISTICS**

Identifying Ashman's phenomenon

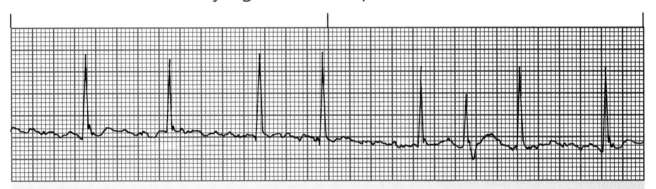

Rhythm
- Atrial: Irregular
- Ventricular: Irregular

Rate
- Reflects the underlying rhythm

P wave
- May be visible
- Abnormal configuration
- Unchanged if present in the underlying rhythm

PR interval
- Commonly changes on the premature beat, if measurable at all

QRS complex
- Altered configuration with right bundle-branch block (RBBB) pattern

T wave
- Deflection opposite that of QRS complex in most leads because of RBBB

QT interval
- Usually changed because of RBBB

Other
- No compensatory pause after an aberrant beat
- Aberrancy may continue for several beats and typically ends a short cycle preceded by a long cycle

Ashman's phenomenon

Use the 8-step method to interpret the following rhythm strip. Place your answers on the blank lines. See the answer key below.

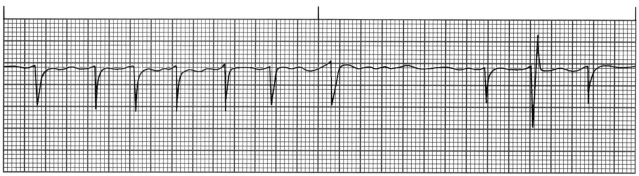

Rhythm: _____

Rate: _____

P wave: _____

PR interval: _____

QRS complex: _____

T wave: _____

QT interval: _____

Other: _____

■ **ANSWER KEY**

Rhythm: Atrial and ventricular—irregular

Rate: Underlying rhythm of 90 beats/minute

P wave: Absent; fibrillatory waves

PR interval: Unmeasurable

QRS complex: 0.12 second; RBBB pattern present on Ashman beat

T wave: Deflection opposite that of QRS complex in the Ashman beat

QT interval: Changed because of RBBB

Other: No compensatory pause after the aberrant beat

Wandering pacemaker

Wandering pacemaker, also called *wandering atrial pacemaker*, is an atrial arrhythmia that results when the site of impulse formation shifts from the SA node to another area above the ventricles. The origin of the impulse may wander beat to beat from the SA node to ectopic sites in the atria or to the AV junctional tissue. The P wave and PR interval vary from beat to beat as the pacemaker site changes. (See *Identifying wandering pacemaker.*)

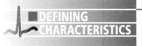

Identifying wandering pacemaker

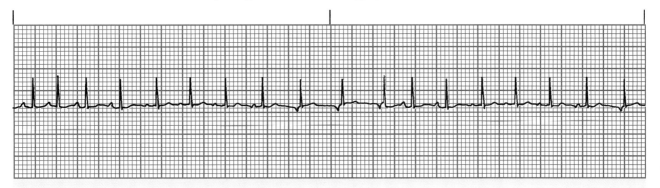

Rhythm
- Atrial: Varies slightly, with an irregular P-P interval
- Ventricular: Varies slightly, with an irregular R-R interval

Rate
- Varies, but usually within normal limits or may be less than 60 beats/minute

P wave
- Altered size and configuration from changing pacemaker site with at least three different P-wave shapes visible
- May be absent or inverted or occur after QRS complex if impulse originates in the AV junction

PR interval
- Varies from beat to beat as pacemaker site changes
- Usually less than 0.20 second
- Less than 0.12 second if impulse originates in the AV junction

QRS complex
- Duration and configuration usually normal because ventricular depolarization is normal

T wave
- Normal size and configuration

QT interval
- Usually within normal limits

Other
- May be difficult to differentiate wandering pacemaker from PACs

Distinguishing wandering pacemaker from PACs

Because premature atrial contractions (PACs) are commonly encountered, it's possible to mistake wandering pacemaker for PACs unless the rhythm strip is carefully examined. In such cases, you may find it helpful to look at a longer (greater than 6 seconds) rhythm strip.

Wandering pacemaker

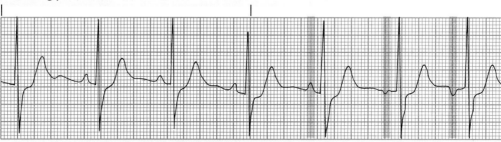

■ Carefully examine the P waves. You must be able to identify at least three different shapes of P waves (see shaded areas above) in wandering pacemaker.

■ Atrial rhythm varies slightly, with an irregular P-P interval. Ventricular rhythm varies slightly, with an irregular R-R interval. These slight variations in rhythm result from the changing site of impulse formation.

PAC

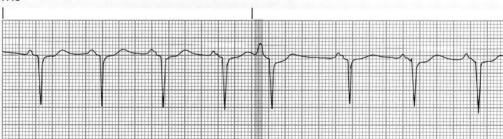

■ The PAC occurs earlier than the sinus P wave, with an abnormal configuration when compared with a sinus P wave (see shaded area above). It's possible, but rare, to see multifocal PACs, which originate from multiple ectopic pacemaker sites in the atria. In this setting, the P waves may have different shapes.

■ With the exception of the irregular atrial and ventricular rhythms as a result of the PAC, the underlying rhythm is usually regular.

At times, it may be difficult to distinguish a wandering pacemaker from a PAC. (See *Distinguishing wandering pacemaker from PACs.*)

PRACTICE Wandering pacemaker

Use the 8-step method to interpret the following rhythm strip. Place your answers on the blank lines. See the answer key below.

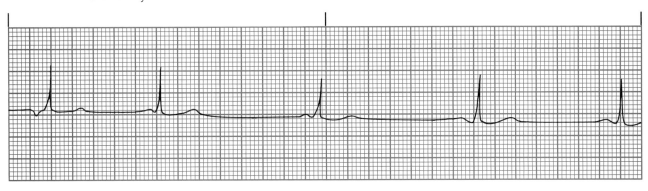

Rhythm: _____

Rate: _____

P wave: _____

PR interval: _____

QRS complex: _____

T wave: _____

QT interval: _____

Other: _____

■ **ANSWER KEY**

Rhythm: **Atrial and ventricular—irregular**

Rate: **Atrial and ventricular—50 beats/minute**

P wave: **Changes in size and shape; first P wave inverted, second upright, fourth flattened**

PR interval: **Variable**

QRS complex: **0.08 second**

T wave: **Normal**

QT interval: **0.44 second**

Other: **None**

■ **PRACTICE STRIPS**

■ **PRACTICE 4-1**

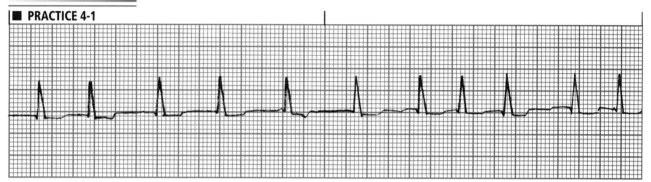

Rhythm: _____   PR interval: _____   QT interval: _____

Rate: _____   QRS complex: _____   Other: _____

P wave: _____   T wave: _____   Interpretation: _____

■ **PRACTICE 4-2**

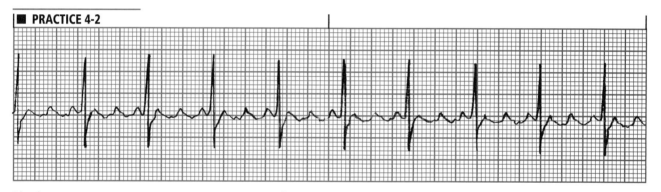

Rhythm: _____   PR interval: _____   QT interval: _____

Rate: _____   QRS complex: _____   Other: _____

P wave: _____   T wave: _____   Interpretation: _____

■ **PRACTICE 4-3**

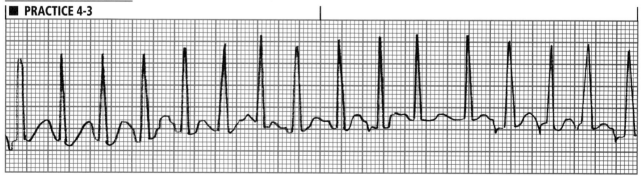

Rhythm: _____   PR interval: _____   QT interval: _____

Rate: _____   QRS complex: _____   Other: _____

P wave: _____   T wave: _____   Interpretation: _____

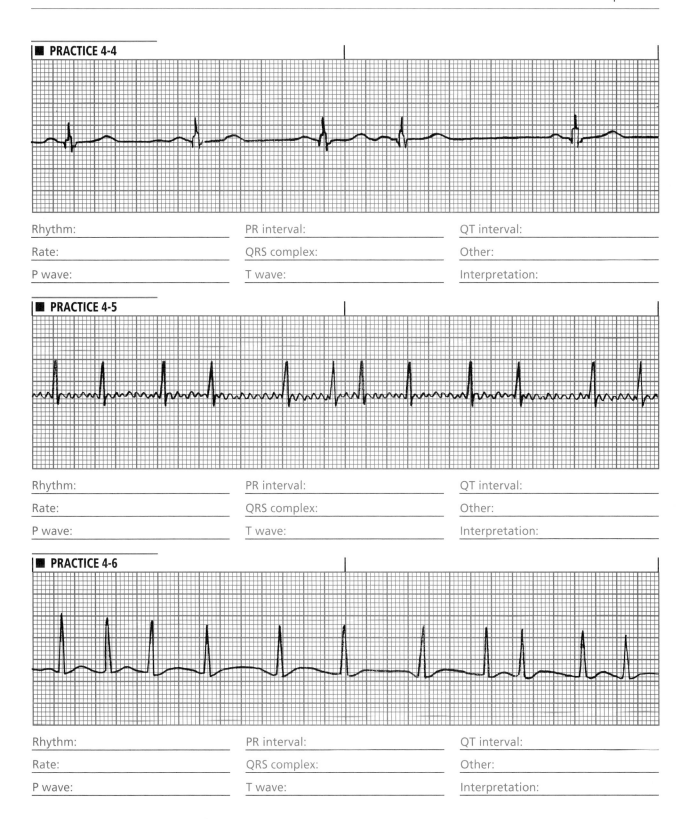

■ **PRACTICE 4-4**

Rhythm: _____   PR interval: _____   QT interval: _____

Rate: _____   QRS complex: _____   Other: _____

P wave: _____   T wave: _____   Interpretation: _____

■ **PRACTICE 4-5**

Rhythm: _____   PR interval: _____   QT interval: _____

Rate: _____   QRS complex: _____   Other: _____

P wave: _____   T wave: _____   Interpretation: _____

■ **PRACTICE 4-6**

Rhythm: _____   PR interval: _____   QT interval: _____

Rate: _____   QRS complex: _____   Other: _____

P wave: _____   T wave: _____   Interpretation: _____

■ PRACTICE 4-7

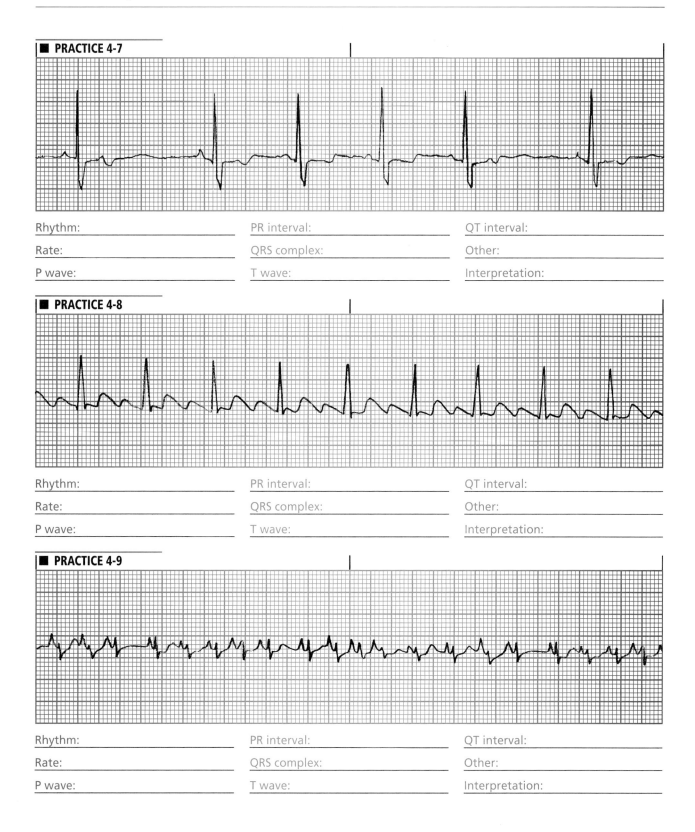

Rhythm: _____   PR interval: _____   QT interval: _____

Rate: _____   QRS complex: _____   Other: _____

P wave: _____   T wave: _____   Interpretation: _____

■ PRACTICE 4-8

Rhythm: _____   PR interval: _____   QT interval: _____

Rate: _____   QRS complex: _____   Other: _____

P wave: _____   T wave: _____   Interpretation: _____

■ PRACTICE 4-9

Rhythm: _____   PR interval: _____   QT interval: _____

Rate: _____   QRS complex: _____   Other: _____

P wave: _____   T wave: _____   Interpretation: _____

■ PRACTICE 4-10

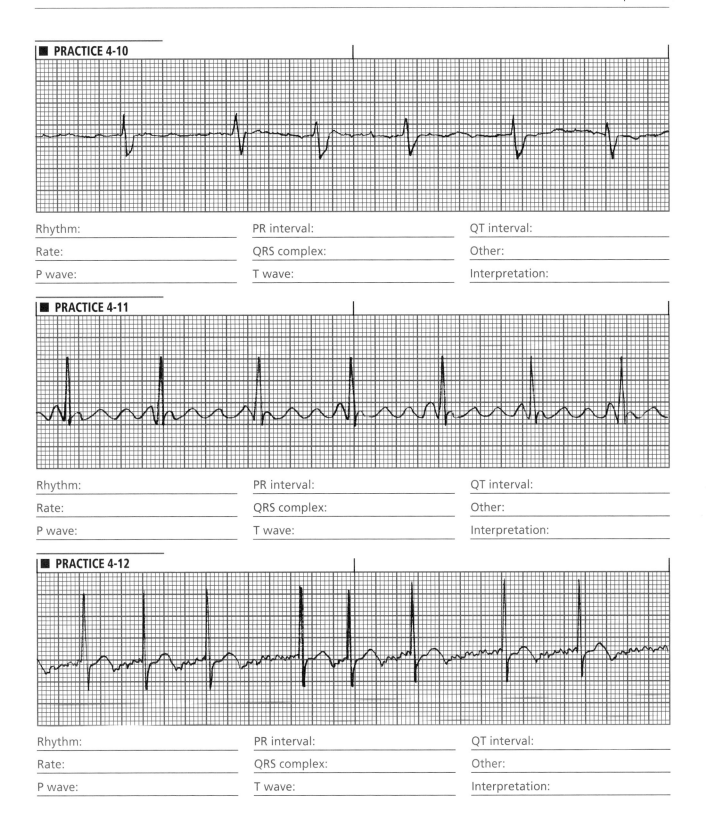

Rhythm: _____

Rate: _____

P wave: _____

PR interval: _____

QRS complex: _____

T wave: _____

QT interval: _____

Other: _____

Interpretation: _____

■ PRACTICE 4-11

Rhythm: _____

Rate: _____

P wave: _____

PR interval: _____

QRS complex: _____

T wave: _____

QT interval: _____

Other: _____

Interpretation: _____

■ PRACTICE 4-12

Rhythm: _____

Rate: _____

P wave: _____

PR interval: _____

QRS complex: _____

T wave: _____

QT interval: _____

Other: _____

Interpretation: _____

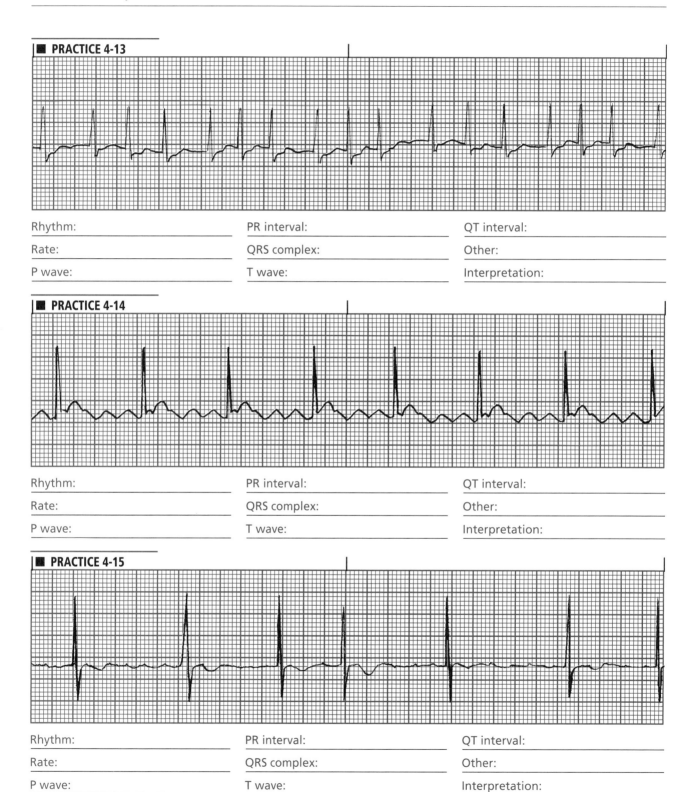

■ PRACTICE 4-13

Rhythm: _____   PR interval: _____   QT interval: _____

Rate: _____   QRS complex: _____   Other: _____

P wave: _____   T wave: _____   Interpretation: _____

■ PRACTICE 4-14

Rhythm: _____   PR interval: _____   QT interval: _____

Rate: _____   QRS complex: _____   Other: _____

P wave: _____   T wave: _____   Interpretation: _____

■ PRACTICE 4-15

Rhythm: _____   PR interval: _____   QT interval: _____

Rate: _____   QRS complex: _____   Other: _____

P wave: _____   T wave: _____   Interpretation: _____

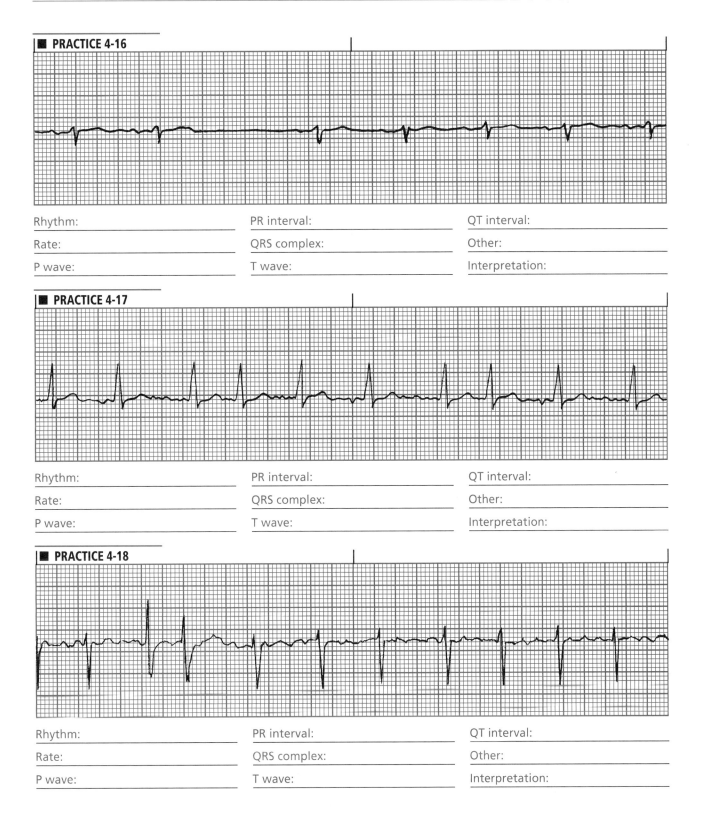

■ **PRACTICE 4-16**

Rhythm: _____   PR interval: _____   QT interval: _____

Rate: _____   QRS complex: _____   Other: _____

P wave: _____   T wave: _____   Interpretation: _____

■ **PRACTICE 4-17**

Rhythm: _____   PR interval: _____   QT interval: _____

Rate: _____   QRS complex: _____   Other: _____

P wave: _____   T wave: _____   Interpretation: _____

■ **PRACTICE 4-18**

Rhythm: _____   PR interval: _____   QT interval: _____

Rate: _____   QRS complex: _____   Other: _____

P wave: _____   T wave: _____   Interpretation: _____

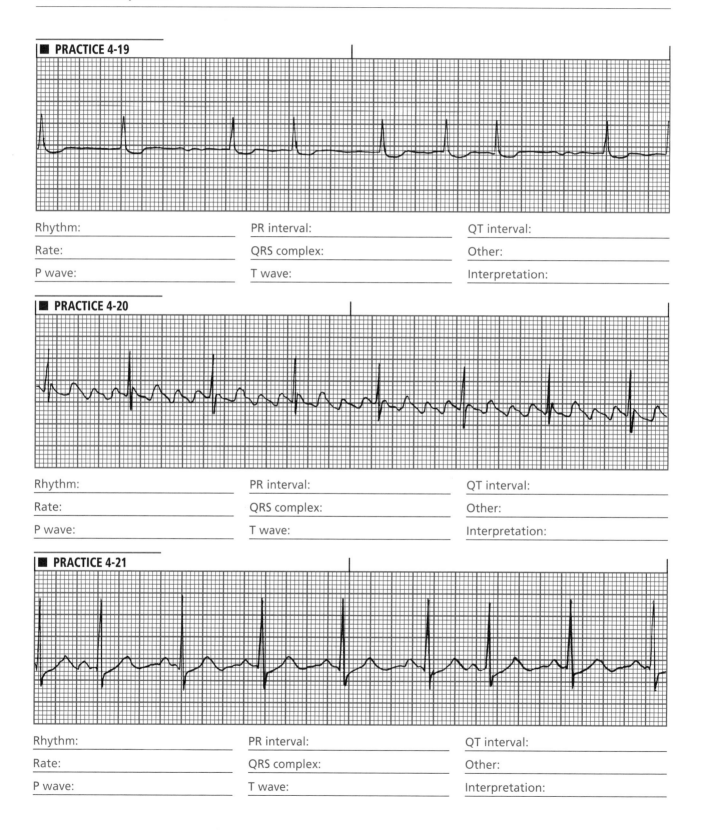

■ **PRACTICE 4-19**

Rhythm: _____   PR interval: _____   QT interval: _____

Rate: _____   QRS complex: _____   Other: _____

P wave: _____   T wave: _____   Interpretation: _____

■ **PRACTICE 4-20**

Rhythm: _____   PR interval: _____   QT interval: _____

Rate: _____   QRS complex: _____   Other: _____

P wave: _____   T wave: _____   Interpretation: _____

■ **PRACTICE 4-21**

Rhythm: _____   PR interval: _____   QT interval: _____

Rate: _____   QRS complex: _____   Other: _____

P wave: _____   T wave: _____   Interpretation: _____

■ PRACTICE 4-22

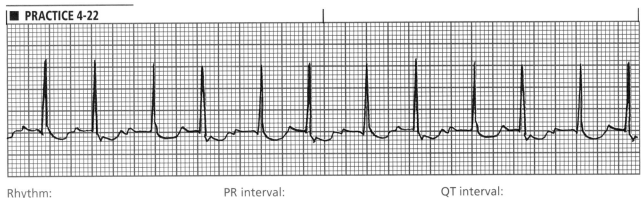

Rhythm: _____   PR interval: _____   QT interval: _____

Rate: _____   QRS complex: _____   Other: _____

P wave: _____   T wave: _____   Interpretation: _____

■ PRACTICE 4-23

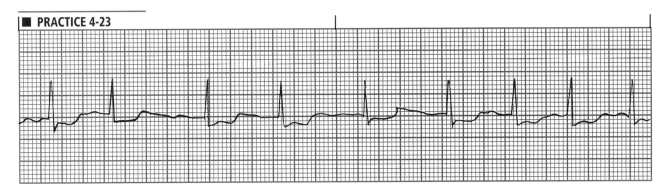

Rhythm: _____   PR interval: _____   QT interval: _____

Rate: _____   QRS complex: _____   Other: _____

P wave: _____   T wave: _____   Interpretation: _____

■ PRACTICE 4-24

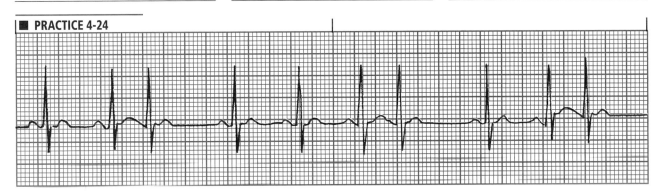

Rhythm: _____   PR interval: _____   QT interval: _____

Rate: _____   QRS complex: _____   Other: _____

P wave: _____   T wave: _____   Interpretation: _____

■ **PRACTICE 4-25**

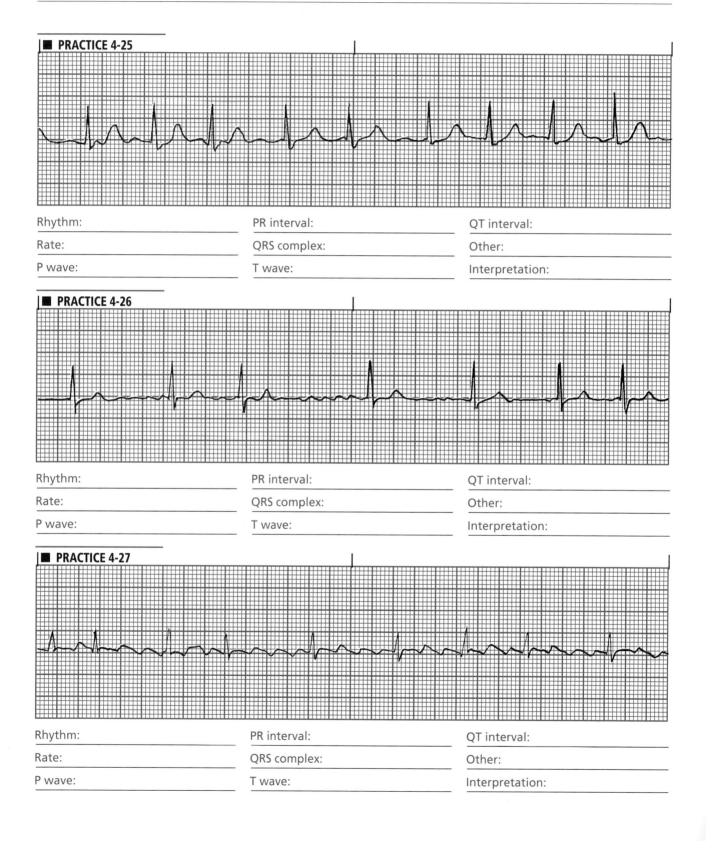

Rhythm: _____

Rate: _____

P wave: _____

PR interval: _____

QRS complex: _____

T wave: _____

QT interval: _____

Other: _____

Interpretation: _____

■ **PRACTICE 4-26**

Rhythm: _____

Rate: _____

P wave: _____

PR interval: _____

QRS complex: _____

T wave: _____

QT interval: _____

Other: _____

Interpretation: _____

■ **PRACTICE 4-27**

Rhythm: _____

Rate: _____

P wave: _____

PR interval: _____

QRS complex: _____

T wave: _____

QT interval: _____

Other: _____

Interpretation: _____

■ PRACTICE 4-28

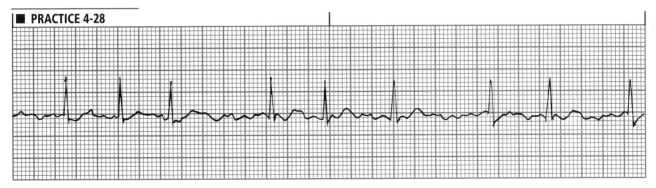

Rhythm:	PR interval:	QT interval:
Rate:	QRS complex:	Other:
P wave:	T wave:	Interpretation:

■ PRACTICE 4-29

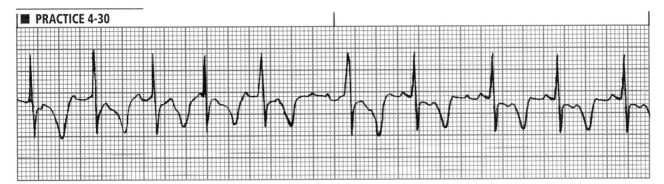

Rhythm:	PR interval:	QT interval:
Rate:	QRS complex:	Other:
P wave:	T wave:	Interpretation:

■ PRACTICE 4-30

Rhythm:	PR interval:	QT interval:
Rate:	QRS complex:	Other:
P wave:	T wave:	Interpretation:

■ PRACTICE 4-31

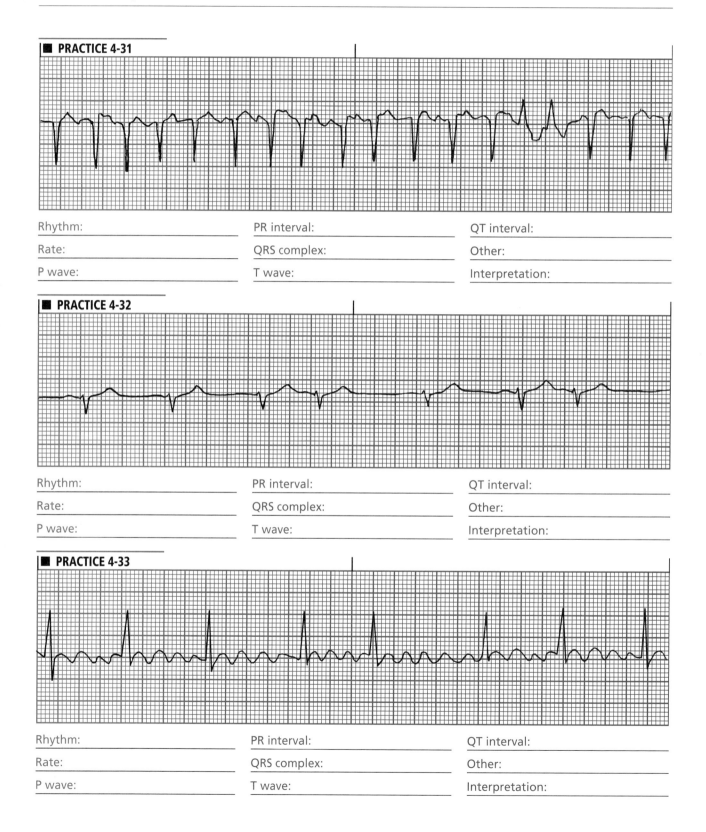

Rhythm: _____

Rate: _____

P wave: _____

PR interval: _____

QRS complex: _____

T wave: _____

QT interval: _____

Other: _____

Interpretation: _____

■ PRACTICE 4-32

Rhythm: _____

Rate: _____

P wave: _____

PR interval: _____

QRS complex: _____

T wave: _____

QT interval: _____

Other: _____

Interpretation: _____

■ PRACTICE 4-33

Rhythm: _____

Rate: _____

P wave: _____

PR interval: _____

QRS complex: _____

T wave: _____

QT interval: _____

Other: _____

Interpretation: _____

■ PRACTICE 4-34

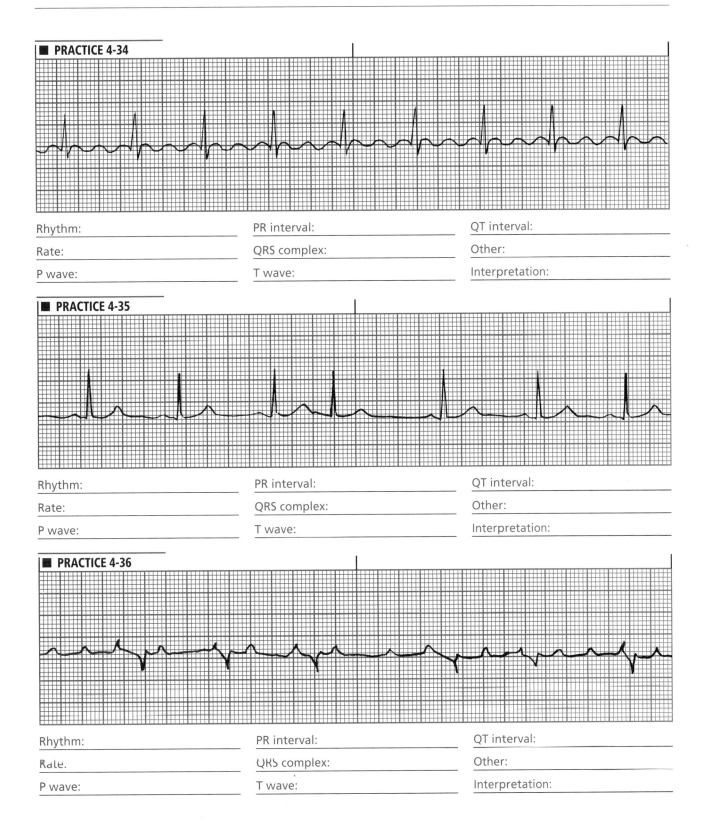

Rhythm: _____

Rate: _____

P wave: _____

PR interval: _____

QRS complex: _____

T wave: _____

QT interval: _____

Other: _____

Interpretation: _____

■ PRACTICE 4-35

Rhythm: _____

Rate: _____

P wave: _____

PR interval: _____

QRS complex: _____

T wave: _____

QT interval: _____

Other: _____

Interpretation: _____

■ PRACTICE 4-36

Rhythm: _____

Rate: _____

P wave: _____

PR interval: _____

QRS complex: _____

T wave: _____

QT interval: _____

Other: _____

Interpretation: _____

■ **PRACTICE 4-37**

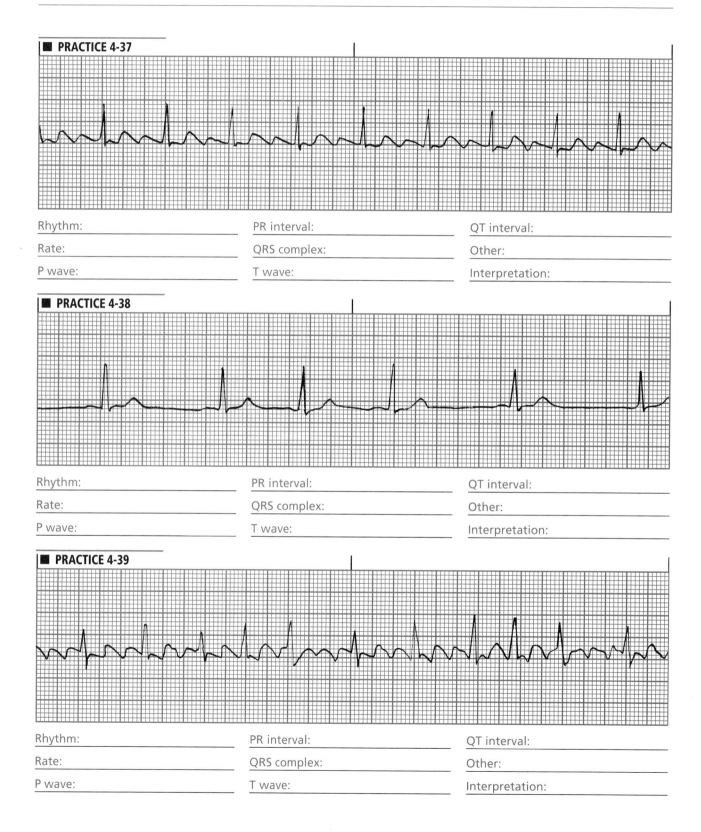

Rhythm: _____

Rate: _____

P wave: _____

PR interval: _____

QRS complex: _____

T wave: _____

QT interval: _____

Other: _____

Interpretation: _____

■ **PRACTICE 4-38**

Rhythm: _____

Rate: _____

P wave: _____

PR interval: _____

QRS complex: _____

T wave: _____

QT interval: _____

Other: _____

Interpretation: _____

■ **PRACTICE 4-39**

Rhythm: _____

Rate: _____

P wave: _____

PR interval: _____

QRS complex: _____

T wave: _____

QT interval: _____

Other: _____

Interpretation: _____

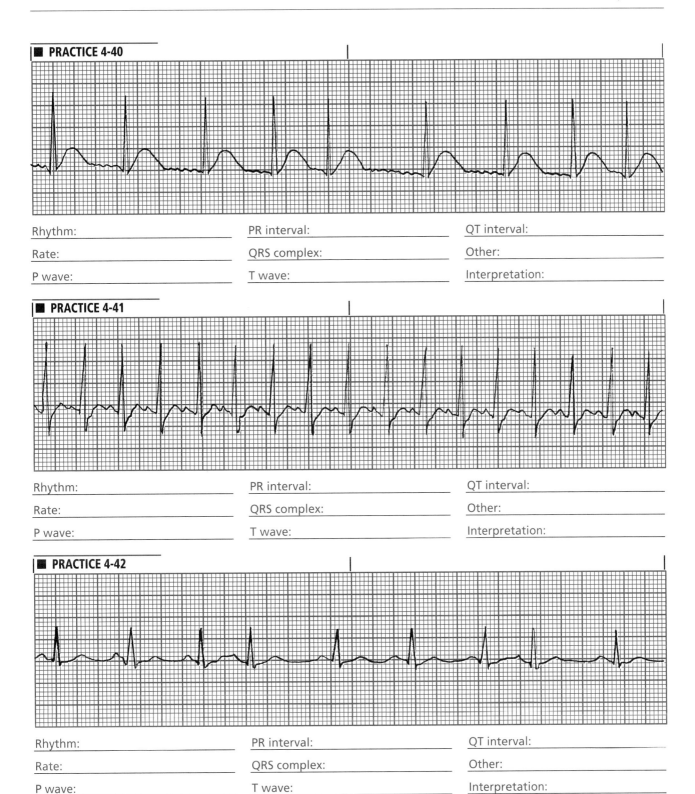

■ PRACTICE 4-40

Rhythm: _____   PR interval: _____   QT interval: _____

Rate: _____   QRS complex: _____   Other: _____

P wave: _____   T wave: _____   Interpretation: _____

■ PRACTICE 4-41

Rhythm: _____   PR interval: _____   QT interval: _____

Rate: _____   QRS complex: _____   Other: _____

P wave: _____   T wave: _____   Interpretation: _____

■ PRACTICE 4-42

Rhythm: _____   PR interval: _____   QT interval: _____

Rate: _____   QRS complex: _____   Other: _____

P wave: _____   T wave: _____   Interpretation: _____

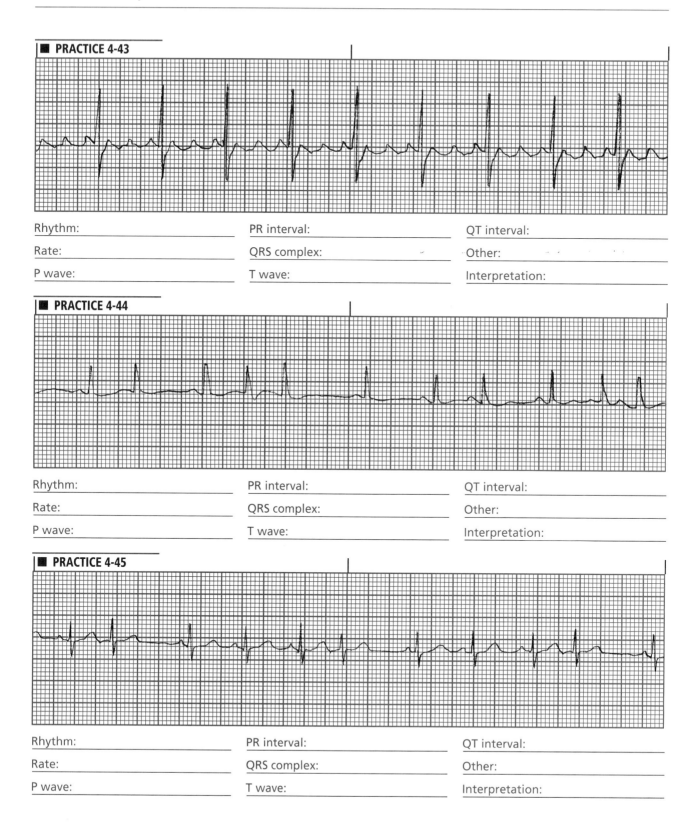

■ PRACTICE 4-43

Rhythm: _____   PR interval: _____   QT interval: _____

Rate: _____   QRS complex: _____   Other: _____

P wave: _____   T wave: _____   Interpretation: _____

■ PRACTICE 4-44

Rhythm: _____   PR interval: _____   QT interval: _____

Rate: _____   QRS complex: _____   Other: _____

P wave: _____   T wave: _____   Interpretation: _____

■ PRACTICE 4-45

Rhythm: _____   PR interval: _____   QT interval: _____

Rate: _____   QRS complex: _____   Other: _____

P wave: _____   T wave: _____   Interpretation: _____

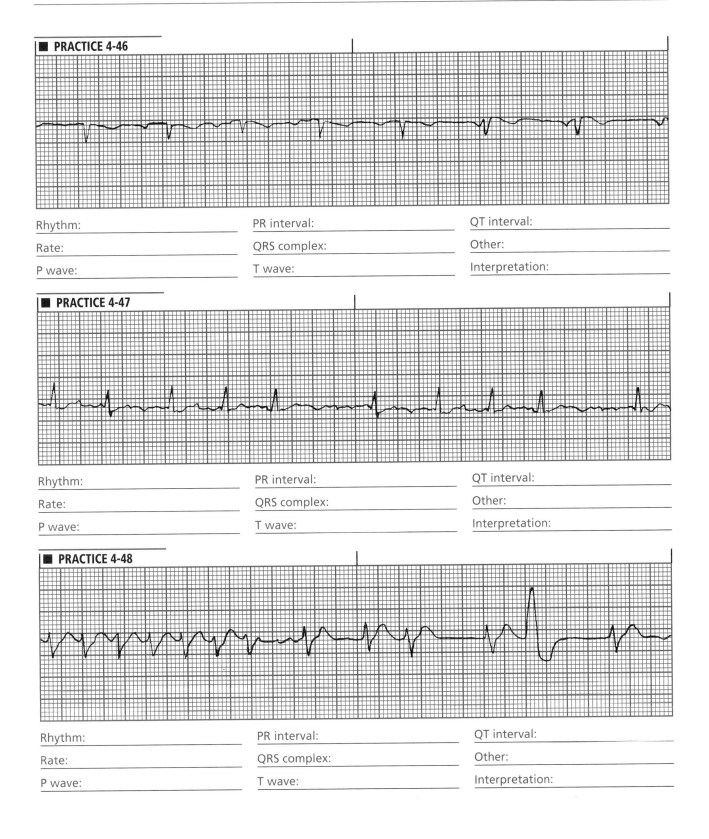

PRACTICE 4-46

Rhythm: _____

Rate: _____

P wave: _____

PR interval: _____

QRS complex: _____

T wave: _____

QT interval: _____

Other: _____

Interpretation: _____

PRACTICE 4-47

Rhythm: _____

Rate: _____

P wave: _____

PR interval: _____

QRS complex: _____

T wave: _____

QT interval: _____

Other: _____

Interpretation: _____

PRACTICE 4-48

Rhythm: _____

Rate: _____

P wave: _____

PR interval: _____

QRS complex: _____

T wave: _____

QT interval: _____

Other: _____

Interpretation: _____

■ PRACTICE 4-49

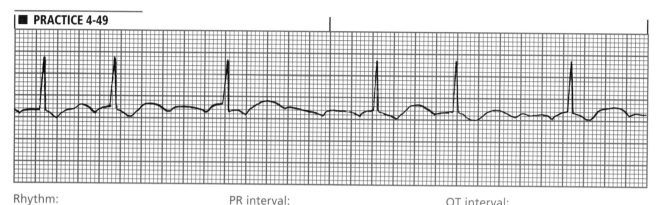

Rhythm: _____   PR interval: _____   QT interval: _____

Rate: _____   QRS complex: _____   Other: _____

P wave: _____   T wave: _____   Interpretation: _____

■ PRACTICE 4-50

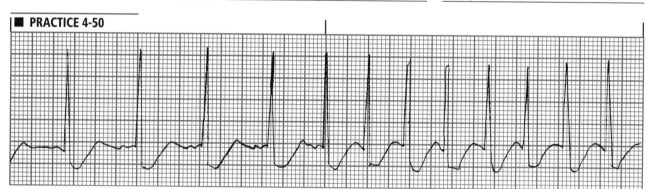

Rhythm: _____   PR interval: _____   QT interval: _____

Rate: _____   QRS complex: _____   Other: _____

P wave: _____   T wave: _____   Interpretation: _____

■ PRACTICE 4-51

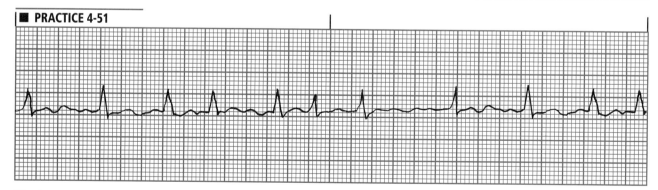

Rhythm: _____   PR interval: _____   QT interval: _____

Rate: _____   QRS complex: _____   Other: _____

P wave: _____   T wave: _____   Interpretation: _____

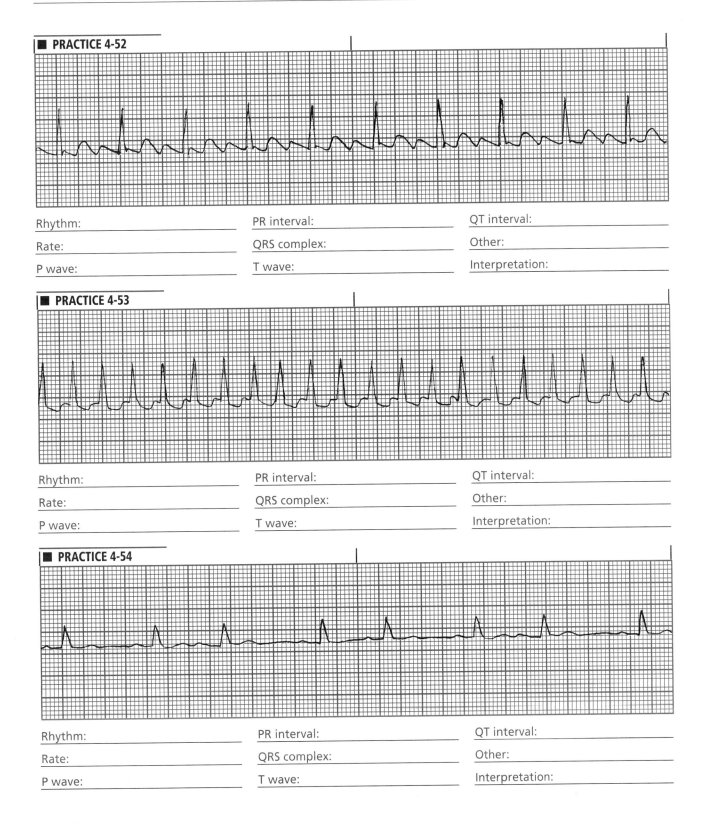

■ PRACTICE 4-52

Rhythm: _____   PR interval: _____   QT interval: _____

Rate: _____   QRS complex: _____   Other: _____

P wave: _____   T wave: _____   Interpretation: _____

■ PRACTICE 4-53

Rhythm: _____   PR interval: _____   QT interval: _____

Rate: _____   QRS complex: _____   Other: _____

P wave: _____   T wave: _____   Interpretation: _____

■ PRACTICE 4-54

Rhythm: _____   PR interval: _____   QT interval: _____

Rate: _____   QRS complex: _____   Other: _____

P wave: _____   T wave: _____   Interpretation: _____

■ **PRACTICE 4-55**

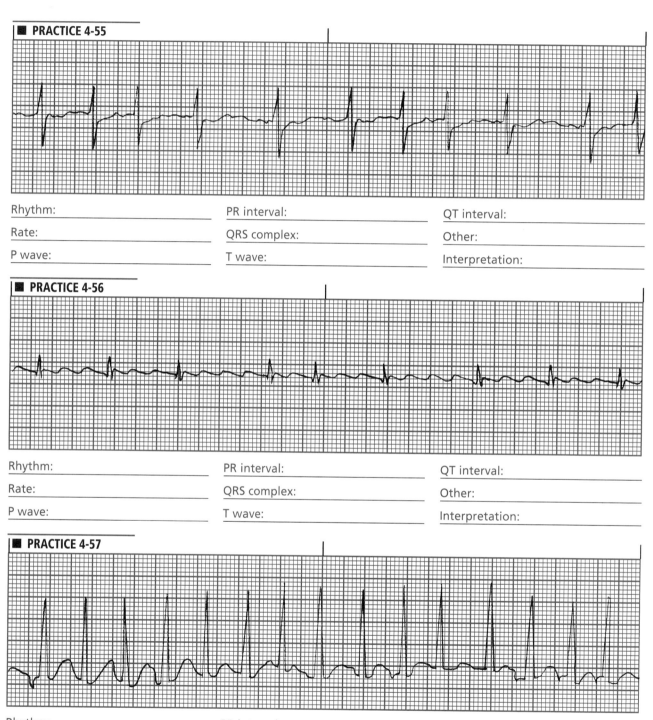

Rhythm: _____   PR interval: _____   QT interval: _____

Rate: _____   QRS complex: _____   Other: _____

P wave: _____   T wave: _____   Interpretation: _____

■ **PRACTICE 4-56**

Rhythm: _____   PR interval: _____   QT interval: _____

Rate: _____   QRS complex: _____   Other: _____

P wave: _____   T wave: _____   Interpretation: _____

■ **PRACTICE 4-57**

Rhythm: _____   PR interval: _____   QT interval: _____

Rate: _____   QRS complex: _____   Other: _____

P wave: _____   T wave: _____   Interpretation: _____

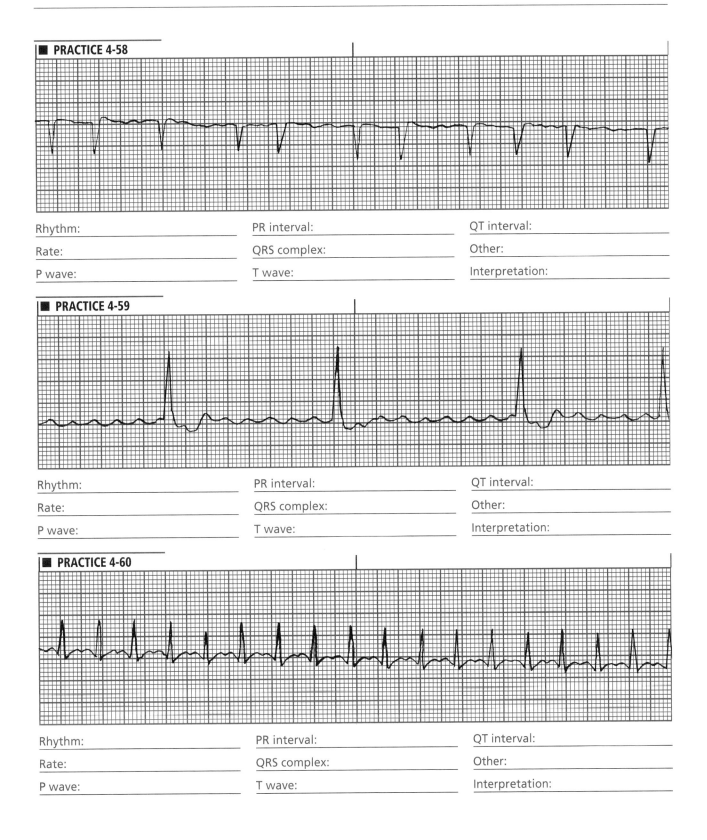

■ **PRACTICE 4-58**

Rhythm: _____   PR interval: _____   QT interval: _____

Rate: _____   QRS complex: _____   Other: _____

P wave: _____   T wave: _____   Interpretation: _____

■ **PRACTICE 4-59**

Rhythm: _____   PR interval: _____   QT interval: _____

Rate: _____   QRS complex: _____   Other: _____

P wave: _____   T wave: _____   Interpretation: _____

■ **PRACTICE 4-60**

Rhythm: _____   PR interval: _____   QT interval: _____

Rate: _____   QRS complex: _____   Other: _____

P wave: _____   T wave: _____   Interpretation: _____

■ PRACTICE 4-61

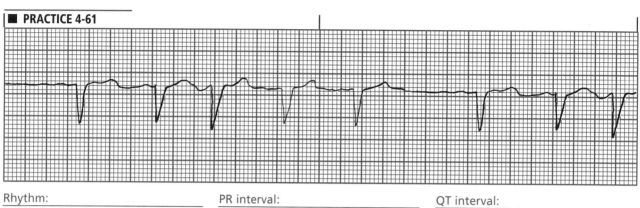

Rhythm: _____   PR interval: _____   QT interval: _____

Rate: _____   QRS complex: _____   Other: _____

P wave: _____   T wave: _____   Interpretation: _____

■ PRACTICE 4-62

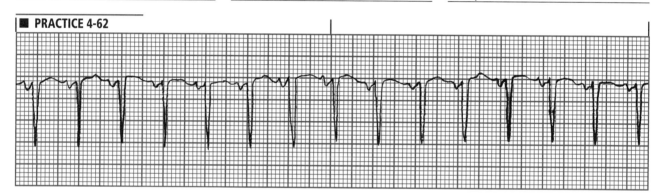

Rhythm: _____   PR interval: _____   QT interval: _____

Rate: _____   QRS complex: _____   Other: _____

P wave: _____   T wave: _____   Interpretation: _____

■ PRACTICE 4-63

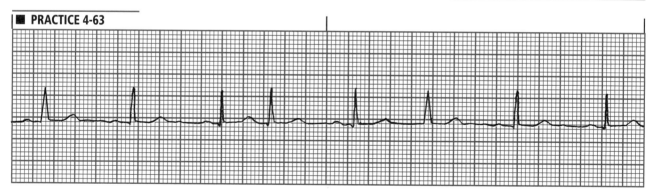

Rhythm: _____   PR interval: _____   QT interval: _____

Rate: _____   QRS complex: _____   Other: _____

P wave: _____   T wave: _____   Interpretation: _____

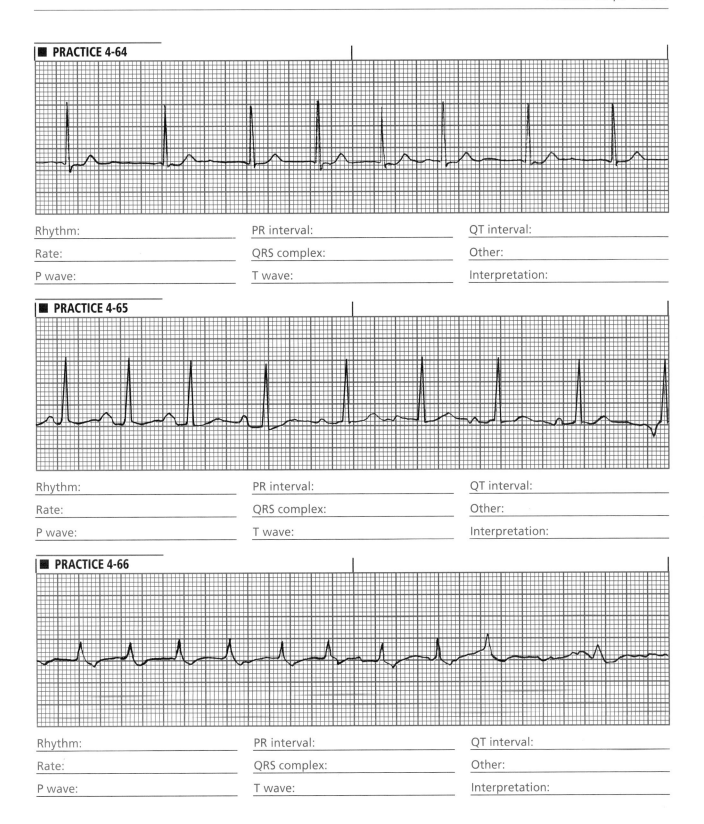

■ **PRACTICE 4-64**

Rhythm: _____   PR interval: _____   QT interval: _____

Rate: _____   QRS complex: _____   Other: _____

P wave: _____   T wave: _____   Interpretation: _____

■ **PRACTICE 4-65**

Rhythm: _____   PR interval: _____   QT interval: _____

Rate: _____   QRS complex: _____   Other: _____

P wave: _____   T wave: _____   Interpretation: _____

■ **PRACTICE 4-66**

Rhythm: _____   PR interval: _____   QT interval: _____

Rate: _____   QRS complex: _____   Other: _____

P wave: _____   T wave: _____   Interpretation: _____

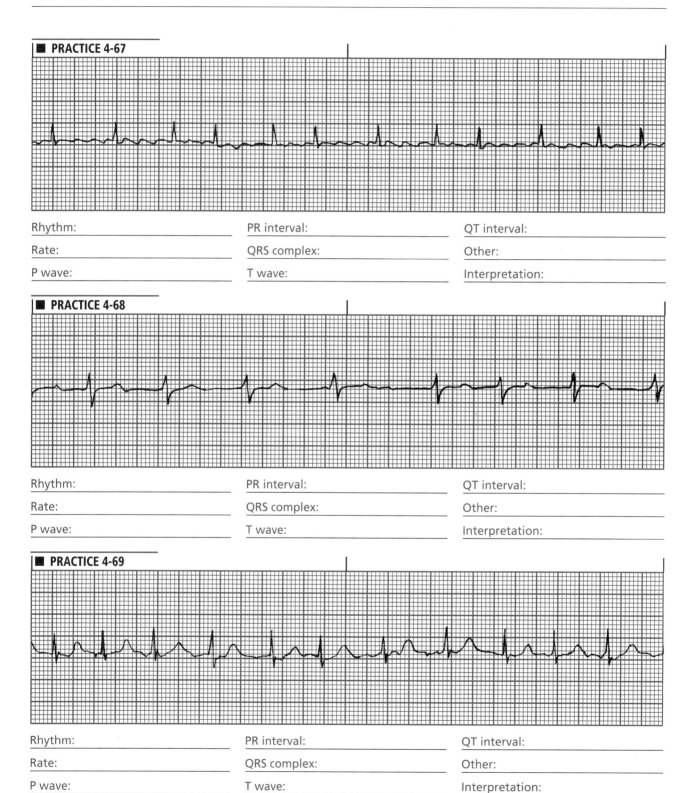

■ PRACTICE 4-67

Rhythm:	PR interval:	QT interval:
Rate:	QRS complex:	Other:
P wave:	T wave:	Interpretation:

■ PRACTICE 4-68

Rhythm:	PR interval:	QT interval:
Rate:	QRS complex:	Other:
P wave:	T wave:	Interpretation:

■ PRACTICE 4-69

Rhythm:	PR interval:	QT interval:
Rate:	QRS complex:	Other:
P wave:	T wave:	Interpretation:

■ **PRACTICE 4-70**

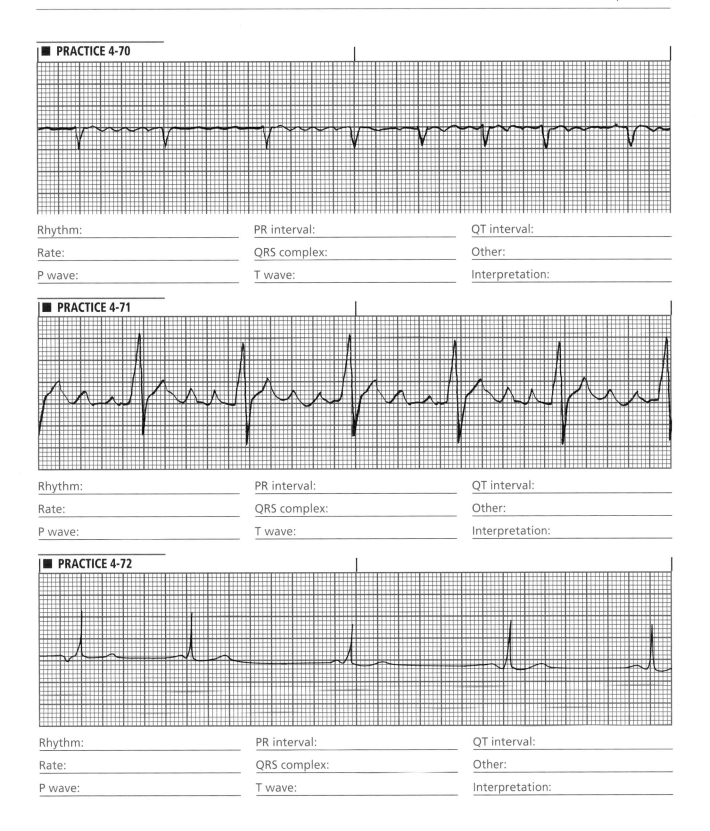

Rhythm: _____   PR interval: _____   QT interval: _____

Rate: _____   QRS complex: _____   Other: _____

P wave: _____   T wave: _____   Interpretation: _____

■ **PRACTICE 4-71**

Rhythm: _____   PR interval: _____   QT interval: _____

Rate: _____   QRS complex: _____   Other: _____

P wave: _____   T wave: _____   Interpretation: _____

■ **PRACTICE 4-72**

Rhythm: _____   PR interval: _____   QT interval: _____

Rate: _____   QRS complex: _____   Other: _____

P wave: _____   T wave: _____   Interpretation: _____

■ **PRACTICE 4-73**

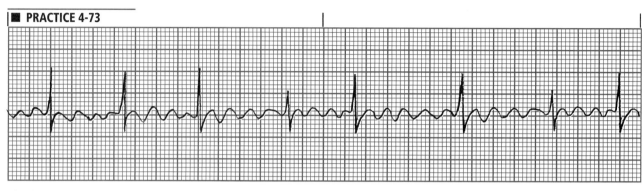

Rhythm: _____   PR interval: _____   QT interval: _____

Rate: _____   QRS complex: _____   Other: _____

P wave: _____   T wave: _____   Interpretation: _____

■ **PRACTICE 4-74**

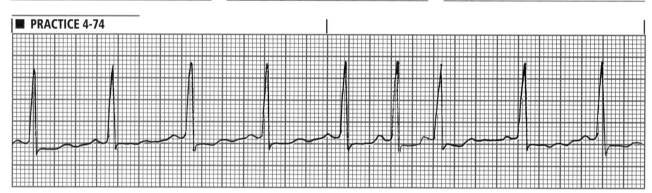

Rhythm: _____   PR interval: _____   QT interval: _____

Rate: _____   QRS complex: _____   Other: _____

P wave: _____   T wave: _____   Interpretation: _____

■ **PRACTICE 4-75**

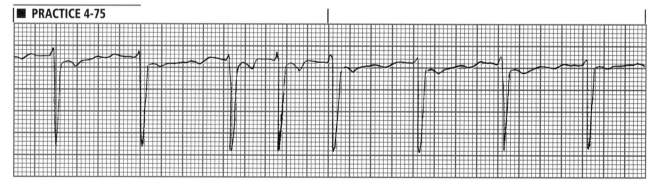

Rhythm: _____   PR interval: _____   QT interval: _____

Rate: _____   QRS complex: _____   Other: _____

P wave: _____   T wave: _____   Interpretation: _____

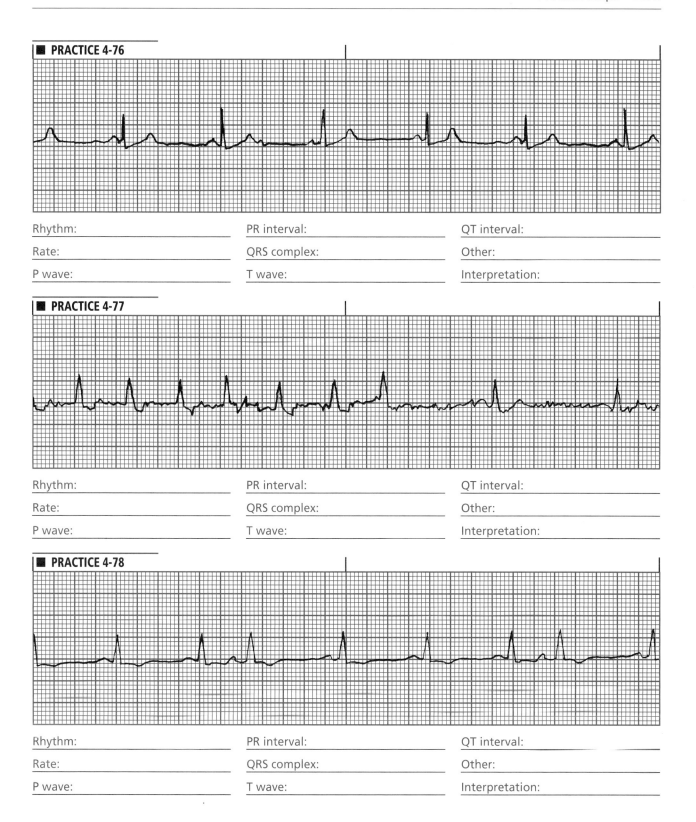

■ PRACTICE 4-76

Rhythm: _____   PR interval: _____   QT interval: _____

Rate: _____   QRS complex: _____   Other: _____

P wave: _____   T wave: _____   Interpretation: _____

■ PRACTICE 4-77

Rhythm: _____   PR interval: _____   QT interval: _____

Rate: _____   QRS complex: _____   Other: _____

P wave: _____   T wave: _____   Interpretation: _____

■ PRACTICE 4-78

Rhythm: _____   PR interval: _____   QT interval: _____

Rate: _____   QRS complex: _____   Other: _____

P wave: _____   T wave: _____   Interpretation: _____

■ **PRACTICE 4-79**

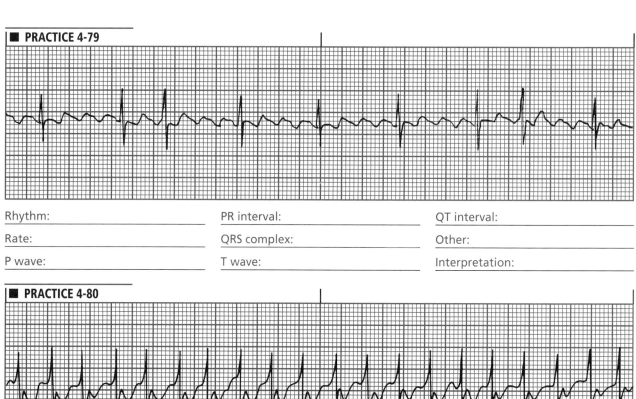

Rhythm:	PR interval:	QT interval:
Rate:	QRS complex:	Other:
P wave:	T wave:	Interpretation:

■ **PRACTICE 4-80**

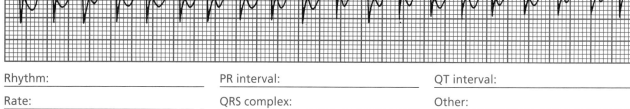

Rhythm:	PR interval:	QT interval:
Rate:	QRS complex:	Other:
P wave:	T wave:	Interpretation:

■ **PRACTICE 4-81**

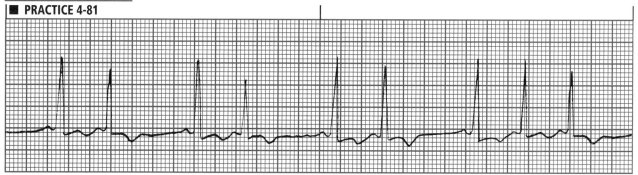

Rhythm:	PR interval:	QT interval:
Rate:	QRS complex:	Other:
P wave:	T wave:	Interpretation:

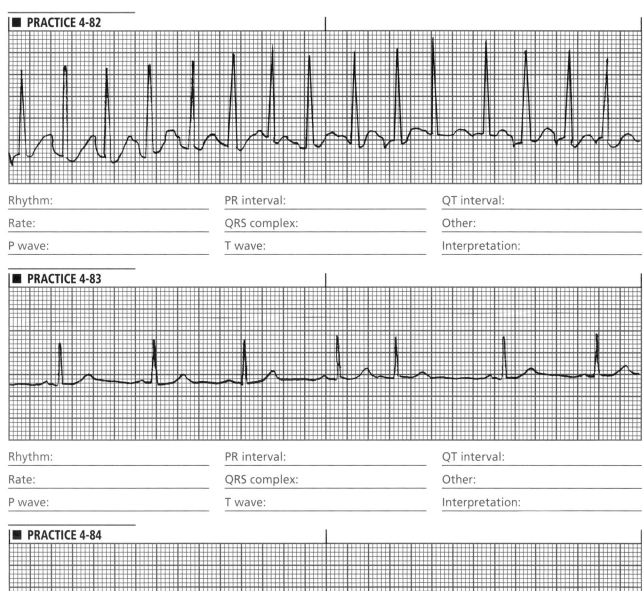

■ PRACTICE 4-82

Rhythm:	PR interval:	QT interval:
Rate:	QRS complex:	Other:
P wave:	T wave:	Interpretation:

■ PRACTICE 4-83

Rhythm:	PR interval:	QT interval:
Rate:	QRS complex:	Other:
P wave:	T wave:	Interpretation:

■ PRACTICE 4-84

Rhythm:	PR interval:	QT interval:
Rate:	QRS complex:	Other:
P wave:	T wave:	Interpretation:

■ **PRACTICE 4-85**

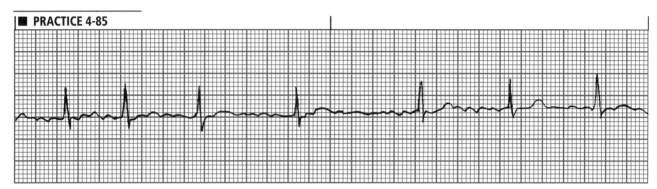

Rhythm: _____   PR interval: _____   QT interval: _____

Rate: _____   QRS complex: _____   Other: _____

P wave: _____   T wave: _____   Interpretation: _____

■ **PRACTICE 4-86**

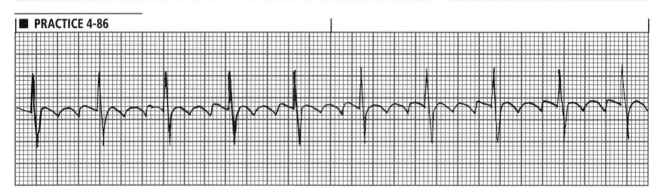

Rhythm: _____   PR interval: _____   QT interval: _____

Rate: _____   QRS complex: _____   Other: _____

P wave: _____   T wave: _____   Interpretation: _____

■ **PRACTICE 4-87**

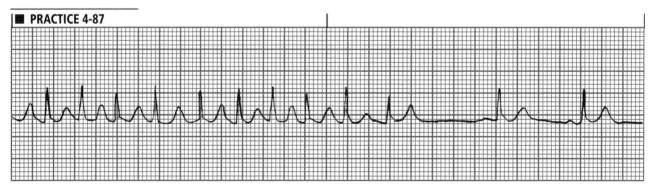

Rhythm: _____   PR interval: _____   QT interval: _____

Rate: _____   QRS complex: _____   Other: _____

P wave: _____   T wave: _____   Interpretation: _____

■ PRACTICE 4-88

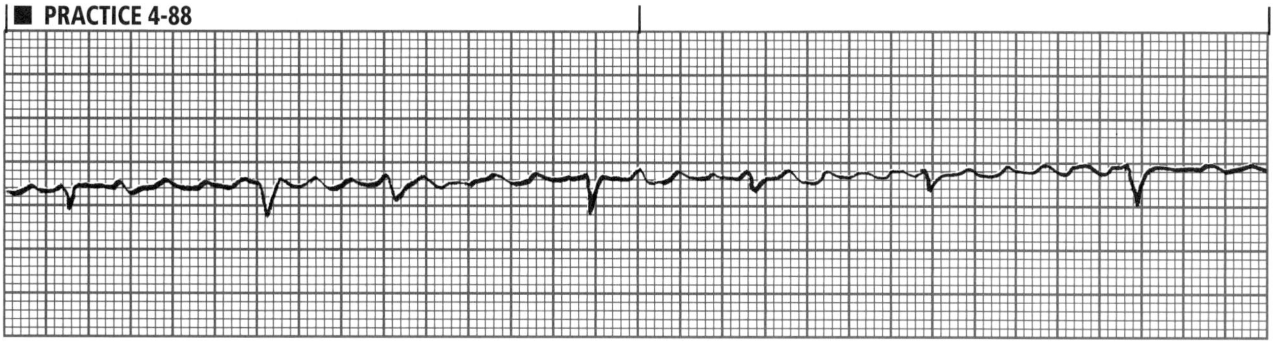

Rhythm: _____   PR interval: _____   QT interval: _____

Rate: _____   QRS complex: _____   Other: _____

P wave: _____   T wave: _____   Interpretation: _____

■ PRACTICE 4-89

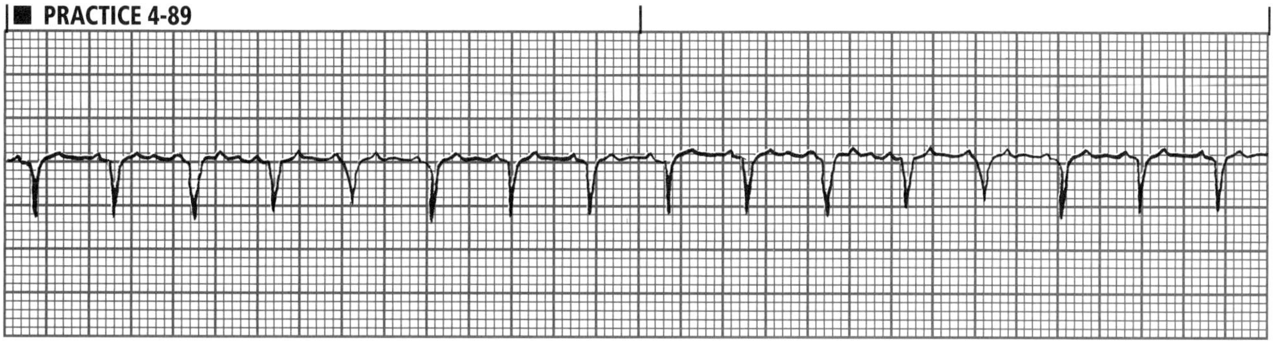

Rhythm: _____   PR interval: _____   QT interval: _____

Rate: _____   QRS complex: _____   Other: _____

P wave: _____   T wave: _____   Interpretation: _____

■ PRACTICE 4-90

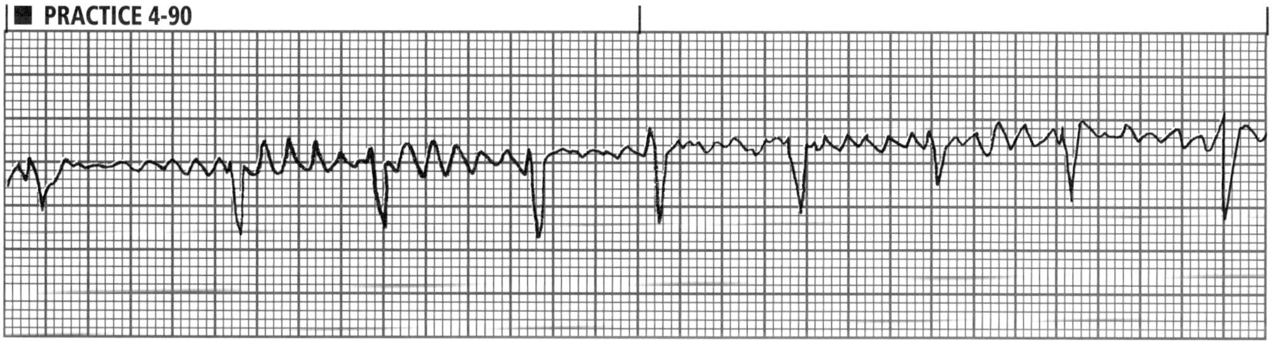

Rhythm: _____   PR interval: _____   QT interval: _____

Rate: _____   QRS complex: _____   Other: _____

P wave: _____   T wave: _____   Interpretation: _____

■ PRACTICE 4-91

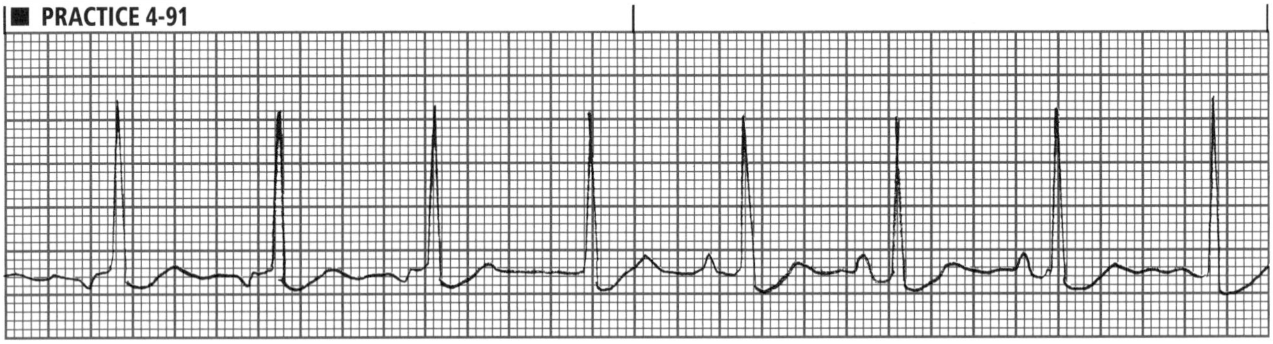

Rhythm: _____   PR interval: _____   QT interval: _____

Rate: _____   QRS complex: _____   Other: _____

P wave: _____   T wave: _____   Interpretation: _____

■ PRACTICE 4-92

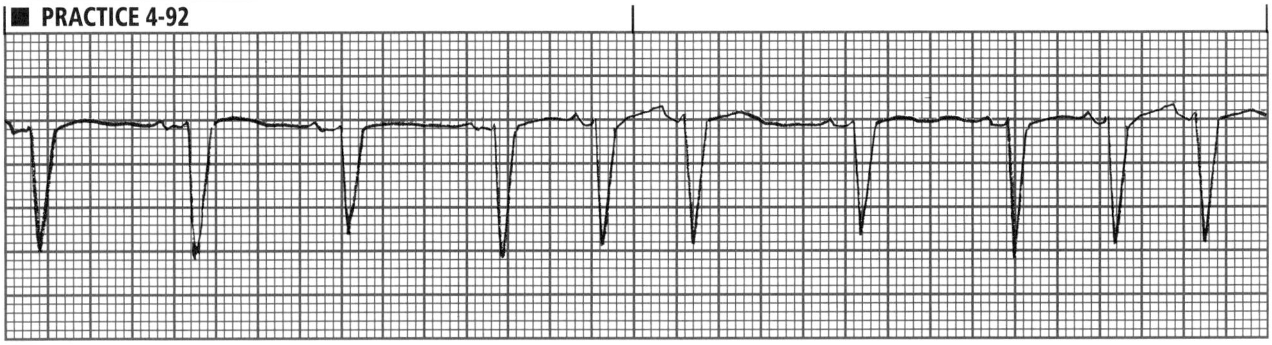

Rhythm: _____   PR interval: _____   QT interval: _____

Rate: _____   QRS complex: _____   Other: _____

P wave: _____   T wave: _____   Interpretation: _____

■ PRACTICE 4-93

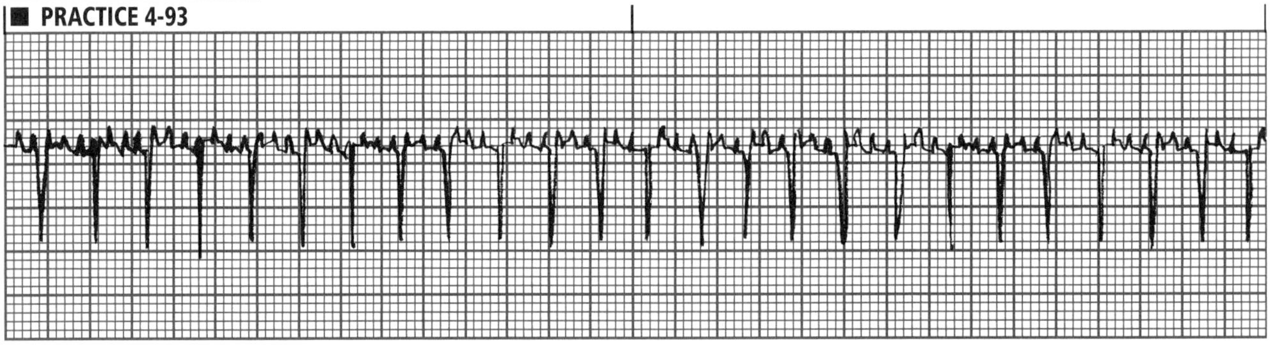

Rhythm: _____   PR interval: _____   QT interval: _____

Rate: _____   QRS complex: _____   Other: _____

P wave: _____   T wave: _____   Interpretation: _____

■ PRACTICE 4-94

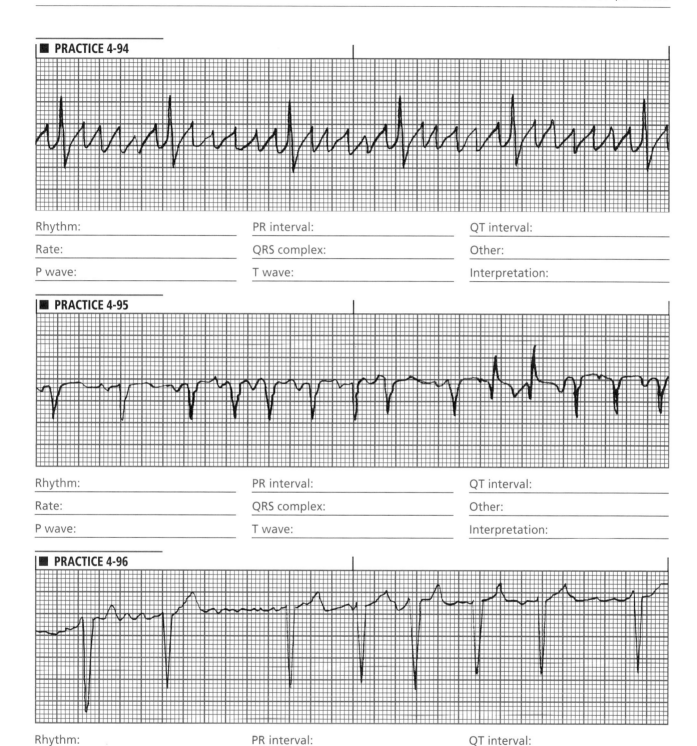

Rhythm: _____   PR interval: _____   QT interval: _____

Rate: _____   QRS complex: _____   Other: _____

P wave: _____   T wave: _____   Interpretation: _____

■ PRACTICE 4-95

Rhythm: _____   PR interval: _____   QT interval: _____

Rate: _____   QRS complex: _____   Other: _____

P wave: _____   T wave: _____   Interpretation: _____

■ PRACTICE 4-96

Rhythm: _____   PR interval: _____   QT interval: _____

Rate: _____   QRS complex: _____   Other: _____

P wave: _____   T wave: _____   Interpretation: _____

■ **PRACTICE 4-97**

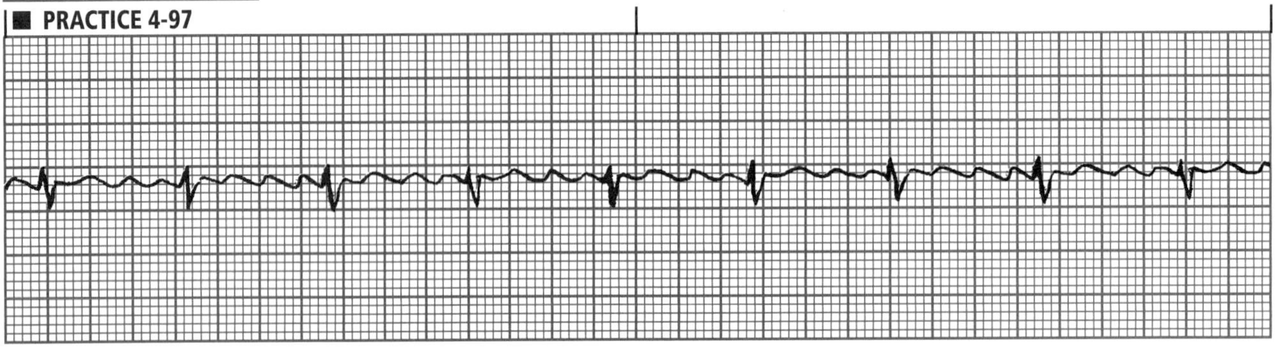

Rhythm: _____

Rate: _____

P wave: _____

PR interval: _____

QRS complex: _____

T wave: _____

QT interval: _____

Other: _____

Interpretation: _____

■ **PRACTICE 4-98**

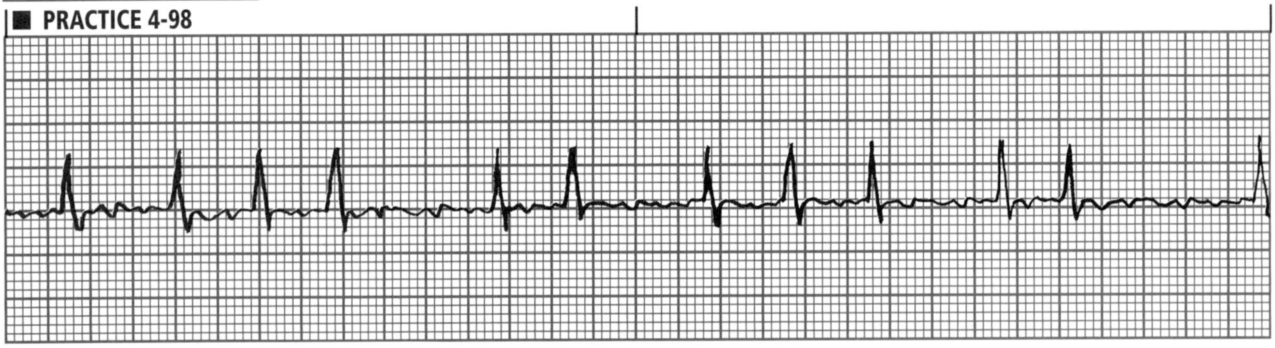

Rhythm: _____

Rate: _____

P wave: _____

PR interval: _____

QRS complex: _____

T wave: _____

QT interval: _____

Other: _____

Interpretation: _____

■ **PRACTICE 4-99**

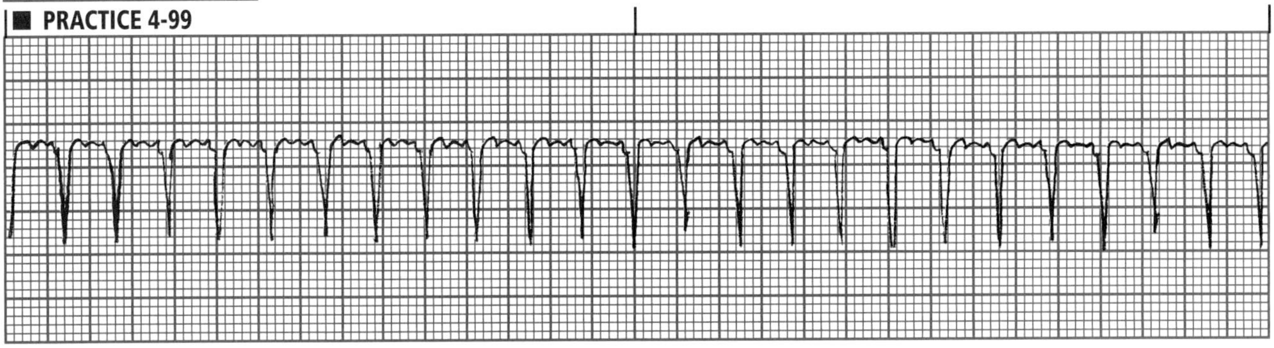

Rhythm: _____

Rate: _____

P wave: _____

PR interval: _____

QRS complex: _____

T wave: _____

QT interval: _____

Other: _____

Interpretation: _____

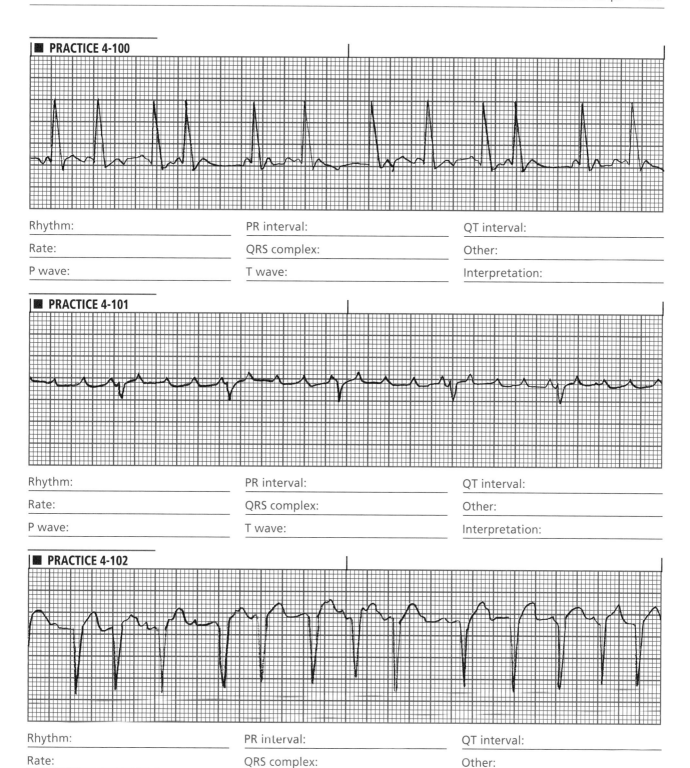

PRACTICE 4-100

Rhythm: _____ PR interval: _____ QT interval: _____

Rate: _____ QRS complex: _____ Other: _____

P wave: _____ T wave: _____ Interpretation: _____

PRACTICE 4-101

Rhythm: _____ PR interval: _____ QT interval: _____

Rate: _____ QRS complex: _____ Other: _____

P wave: _____ T wave: _____ Interpretation: _____

PRACTICE 4-102

Rhythm: _____ PR interval: _____ QT interval: _____

Rate: _____ QRS complex: _____ Other: _____

P wave: _____ T wave: _____ Interpretation: _____

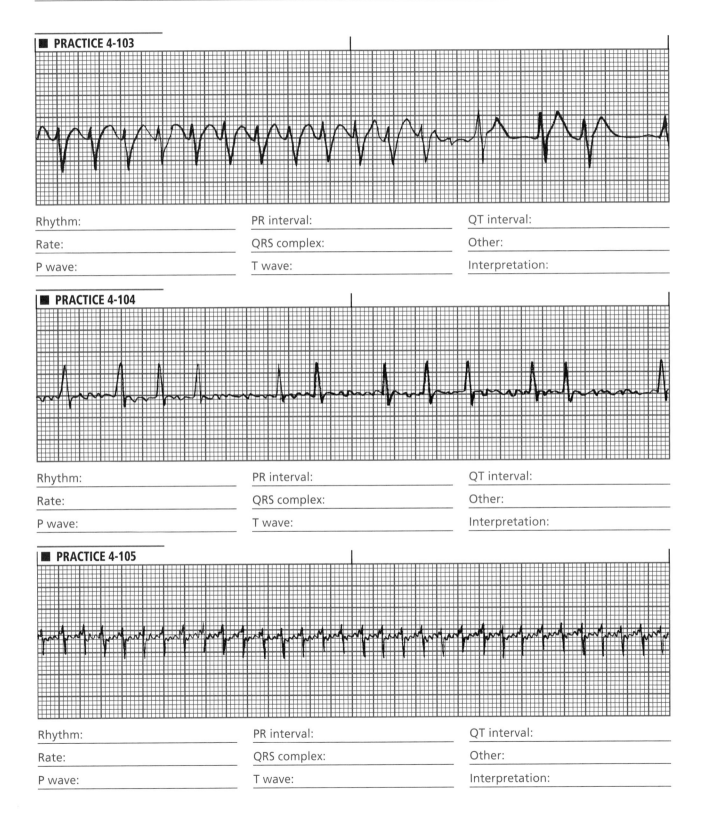

■ PRACTICE 4-103

Rhythm: _____ PR interval: _____ QT interval: _____

Rate: _____ QRS complex: _____ Other: _____

P wave: _____ T wave: _____ Interpretation: _____

■ PRACTICE 4-104

Rhythm: _____ PR interval: _____ QT interval: _____

Rate: _____ QRS complex: _____ Other: _____

P wave: _____ T wave: _____ Interpretation: _____

■ PRACTICE 4-105

Rhythm: _____ PR interval: _____ QT interval: _____

Rate: _____ QRS complex: _____ Other: _____

P wave: _____ T wave: _____ Interpretation: _____

■ **PRACTICE 4-106**

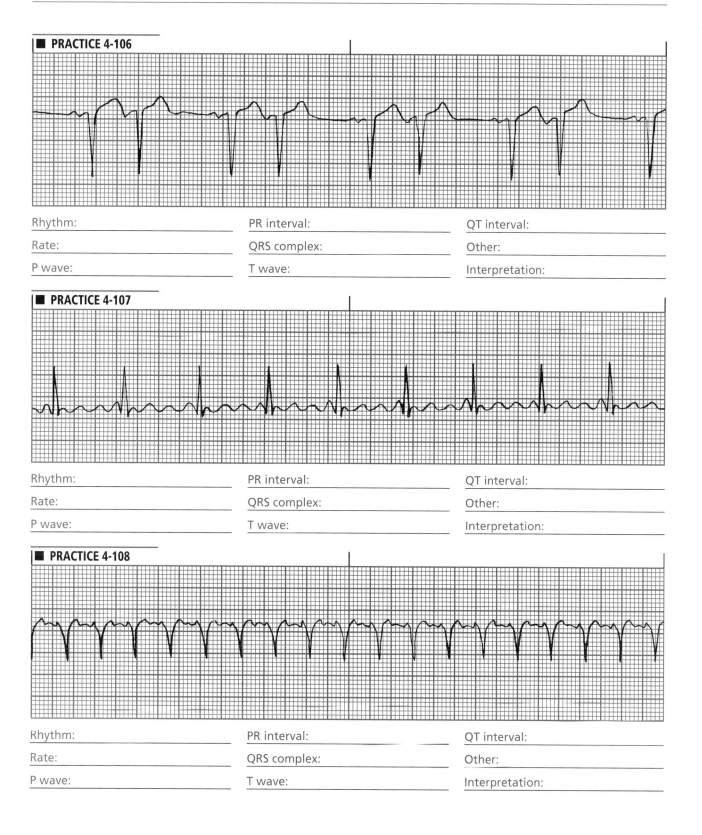

Rhythm: _____ PR interval: _____ QT interval: _____

Rate: _____ QRS complex: _____ Other: _____

P wave: _____ T wave: _____ Interpretation: _____

■ **PRACTICE 4-107**

Rhythm: _____ PR interval: _____ QT interval: _____

Rate: _____ QRS complex: _____ Other: _____

P wave: _____ T wave: _____ Interpretation: _____

■ **PRACTICE 4-108**

Rhythm: _____ PR interval: _____ QT interval: _____

Rate: _____ QRS complex: _____ Other: _____

P wave: _____ T wave: _____ Interpretation: _____

■ **PRACTICE 4-109**

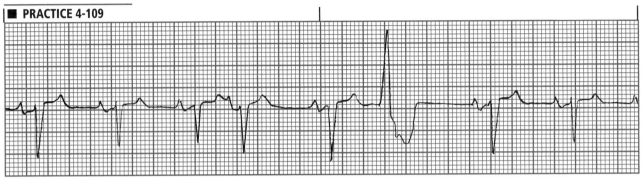

Rhythm: _____   PR interval: _____   QT interval: _____

Rate: _____   QRS complex: _____   Other: _____

P wave: _____   T wave: _____   Interpretation: _____

■ **PRACTICE 4-110**

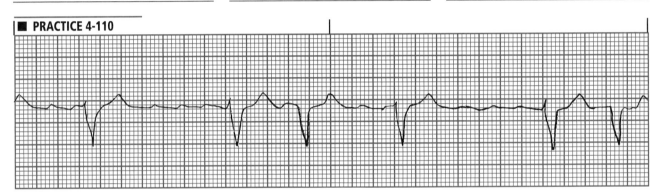

Rhythm: _____   PR interval: _____   QT interval: _____

Rate: _____   QRS complex: _____   Other: _____

P wave: _____   T wave: _____   Interpretation: _____

■ **PRACTICE 4-111**

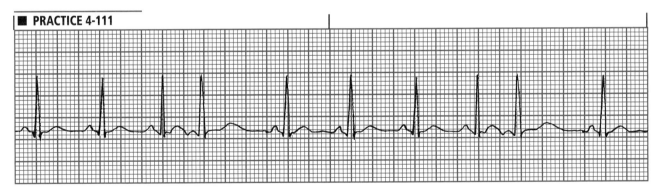

Rhythm: _____   PR interval: _____   QT interval: _____

Rate: _____   QRS complex: _____   Other: _____

P wave: _____   T wave: _____   Interpretation: _____

■ **PRACTICE 4-112**

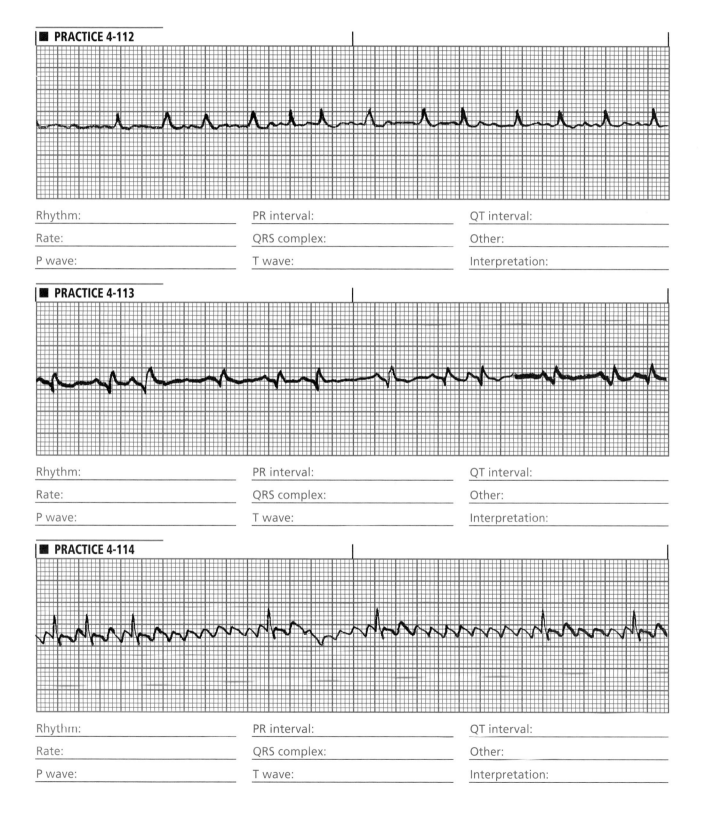

Rhythm: _____   PR interval: _____   QT interval: _____

Rate: _____   QRS complex: _____   Other: _____

P wave: _____   T wave: _____   Interpretation: _____

■ **PRACTICE 4-113**

Rhythm: _____   PR interval: _____   QT interval: _____

Rate: _____   QRS complex: _____   Other: _____

P wave: _____   T wave: _____   Interpretation: _____

■ **PRACTICE 4-114**

Rhythm: _____   PR interval: _____   QT interval: _____

Rate: _____   QRS complex: _____   Other: _____

P wave: _____   T wave: _____   Interpretation: _____

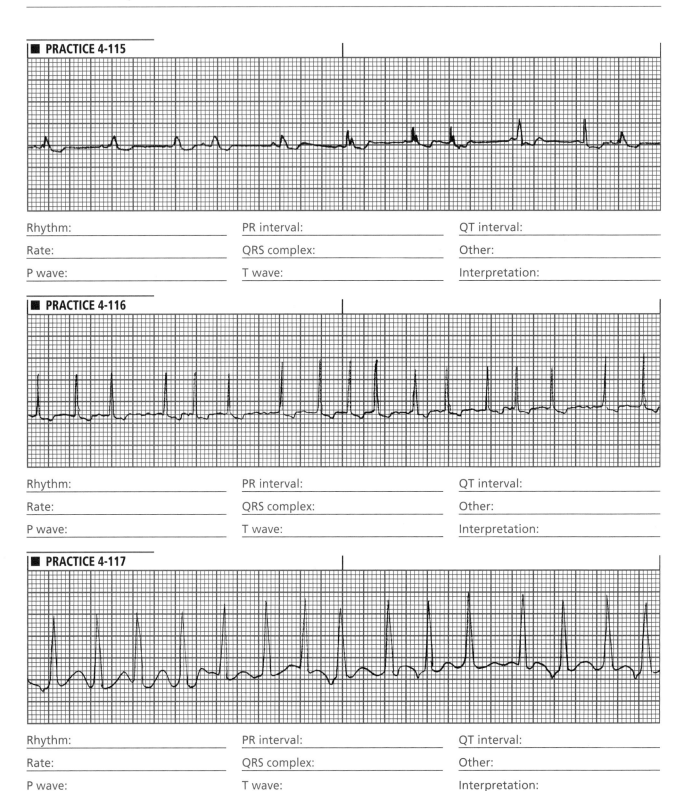

■ PRACTICE 4-115

Rhythm:	PR interval:	QT interval:
Rate:	QRS complex:	Other:
P wave:	T wave:	Interpretation:

■ PRACTICE 4-116

Rhythm:	PR interval:	QT interval:
Rate:	QRS complex:	Other:
P wave:	T wave:	Interpretation:

■ PRACTICE 4-117

Rhythm:	PR interval:	QT interval:
Rate:	QRS complex:	Other:
P wave:	T wave:	Interpretation:

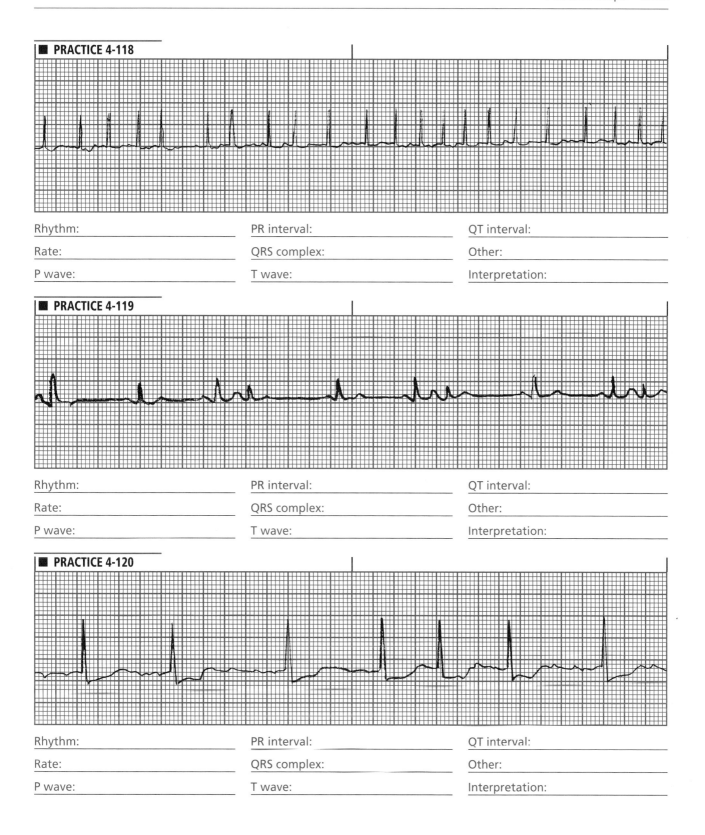

PRACTICE 4-118

Rhythm: _____ PR interval: _____ QT interval: _____

Rate: _____ QRS complex: _____ Other: _____

P wave: _____ T wave: _____ Interpretation: _____

PRACTICE 4-119

Rhythm: _____ PR interval: _____ QT interval: _____

Rate: _____ QRS complex: _____ Other: _____

P wave: _____ T wave: _____ Interpretation: _____

PRACTICE 4-120

Rhythm: _____ PR interval: _____ QT interval: _____

Rate: _____ QRS complex: _____ Other: _____

P wave: _____ T wave: _____ Interpretation: _____

■ PRACTICE STRIP ANSWERS

PRACTICE 4-1
- Rhythm: Irregular
- Rate: 110 beats/minute
- P wave: Not present
- PR interval: Unmeasurable
- QRS complex: 0.10 second
- T wave: Inverted
- QT interval: 0.28 second
- Other: None
- Interpretation: Uncontrolled atrial fibrillation

PRACTICE 4-2
- Rhythm: Regular
- Rate: 100 beats/minute
- P wave: Flutter waves
- PR interval: Unmeasurable
- QRS complex: 0.08 second
- T wave: Not discernible
- QT interval: Unmeasurable
- Other: None
- Interpretation: 3:1 atrial flutter

PRACTICE 4-3
- Rhythm: Irregular
- Rate: 160 beats/minute
- P wave: Not discernible
- PR interval: Unmeasurable
- QRS complex: 0.08 second
- T wave: Not discernible
- QT interval: Unmeasurable
- Other: None
- Interpretation: Uncontrolled atrial fibrillation

PRACTICE 4-4
- Rhythm: Irregular
- Rate: 50 beats/minute
- P wave: Normal
- PR interval: 0.20 second
- QRS complex: 0.08 second
- T wave: Normal
- QT interval: 0.52 second
- Other: None
- Interpretation: Sinus bradycardia with PAC

PRACTICE 4-5
- Rhythm: Irregular
- Rate: 120 beats/minute
- P wave: Fibrillatory waves
- PR interval: Unmeasurable
- QRS complex: 0.08 second
- T wave: Not discernible
- QT interval: Unmeasurable
- Other: None
- Interpretation: Uncontrolled atrial fibrillation

PRACTICE 4-6
- Rhythm: Irregular
- Rate: 110 beats/minute
- P wave: Not present
- PR interval: Unmeasurable
- QRS complex: 0.06 second
- T wave: Not discernible
- QT interval: Unmeasurable
- Other: None
- Interpretation: Uncontrolled atrial fibrillation

PRACTICE 4-7
- Rhythm: Irregular
- Rate: 60 beats/minute
- P wave: Variable
- PR interval: 0.16 second
- QRS complex: 0.10 second
- T wave: Inverted
- QT interval: 0.36 second
- Other: None
- Interpretation: Wandering pacemaker

PRACTICE 4-8
- Rhythm: Regular
- Rate: 94 beats/minute
- P wave: Flutter waves
- PR interval: Unmeasurable
- QRS complex: 0.08 second
- T wave: Not discernible
- QT interval: Unmeasurable
- Other: None
- Interpretation: 3:1 atrial flutter

PRACTICE 4-9
- Rhythm: Irregular
- Rate: 200 beats/minute
- P wave: Normal
- PR interval: 0.12 second
- QRS complex: 0.06 second
- T wave: Inverted
- QT interval: 0.16 second
- Other: None
- Interpretation: Atrial tachycardia with PACs

PRACTICE 4-10
- Rhythm: Irregular
- Rate: 60 beats/minute
- P wave: Not discernible
- PR interval: Unmeasurable
- QRS complex: 0.12 second
- T wave: Not discernible
- QT interval: Unmeasurable
- Other: None
- Interpretation: Controlled atrial fibrillation

PRACTICE 4-11
- Rhythm: Regular
- Rate: 70 beats/minute
- P wave: Flutter waves
- PR interval: Unmeasurable
- QRS complex: 0.12 second
- T wave: Not discernible
- QT interval: Unmeasurable
- Other: None
- Interpretation: 4:1 atrial flutter

PRACTICE 4-12
- Rhythm: Irregular
- Rate: 80 beats/minute
- P wave: Not discernible
- PR interval: Unmeasurable
- QRS complex: 0.08 second
- T wave: Normal
- QT interval: 0.32 second
- Other: None
- Interpretation: Controlled atrial fibrillation

PRACTICE 4-13
- Rhythm: Irregular
- Rate: 170 beats/minute
- P wave: Not discernible
- PR interval: Unmeasurable
- QRS complex: 0.08 second
- T wave: Not discernible
- QT interval: Unmeasurable
- Other: None
- Interpretation: Uncontrolled atrial fibrillation

PRACTICE 4-14
- Rhythm: Regular
- Rate: 79 beats/minute
- P wave: Flutter waves
- PR interval: Unmeasurable
- QRS complex: 0.08 second
- T wave: Not discernible
- QT interval: Unmeasurable
- Other: None
- Interpretation: 4:1 atrial flutter

PRACTICE 4-15
- Rhythm: Irregular
- Rate: 70 beats/minute
- P wave: Not discernible
- PR interval: Unmeasurable
- QRS complex: 0.08 second
- T wave: Inverted
- QT interval: 0.36 second
- Other: None
- Interpretation: Controlled atrial fibrillation

PRACTICE 4-16
- Rhythm: Irregular
- Rate: 70 beats/minute
- P wave: Normal
- PR interval: 0.20 second
- QRS complex: 0.08 second
- T wave: Normal
- QT interval: 0.32 second
- Other: None
- Interpretation: NSR with blocked PAC

PRACTICE 4-17
- Rhythm: Irregular
- Rate: 100 beats/minute
- P wave: Fibrillatory waves
- PR interval: Unmeasurable
- QRS complex: 0.12 second
- T wave: Normal
- QT interval: 0.32 second
- Other: None
- Interpretation: Uncontrolled atrial fibrillation

PRACTICE 4-18
- Rhythm: Irregular
- Rate: 100 beats/minute
- P wave: Fibrillatory waves
- PR interval: Unmeasurable
- QRS complex: 0.10 second
- T wave: Not discernible
- QT interval: Unmeasurable
- Other: None
- Interpretation: Uncontrolled atrial fibrillation

PRACTICE 4-19
- Rhythm: Irregular
- Rate: 90 beats/minute
- P wave: Not discernible
- PR interval: Unmeasurable
- QRS complex: 0.06 second
- T wave: Not discernible
- QT interval: Unmeasurable
- Other: None
- Interpretation: Controlled atrial fibrillation

PRACTICE 4-20
- Rhythm: Regular
- Rate: 75 beats/minute
- P wave: Flutter waves
- PR interval: Unmeasurable
- QRS complex: 0.08 second
- T wave: Not discernible
- QT interval: Unmeasurable
- Other: None
- Interpretation: 4:1 atrial flutter

PRACTICE 4-21
- Rhythm: Irregular
- Rate: 90 beats/minute
- P wave: Normal
- PR interval: 0.20 second
- QRS complex: 0.08 second
- T wave: Normal
- QT interval: 0.40 second
- Other: None
- Interpretation: NSR with PACs

PRACTICE 4-22
- Rhythm: Irregular
- Rate: 120 beats/minute
- P wave: Variable
- PR interval: Variable
- QRS complex: 0.08 second
- T wave: Distorted
- QT interval: Variable
- Other: None
- Interpretation: MAT

PRACTICE 4-23
- Rhythm: Irregular
- Rate: 90 beats/minute
- P wave: Not discernible
- PR interval: Unmeasurable
- QRS complex: 0.08 second
- T wave: Inverted
- QT interval: 0.32 second
- Other: None
- Interpretation: Controlled atrial fibrillation

PRACTICE 4-24
- Rhythm: Irregular
- Rate: 100 beats/minute
- P wave: Normal
- PR interval: 0.16 second
- QRS complex: 0.08 second
- T wave: Normal
- QT interval: 0.28 second
- Other: None P wave buried with PAC
- Interpretation: NSR with PACs

PRACTICE 4-25
- Rhythm: Irregular
- Rate: 90 beats/minute
- P wave: Not discernible
- PR interval: Unmeasurable
- QRS complex: 0.08 second
- T wave: Normal
- QT interval: 0.36 second
- Other: ST-segment depression
- Interpretation: Controlled atrial fibrillation

PRACTICE 4-26
- Rhythm: Irregular
- Rate: 70 beats/minute
- P wave: Fibrillatory waves
- PR interval: Unmeasurable
- QRS complex: 0.08 second
- T wave: Normal
- QT interval: 0.36 second
- Other: None
- Interpretation: Controlled atrial fibrillation

PRACTICE 4-27
- Rhythm: Irregular
- Rate: 90 beats/minute
- P wave: Flutter waves
- PR interval: Unmeasurable
- QRS complex: 0.08 second
- T wave: Indiscernible
- QT interval: Unmeasurable
- Other: None
- Interpretation: Atrial flutter with variable block

PRACTICE 4-28
- Rhythm: Irregular
- Rate: 90 beats/minute
- P wave: Fibrillatory waves
- PR interval: Unmeasurable
- QRS complex: 0.06 second
- T wave: Not discernible
- QT interval: Unmeasurable
- Other: None
- Interpretation: Controlled atrial fibrillation

PRACTICE 4-29
- Rhythm: Irregular
- Rate: 80 beats/minute
- P wave: Normal
- PR interval: 0.16 second
- QRS complex: 0.08 second
- T wave: Normal
- QT interval: 0.40 second
- Other: None
- Interpretation: NSR with PACs

PRACTICE 4-30
- Rhythm: Irregular
- Rate: 90 beats/minute
- P wave: Variable
- PR interval: Variable
- QRS complex: 0.08 second
- T wave: Inverted
- QT interval: 0.36 second
- Other: None
- Interpretation: PAT leading back to NSR

PRACTICE 4-31
- Rhythm: Irregular
- Rate: 180 beats/minute
- P wave: Not discernible
- PR interval: Unmeasurable
- QRS complex: 0.08 second
- T wave: Not discernible
- QT interval: Unmeasurable
- Other: None
- Interpretation: Uncontrolled atrial fibrillation (with a pair of PVCs)

PRACTICE 4-32
- Rhythm: Irregular
- Rate: 70 beats/minute
- P wave: Slightly flattened
- PR interval: 0.18 second
- QRS complex: 0.10 second
- T wave: Normal
- QT interval: 0.36 second
- Other: None
- Interpretation: NSR with PACs

PRACTICE 4-33
- Rhythm: Irregular
- Rate: 80 beats/minute
- P wave: Flutter waves
- PR interval: Unmeasurable
- QRS complex: 0.10 second
- T wave: Not discernible
- QT interval: Unmeasurable
- Other: None
- Interpretation: Atrial flutter with variable block

PRACTICE 4-34
- Rhythm: Regular
- Rate: 88 beats/minute
- P wave: Flutter waves
- PR interval: Unmeasurable
- QRS complex: 0.10 second
- T wave: Not discernible
- QT interval: Unmeasurable
- Other: None
- Interpretation: 3:1 atrial flutter

PRACTICE 4-35
- Rhythm: Irregular
- Rate: 70 beats/minute
- P wave: Normal
- PR interval: 0.16 second
- QRS complex: 0.08 second
- T wave: Normal
- QT interval: 0.36 second
- Other: None
- Interpretation: NSR with PAC

PRACTICE 4-36
- Rhythm: Irregular
- Rate: 60 beats/minute
- P wave: Flutter waves
- PR interval: Unmeasurable
- QRS complex: 0.12 second
- T wave: Not discernible
- QT interval: 0.36 second
- Other: None
- Interpretation: Atrial flutter with variable block

PRACTICE 4-37
- Rhythm: Regular
- Rate: 94 beats/minute
- P wave: Flutter waves
- PR interval: Unmeasurable
- QRS complex: 0.08 second
- T wave: Not discernible
- QT interval: Unmeasurable
- Other: None
- Interpretation: 2:1 atrial flutter

PRACTICE 4-38
- Rhythm: Irregular
- Rate: 60 beats/minute
- P wave: Normal
- PR interval: 0.16 second
- QRS complex: 0.08 second
- T wave: Normal
- QT interval: 0.40 second
- Other: None
- Interpretation: NSR with PACs

PRACTICE 4-39
- Rhythm: Irregular
- Rate: 110 beats/minute
- P wave: Flutter waves
- PR interval: Unmeasurable
- QRS complex: 0.08 second
- T wave: Not discernible
- QT interval: Unmeasurable
- Other: None
- Interpretation: Atrial flutter with variable block

PRACTICE 4-40
- Rhythm: Irregular
- Rate: 90 beats/minute
- P wave: Fibrillatory waves
- PR interval: Unmeasurable
- QRS complex: 0.08 second
- T wave: Normal
- QT interval: 0.36 second
- Other: None
- Interpretation: Controlled atrial fibrillation

PRACTICE 4-41
- Rhythm: Regular
- Rate: 167 beats/minute
- P wave: Normal
- PR interval: 0.12 second
- QRS complex: 0.10 second
- T wave: Normal
- QT interval: 0.24 second
- Other: None
- Interpretation: Atrial tachycardia

PRACTICE 4-42
- Rhythm: Irregular
- Rate: 90 beats/minute
- P wave: Variable
- PR interval: Variable
- QRS complex: 0.08 second
- T wave: Normal
- QT interval: 0.36 second
- Other: None
- Interpretation: Wandering atrial pacemaker

PRACTICE 4-43
- Rhythm: Regular
- Rate: 94 beats/minute
- P wave: Flutter waves
- PR interval: Unmeasurable
- QRS complex: 0.08 second
- T wave: Not discernible
- QT interval: Unmeasurable
- Other: None
- Interpretation: 3:1 atrial flutter

PRACTICE 4-44
- Rhythm: Irregular
- Rate: 110 beats/minute
- P wave: Variable
- PR interval: 0.16 second
- QRS complex: 0.08 second
- T wave: Not discernible
- QT interval: Unmeasurable
- Other: None
- Interpretation: MAT

PRACTICE 4-45
- Rhythm: Irregular
- Rate: 110 beats/minute
- P wave: Normal
- PR interval: 0.12 second
- QRS complex: 0.08 second
- T wave: Normal
- QT interval: 0.32 second
- Other: None
- Interpretation: Sinus tachycardia with PACs

PRACTICE 4-46
- Rhythm: Irregular
- Rate: 70 to 80 beats/minute
- P wave: Variable
- PR interval: Variable
- QRS complex: 0.08 second
- T wave: Inverted
- QT interval: 0.36 second
- Other: None
- Interpretation: Wandering atrial pacemaker

PRACTICE 4-47
- Rhythm: Irregular
- Rate: 100 beats/minute
- P wave: Fibrillatory waves
- PR interval: Unmeasurable
- QRS complex: 0.08 second
- T wave: Not discernible
- QT interval: Unmeasurable
- Other: None
- Interpretation: Uncontrolled atrial fibrillation

PRACTICE 4-48
- Rhythm: Irregular
- Rate: 214 down to 50 beats/minute
- P wave: Not discernible
- PR interval: Unmeasurable
- QRS complex: 0.12 second
- T wave: Normal
- QT interval: 0.28 second
- Other: None
- Interpretation: Atrial tachycardia changing to atrial fibrillation with PVCs

PRACTICE 4-49
- Rhythm: Irregular
- Rate: 60 beats/minute
- P wave: Not discernible
- PR interval: Unmeasurable
- QRS complex: 0.08 second
- T wave: Not discernible
- QT interval: Unmeasurable
- Other: None
- Interpretation: Controlled atrial fibrillation

PRACTICE 4-50
- Rhythm: Irregular
- Rate: 120 beats/minute
- P wave: Normal to absent
- PR interval: 0.12 second when present
- QRS complex: 0.08 second
- T wave: Depressed
- QT interval: Variable
- Other: None
- Interpretation: Sinus tachycardia changing to atrial tachycardia

PRACTICE 4-51
- Rhythm: Irregular
- Rate: 110 beats/minute
- P wave: Fibrillatory waves
- PR interval: Unmeasurable
- QRS complex: 0.12 second
- T wave: Not discernible
- QT interval: Unmeasurable
- Other: None
- Interpretation: Uncontrolled atrial fibrillation

PRACTICE 4-52
- Rhythm: Regular
- Rate: 100 beats/minute
- P wave: Flutter waves
- PR interval: Unmeasurable
- QRS complex: 0.08 second
- T wave: Not discernible
- QT interval: Unmeasurable
- Other: None
- Interpretation: 2:1 atrial flutter

PRACTICE 4-53
- Rhythm: Regular
- Rate: 214 beats/minute
- P wave: Not discernible
- PR interval: Unmeasurable
- QRS complex: 0.08 second
- T wave: Not discernible
- QT interval: Unmeasurable
- Other: None
- Interpretation: Atrial tachycardia

PRACTICE 4-54
- Rhythm: Irregular
- Rate: 80 beats/minute
- P wave: Normal
- PR interval: 0.22 second
- QRS complex: 0.10 second
- T wave: Normal
- QT interval: 0.38 second
- Other: None
- Interpretation: First-degree AV block with bigeminal PACs

PRACTICE 4-55
- Rhythm: Irregular
- Rate: 110 beats/minute
- P wave: Fibrillatory waves
- PR interval: Unmeasurable
- QRS complex: 0.08 second
- T wave: Not discernible
- QT interval: Unmeasurable
- Other: None
- Interpretation: Uncontrolled atrial fibrillation

PRACTICE 4-56
- Rhythm: Irregular
- Rate: 90 beats/minute
- P wave: Flutter waves
- PR interval: Unmeasurable
- QRS complex: 0.08 second
- T wave: Not discernible
- QT interval: Unmeasurable
- Other: None
- Interpretation: Atrial flutter with variable block

PRACTICE 4-57
- Rhythm: Regular
- Rate: 167 beats/minute
- P wave: Not discernible
- PR interval: Unmeasurable
- QRS complex: 0.08 second
- T wave: Not discernible
- QT interval: Unmeasurable
- Other: None
- Interpretation: Atrial tachycardia

PRACTICE 4-58
- Rhythm: Irregular
- Rate: 110 beats/minute
- P wave: Not discernible
- PR interval: Unmeasurable
- QRS complex: 0.08 second
- T wave: Not discernible
- QT interval: Unmeasurable
- Other: None
- Interpretation: Uncontrolled atrial fibrillation

PRACTICE 4-59
- Rhythm: Irregular
- Rate: 40 beats/minute
- P wave: Flutter waves
- PR interval: Unmeasurable
- QRS complex: 0.12 second
- T wave: Not discernible
- QT interval: Unmeasurable
- Other: None
- Interpretation: Atrial flutter with variable block

PRACTICE 4-60
- Rhythm: Regular
- Rate: 188 beats/minute
- P wave: Normal
- PR interval: 0.12 second
- QRS complex: 0.06 second
- T wave: Normal
- QT interval: 0.20 second
- Other: None
- Interpretation: Atrial tachycardia

PRACTICE 4-61
- Rhythm: Irregular
- Rate: 80 beats/minute
- P wave: Not discernible
- PR interval: Unmeasurable
- QRS complex: 0.10 second
- T wave: Variable
- QT interval: Variable
- Other: None
- Interpretation: Controlled atrial fibrillation

PRACTICE 4-62
- Rhythm: Regular
- Rate: 150 beats/minute
- P wave: Peaked
- PR interval: 0.12 second
- QRS complex: 0.08 second
- T wave: Flattened
- QT interval: 0.24 second
- Other: None
- Interpretation: Atrial tachycardia

PRACTICE 4-63
- Rhythm: Irregular
- Rate: 80 beats/minute
- P wave: Normal
- PR interval: 0.20 second
- QRS complex: 0.08 second
- T wave: Normal
- QT interval: 0.36 second
- Other: None
- Interpretation: NSR with PACs

PRACTICE 4-64
- Rhythm: Irregular
- Rate: 80 beats/minute
- P wave: Not discernible
- PR interval: Unmeasurable
- QRS complex: 0.08 second
- T wave: Normal
- QT interval: 0.32 second
- Other: None
- Interpretation: Controlled atrial fibrillation

PRACTICE 4-65
- Rhythm: Irregular
- Rate: 90 beats/minute
- P wave: Variable
- PR interval: 0.20 second
- QRS complex: 0.08 second
- T wave: Normal
- QT interval: 0.36 second
- Other: None
- Interpretation: Wandering atrial pacemaker

PRACTICE 4-66
- Rhythm: Irregular
- Rate: 100 beats/minute
- P wave: Not discernible
- PR interval: Unmeasurable
- QRS complex: 0.08 second
- T wave: Flattened
- QT interval: Unmeasurable
- Other: None
- Interpretation: Uncontrolled atrial fibrillation

PRACTICE 4-67
- Rhythm: Irregular
- Rate: 120 beats/minute
- P wave: Flutter waves
- PR interval: Unmeasurable
- QRS complex: 0.04 second
- T wave: Not discernible
- QT interval: Unmeasurable
- Other: None
- Interpretation: Atrial flutter with variable block

PRACTICE 4-68
- Rhythm: Irregular
- Rate: 80 beats/minute
- P wave: Not discernible
- PR interval: Unmeasurable
- QRS complex: 0.12 second
- T wave: Normal
- QT interval: 0.40 second
- Other: None
- Interpretation: Controlled atrial fibrillation

PRACTICE 4-69
- Rhythm: Irregular
- Rate: 110 beats/minute
- P wave: Not discernible
- PR interval: Unmeasurable
- QRS complex: 0.08 second
- T wave: Normal
- QT interval: 0.32 second
- Other: None
- Interpretation: Uncontrolled atrial fibrillation

PRACTICE 4-70
- Rhythm: Irregular
- Rate: 80 beats/minute
- P wave: Some flutter waves
- PR interval: Unmeasurable
- QRS complex: 0.08 second
- T wave: Not discernible
- QT interval: Unmeasurable
- Other: None
- Interpretation: Atrial fibrillation/atrial flutter

PRACTICE 4-71
- Rhythm: Regular
- Rate: 65 beats/minute
- P wave: Flutter waves
- PR interval: Unmeasurable
- QRS complex: 0.16 second
- T wave: Not discernible
- QT interval: Unmeasurable
- Other: None
- Interpretation: 3:1 atrial flutter

PRACTICE 4-72
- Rhythm: Irregular
- Rate: 50 beats/minute
- P wave: Variable
- PR interval: 0.16 second in most complexes
- QRS complex: 0.08 second
- T wave: Normal
- QT interval: 0.42 second
- Other: None
- Interpretation: Wandering pacemaker

PRACTICE 4-73
- Rhythm: Irregular
- Rate: 80 beats/minute
- P wave: Flutter waves
- PR interval: Unmeasurable
- QRS complex: 0.08 second
- T wave: Not discernible
- QT interval: Unmeasurable
- Other: None
- Interpretation: Atrial flutter with variable block

PRACTICE 4-74
- Rhythm: Irregular
- Rate: 90 beats/minute
- P wave: Normal
- PR interval: 0.16 second
- QRS complex: 0.10 second
- T wave: Flattened
- QT interval: 0.40 second
- Other: Slight ST-segment depression
- Interpretation: NSR with PACs

PRACTICE 4-75
- Rhythm: Irregular
- Rate: 80 beats/minute
- P wave: Not discernible
- PR interval: Unmeasurable
- QRS complex: 0.10 second
- T wave: Inverted
- QT interval: 0.30 second
- Other: None
- Interpretation: Controlled atrial fibrillation

PRACTICE 4-76
- Rhythm: Regular
- Rate: 63 beats/minute
- P wave: Normal
- PR interval: 0.16 second
- QRS complex: 0.04 second
- T wave: Normal
- QT interval: 0.36 second
- Other: None
- Interpretation: NSR with one nonconducted PAC

PRACTICE 4-77
- Rhythm: Irregular
- Rate: 90 beats/minute
- P wave: Fibrillatory waves
- PR interval: Unmeasurable
- QRS complex: 0.08 second
- T wave: Not discernible
- QT interval: Unmeasurable
- Other: None
- Interpretation: Controlled atrial fibrillation

PRACTICE 4-78
- Rhythm: Irregular
- Rate: 90 beats/minute
- P wave: Normal
- PR interval: 0.16 second
- QRS complex: 0.08 second
- T wave: Inverted
- QT interval: 0.36 second
- Other: None
- Interpretation: NSR with PACs

PRACTICE 4-79
- Rhythm: Irregular
- Rate: 90 beats/minute
- P wave: Flutter waves
- PR interval: Unmeasurable
- QRS complex: 0.06 second
- T wave: Not discernible
- QT interval: Unmeasurable
- Other: None
- Interpretation: Atrial flutter with variable block

PRACTICE 4-80
- Rhythm: Regular
- Rate: 188 beats/minute
- P wave: Not discernible
- PR interval: Unmeasurable
- QRS complex: 0.10 second
- T wave: Inverted
- QT interval: 0.20 second
- Other: None
- Interpretation: Atrial tachycardia

PRACTICE 4-81
- Rhythm: Irregular
- Rate: 90 beats/minute
- P wave: Normal
- PR interval: 0.12 second
- QRS complex: 0.08 second
- T wave: Inverted
- QT interval: 0.36 second
- Other: None
- Interpretation: NSR with PACs

PRACTICE 4-82
- Rhythm: Slightly irregular
- Rate: 150 beats/minute
- P wave: Not discernible
- PR interval: Unmeasurable
- QRS complex: 0.08 second
- T wave: Not discernible
- QT interval: Unmeasurable
- Other: None
- Interpretation: Atrial tachycardia

PRACTICE 4-83
- Rhythm: Irregular
- Rate: 70 beats/minute
- P wave: Normal
- PR interval: 0.20 second
- QRS complex: 0.06 second
- T wave: Normal
- QT interval: 0.36 second
- Other: None
- Interpretation: NSR with PAC

PRACTICE 4-84
- Rhythm: Irregular
- Rate: 100 beats/minute
- P wave: Flutter waves
- PR interval: Unmeasurable
- QRS complex: 0.12 second
- T wave: Not discernible
- QT interval: Unmeasurable
- Other: None
- Interpretation: Atrial flutter with variable block

PRACTICE 4-85
- Rhythm: Irregular
- Rate: 70 beats/minute
- P wave: Fibrillatory waves
- PR interval: Unmeasurable
- QRS complex: 0.08 second
- T wave: Not discernible
- QT interval: Unmeasurable
- Other: None
- Interpretation: Controlled atrial fibrillation

PRACTICE 4-86
- Rhythm: Regular
- Rate: 94 beats/minute
- P wave: Flutter waves
- PR interval: Unmeasurable
- QRS complex: 0.08 second
- T wave: Not discernible
- QT interval: Unmeasurable
- Other: None
- Interpretation: 3:1 atrial flutter

PRACTICE 4-87
- Rhythm: Irregular
- Rate: 120 beats/minute
- P wave: Normal when NSR
- PR interval: 0.16 second
- QRS complex: 0.06 second
- T wave: Normal
- QT interval: 0.32 second
- Other: None
- Interpretation: Atrial tachycardia converting to NSR

PRACTICE 4-88
- Rhythm: Irregular
- Rate: 70 beats/minute
- P wave: Flutter waves
- PR interval: Unmeasurable
- QRS complex: 0.08 second
- T wave: Not discernible
- QT interval: Unmeasurable
- Other: None
- Interpretation: Atrial flutter with variable block

PRACTICE 4-89
- Rhythm: Regular
- Rate: 150 beats/minute
- P wave: Mostly normal
- PR interval: 0.10 second
- QRS complex: 0.08 second
- T wave: Normal
- QT interval: 0.16 second
- Other: None
- Interpretation: Atrial tachycardia

PRACTICE 4-90
- Rhythm: Irregular
- Rate: 90 beats/minute
- P wave: Fibrillatory and flutter waves
- PR interval: Unmeasurable
- QRS complex: 0.10 second
- T wave: Not discernible
- QT interval: Unmeasurable
- Other: None
- Interpretation: Atrial fibrillation/atrial flutter

PRACTICE 4-91
- Rhythm: Regular
- Rate: 83 beats/minute
- P wave: Variable
- PR interval: 0.18 second
- QRS complex: 0.08 second
- T wave: Normal
- QT interval: 0.36 second
- Other: ST-segment depression
- Interpretation: Wandering atrial pacemaker

PRACTICE 4-92
- Rhythm: Irregular
- Rate: 100 beats/minute
- P wave: Normal
- PR interval: 0.16 second
- QRS complex: 0.12 second
- T wave: Flattened
- QT interval: 0.36 second
- Other: None
- Interpretation: NSR with PAC couplets

PRACTICE 4-93
- Rhythm: Regular
- Rate: 250 beats/minute
- P wave: Not discernible
- PR interval: Unmeasurable
- QRS complex: 0.06 second
- T wave: Not discernible
- QT interval: Unmeasurable
- Other: None
- Interpretation: Atrial tachycardia

PRACTICE 4-94
- Rhythm: Irregular
- Rate: 60 beats/minute
- P wave: Flutter waves
- PR interval: Unmeasurable
- QRS complex: 0.12 second
- T wave: Not discernible
- QT interval: Unmeasurable
- Other: None
- Interpretation: Atrial flutter with variable block

PRACTICE 4-95
- Rhythm: Irregular
- Rate: 140 beats/minute
- P wave: Occasionally normal
- PR interval: 0.20 second
- QRS complex: 0.10 second
- T wave: Variable
- QT interval: Variable
- Other: None
- Interpretation: NSR with run of atrial tachycardia

PRACTICE 4-96
- Rhythm: Irregular
- Rate: 80 beats/minute
- P wave: Fibrillatory waves
- PR interval: Unmeasurable
- QRS complex: 0.12 second
- T wave: Normal
- QT interval: 0.36 second
- Other: None
- Interpretation: Controlled atrial fibrillation

PRACTICE 4-97
- Rhythm: Regular
- Rate: 88 beats/minute
- P wave: Flutter waves
- PR interval: Unmeasurable
- QRS complex: 0.08 second
- T wave: Not discernible
- QT interval: Unmeasurable
- Other: None
- Interpretation: 4:1 atrial flutter

PRACTICE 4-98
- Rhythm: Irregular
- Rate: 120 beats/minute
- P wave: Fibrillatory waves
- PR interval: Unmeasurable
- QRS complex: 0.08 second
- T wave: Not discernible
- QT interval: Unmeasurable
- Other: None
- Interpretation: Uncontrolled atrial fibrillation

PRACTICE 4-99
- Rhythm: Regular
- Rate: 250 beats/minute
- P wave: Normal
- PR interval: 0.08 second
- QRS complex: 0.08 second
- T wave: Inverted
- QT interval: 0.16 second
- Other: None
- Interpretation: Atrial tachycardia

PRACTICE 4-100
- Rhythm: Irregular
- Rate: 120 beats/minute
- P wave: Not discernible
- PR interval: Unmeasurable
- QRS complex: 0.12 second
- T wave: Not discernible
- QT interval: Unmeasurable
- Other: None
- Interpretation: Uncontrolled atrial fibrillation

PRACTICE 4-101
- Rhythm: Regular
- Rate: 58 beats/minute
- P wave: Flutter waves
- PR interval: Unmeasurable
- QRS complex: 0.08 second
- T wave: Not discernible
- QT interval: Unmeasurable
- Other: None
- Interpretation: 4:1 atrial flutter

PRACTICE 4-102
- Rhythm: Irregular
- Rate: 130 beats/minute
- P wave: Not discernible
- PR interval: Unmeasurable
- QRS complex: 0.10 second
- T wave: Variable
- QT interval: Unmeasurable
- Other: None
- Interpretation: Uncontrolled atrial fibrillation

PRACTICE 4-103
- Rhythm: Irregular
- Rate: 160 beats/minute
- P wave: Not discernible
- PR interval: Unmeasurable
- QRS complex: 0.12 second
- T wave: Normal
- QT interval: 0.28 second
- Other: None
- Interpretation: Atrial tachycardia

PRACTICE 4-104
- Rhythm: Irregular
- Rate: 120 beats/minute
- P wave: Fibrillatory waves
- PR interval: Unmeasurable
- QRS complex: 0.08 second
- T wave: Not discernible
- QT interval: Unmeasurable
- Other: None
- Interpretation: Uncontrolled atrial fibrillation

PRACTICE 4-105
- Rhythm: Regular
- Rate: 320 beats/minute
- P wave: Not discernible
- PR interval: Unmeasurable
- QRS complex: 0.04 second
- T wave: Not discernible
- QT interval: Unmeasurable
- Other: None
- Interpretation: Atrial tachycardia

PRACTICE 4-106
- Rhythm: Irregular
- Rate: 90 beats/minute
- P wave: Normal in every other complex
- PR interval: 0.16 second
- QRS complex: 0.08 second
- T wave: Normal
- QT interval: 0.34 second
- Other: None
- Interpretation: NSR with bigeminal PACs

PRACTICE 4-107
- Rhythm: Regular
- Rate: 94 beats/minute
- P wave: Flutter waves
- PR interval: Unmeasurable
- QRS complex: 0.08 second
- T wave: Not discernible
- QT interval: Unmeasurable
- Other: None
- Interpretation: 4:1 atrial flutter

PRACTICE 4-108
- Rhythm: Regular
- Rate: 188 beats/minute
- P wave: Normal
- PR interval: 0.12 second
- QRS complex: 0.08 second
- T wave: Normal
- QT interval: 0.20 second
- Other: None
- Interpretation: Atrial tachycardia

PRACTICE 4-109
- Rhythm: Irregular
- Rate: 80 beats/minute
- P wave: Normal in most complexes
- PR interval: 0.16 second
- QRS complex: 0.10 second
- T wave: Normal
- QT interval: 0.32 second
- Other: None
- Interpretation: NSR with PAC and PVCs

PRACTICE 4-110
- Rhythm: Irregular
- Rate: 60 beats/minute
- P wave: Some flutter waves
- PR interval: Unmeasurable
- QRS complex: 0.14 second
- T wave: Normal
- QT interval: 0.44 second
- Other: None
- Interpretation: Atrial fibrillation/atrial flutter

PRACTICE 4-111
- Rhythm: Irregular
- Rate: 100 beats/minute
- P wave: Normal
- PR interval: 0.12 second
- QRS complex: 0.08 second
- T wave: Normal
- QT interval: 0.30 second
- Other: None
- Interpretation: NSR with PACs

PRACTICE 4-112
- Rhythm: Irregular
- Rate: 130 beats/minute
- P wave: Not discernible
- PR interval: Unmeasurable
- QRS complex: 0.12 second
- T wave: Not discernible
- QT interval: Unmeasurable
- Other: None
- Interpretation: Uncontrolled atrial fibrillation

PRACTICE 4-113
- Rhythm: Irregular
- Rate: 120 beats/minute
- P wave: Normal
- PR interval: 0.12 second
- QRS complex: 0.08 second
- T wave: Flattened
- QT interval: Unmeasurable
- Other: None
- Interpretation: Sinus tachycardia with PACs

PRACTICE 4-114
- Rhythm: Irregular
- Rate: 70 beats/minute
- P wave: Flutter waves
- PR interval: Unmeasurable
- QRS complex: 0.08 second
- T wave: Not discernible
- QT interval: Unmeasurable
- Other: None
- Interpretation: Atrial flutter with variable block

PRACTICE 4-115
- Rhythm: Irregular
- Rate: 110 beats/minute
- P wave: Normal
- PR interval: 0.12 second
- QRS complex: 0.08 second
- T wave: Inverted
- QT interval: 0.20 second
- Other: Artifact present
- Interpretation: Sinus tachycardia with PACs

PRACTICE 4-116
- Rhythm: Irregular
- Rate: 170 beats/minute
- P wave: Not discernible
- PR interval: Unmeasurable
- QRS complex: 0.06 second
- T wave: Not discernible
- QT interval: Unmeasurable
- Other: None
- Interpretation: Uncontrolled atrial fibrillation

PRACTICE 4-117
- Rhythm: Irregular
- Rate: 150 beats/minute
- P wave: Not discernible
- PR interval: Unmeasurable
- QRS complex: 0.08 second
- T wave: Not discernible
- QT interval: Unmeasurable
- Other: None
- Interpretation: Uncontrolled atrial fibrillation

PRACTICE 4-118
- Rhythm: Irregular
- Rate: 220 beats/minute
- P wave: Not discernible
- PR interval: Unmeasurable
- QRS complex: 0.04 second
- T wave: Not discernible
- QT interval: Unmeasurable
- Other: None
- Interpretation: Uncontrolled atrial fibrillation

PRACTICE 4-119
- Rhythm: Irregular
- Rate: 100 beats/minute
- P wave: Normal
- PR interval: 0.12 second
- QRS complex: 0.08 second
- T wave: Normal
- QT interval: 0.28 second
- Other: None
- Interpretation: NSR with trigeminal PACs

PRACTICE 4-120
- Rhythm: Irregular
- Rate: 70 beats/minute
- P wave: Not discernible
- PR interval: Unmeasurable
- QRS complex: 0.06 second
- T wave: Not discernible
- QT interval: Unmeasurable
- Other: None
- Interpretation: Controlled atrial fibrillation

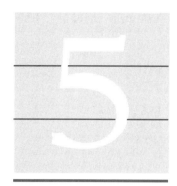

Junctional arrhythmias

Junctional arrhythmias originate in the atrioventricular (AV) junction—the area in and around the AV node and the bundle of His. The specialized pacemaker cells in the AV junction take over as the heart's pacemaker if the sinoatrial (SA) node fails to function properly or if the electrical impulses originating in the SA node are blocked. These junctional pacemaker cells have an inherent firing rate of 40 to 60 beats/minute.

In normal impulse conduction, the AV node slows transmission of the impulse from the atria to the ventricles, which allows the ventricles to fill as much as possible before they contract. However, these impulses don't always follow the normal conduction pathway.

Because of the location of the AV junction within the conduction pathway, electrical impulses originating in this area cause abnormal depolarization of the heart. The impulse is conducted in a retrograde (backward) fashion to depolarize the atria and antegrade (forward) to depolarize the ventricles.

Depolarization of the atria can precede depolarization of the ventricles, or the ventricles can be depolarized before the atria. Depolarization of the atria and ventricles can also occur simultaneously. (See *Locating the P wave.*)

Retrograde depolarization of the atria results in inverted P waves in leads II, III, and aV$_F$, leads in which you would normally see upright P waves appear.

Keep in mind that arrhythmias causing inverted P waves on an electrocardiogram may originate in the atria or AV junction. Atrial arrhythmias are sometimes mistaken for junctional arrhythmias because impulses

Junctional arrhythmias

In junctional arrhythmias, impulses originate in the atrioventricular (AV) junction, the area in and around the AV node and bundle of His.

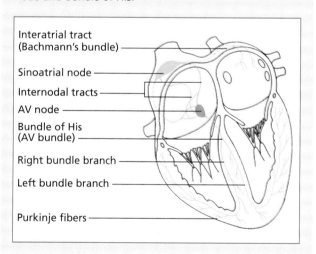

- Interatrial tract (Bachmann's bundle)
- Sinoatrial node
- Internodal tracts
- AV node
- Bundle of His (AV bundle)
- Right bundle branch
- Left bundle branch
- Purkinje fibers

are generated so low in the atria that they cause retrograde depolarization and inverted P waves. Looking at the PR interval will help you determine whether an arrhythmia is atrial or junctional.

134

Locating the P wave

When the specialized pacemaker cells in the atrioventricular junction take over as the dominant pacemaker of the heart:
■ depolarization of the atria can precede depolarization of the ventricles
■ the ventricles can be depolarized before the atria
■ simultaneous depolarization of the atria and ventricles can occur.
 The rhythm strips shown here demonstrate the various locations of the P waves in junctional arrhythmias, depending on the direction of depolarization.

Inverted P wave
If the atria depolarize first, the P wave will occur before the QRS complex.

Retrograde P wave
If the ventricles depolarize first, the P wave will occur after the QRS complex.

Inverted P wave (hidden)
If the ventricles and atria depolarize simultaneously, the P wave will be hidden in the QRS complex.

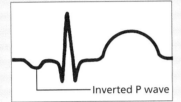

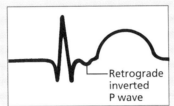

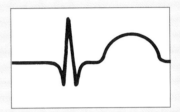

 An arrhythmia with an inverted P wave before the QRS complex and with a normal PR interval (0.12 to 0.20 second) originates in the atria. An arrhythmia with a PR interval less than 0.12 second originates in the AV junction.

Premature junctional contractions

A premature junctional contraction (PJC) is a junctional beat that occurs before a normal sinus beat, interrupting the underlying rhythm and causing an irregular rhythm. These ectopic beats commonly occur as a result of enhanced automaticity in the junctional tissue or bundle of His. As with all impulses generated in the AV junction, the atria are depolarized in a retrograde fashion, causing an inverted P wave. The ventricles are depolarized normally. (See *Identifying premature junctional contractions.*)

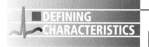

Identifying premature junctional contractions

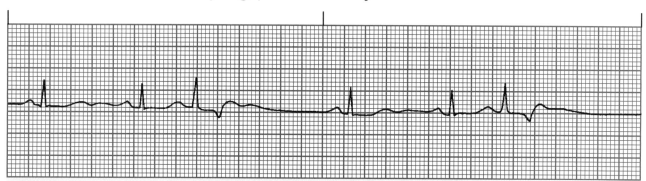

Rhythm

- Atrial: Irregular during PJCs
- Ventricular: Irregular during PJCs
- Underlying rhythm possibly regular

Rate

- Atrial: Reflects underlying rhythm
- Ventricular: Reflects underlying rhythm

P wave

- Usually inverted (leads II, III, and aV$_F$)
- May occur before, during, or after QRS complex, depending on initial direction of depolarization
- May be hidden in QRS complex

PR interval

- Shortened (less than 0.12 second) if P wave precedes QRS complex
- Unmeasurable if P wave doesn't precede QRS complex

QRS complex

- Usually normal configuration and duration because ventricles usually depolarize normally

T wave

- Usually normal configuration

QT interval

- Usually within normal limits

Other

- Commonly accompanied by a compensatory pause reflecting retrograde atrial conduction

PRACTICE

Premature junctional contractions

Use the 8-step method to interpret the following rhythm strip. Place your answers on the blank lines. See the answer key below.

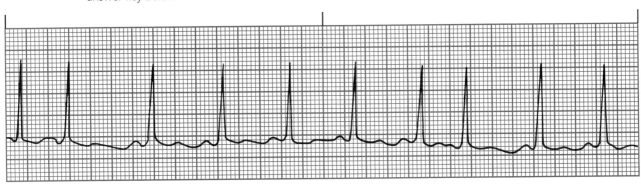

Rhythm: _____

Rate: _____

P wave: _____

PR interval: _____

QRS complex: _____

T wave: _____

QT interval: _____

Other: _____

■ **ANSWER KEY**

Rhythm: Irregular atrial and ventricular rhythms during PJCs

Rate: 100 beats/minute

P wave: Inverted and precedes the QRS complex

PR interval: 0.14 second for the underlying rhythm and 0.06 second for the PJC

QRS complex: 0.06 second

T wave: Normal configuration

QT interval: 0.36 second

Other: Compensatory pause after PJCs

Junctional escape rhythm

Junctional escape rhythm, also referred to as *junctional rhythm*, is an arrhythmia originating in the AV junction. In this arrhythmia, the AV junction takes over as a secondary, or "escape," pacemaker. This usually occurs only when a higher pacemaker site in the atria, usually the SA node, fails as the heart's dominant pacemaker. Remember that the AV junction can take over as the heart's dominant pacemaker if the firing rate of the higher pacemaker sites falls below the AV junction's intrinsic firing rate, if the pacemaker fails to generate an impulse, or if the conduction of the impulses is blocked.

In junctional escape rhythm, as in all junctional arrhythmias, the atria depolarize by means of retrograde conduction. The P waves are inverted, and impulse conduction through the ventricles is normal. The normal intrinsic firing rate for cells in the AV junction is 40 to 60 beats/minute. (See *Identifying junctional escape rhythm.*)

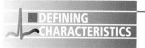
DEFINING CHARACTERISTICS

Identifying junctional escape rhythm

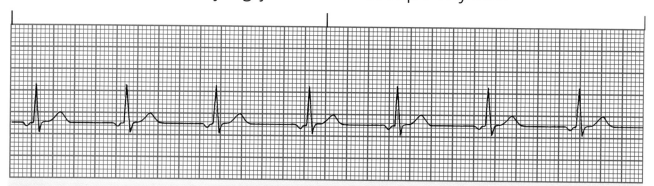

Rhythm

- Atrial: Regular
- Ventricular: Regular

Rate

- Atrial: 40 to 60 beats/minute
- Ventricular: 40 to 60 beats/minute

P wave

- Usually inverted (leads II, III, and aV$_F$)
- May occur before, during, or after QRS complex
- May be hidden in QRS complex

PR interval

- Shortened (less than 0.12 second) if P wave precedes QRS complex
- Unmeasurable if no P wave precedes QRS complex

QRS complex

- Duration: Usually within normal limits
- Configuration: Usually normal

T wave

- Configuration: Usually normal

QT interval

- Usually within normal limits

Other

- Important to differentiate junctional rhythm from idioventricular rhythm (a life-threatening arrhythmia)

PRACTICE Junctional escape rhythm

Use the 8-step method to interpret the following rhythm strip. Place your answers on the blank lines. See the answer key below.

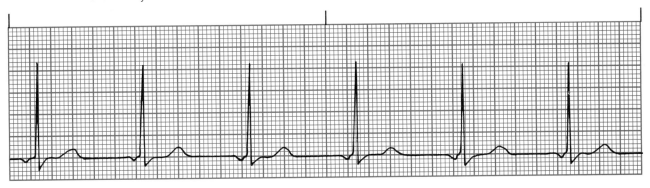

Rhythm: _____

Rate: _____

P wave: _____

PR interval: _____

QRS complex: _____

T wave: _____

QT interval: _____

Other: _____

■ **ANSWER KEY**

Rhythm: **Regular**

Rate: **60 beats/minute**

P wave: **Inverted and preceding each QRS complex**

PR interval: **0.10 second**

QRS complex: **0.10 second**

T wave: **Normal**

QT interval: **0.44 second**

Other: **None**

Accelerated junctional rhythm

An accelerated junctional rhythm is an arrhythmia that originates in the AV junction and is usually caused by enhanced automaticity of the AV junctional tissue. It's called *accelerated* because it occurs at a rate of 60 to 100 beats/minute, exceeding the inherent junctional escape rate of 40 to 60 beats/minute. Because the rate is below 100 beats/minute, the arrhythmia isn't classified as junctional tachycardia. The atria depolarize by means of retrograde conduction, and the ventricles depolarize normally.

The AV nodal escape rhythm in infants and toddlers younger than age 3 is 50 to 80 beats/minute. Consequently, for them, a junctional rhythm is considered accelerated only when greater than 80 beats/minute. (See *Identifying accelerated junctional rhythm.*)

Accelerated junctional rhythm can sometimes be difficult to distinguish from accelerated idioventricular rhythm.

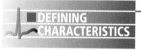

Identifying accelerated junctional rhythm

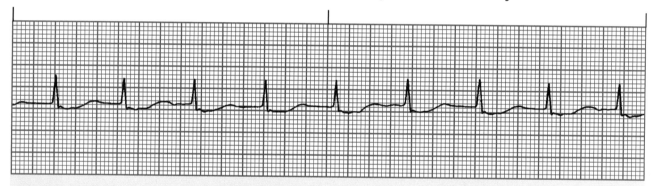

Rhythm

- Atrial: Regular
- Ventricular: Regular

Rate

- Atrial: 60 to 100 beats/minute
- Ventricular: 60 to 100 beats/minute

P wave

- If present, inverted in leads II, III, and aV$_F$
- May occur before, during, or after QRS complex
- May be hidden in QRS complex

PR interval

- Shortened (less than 0.12 second) if P wave precedes QRS complex
- Unmeasurable if no P wave precedes QRS complex

QRS complex

- Duration: Usually within normal limits
- Configuration: Usually normal

T wave

- Usually within normal limits

QT interval

- Usually within normal limits

Other

- Important to differentiate accelerated junctional rhythm from accelerated idioventricular rhythm (a possibly life-threatening arrhythmia)

Accelerated junctional rhythm

Use the 8-step method to interpret the following rhythm strip. Place your answers on the blank lines. See the answer key below.

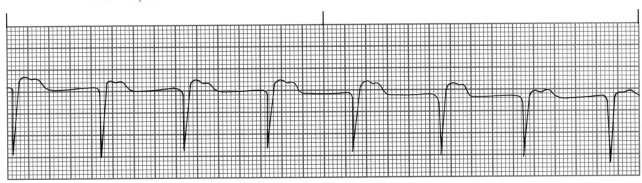

Rhythm: _____

Rate: _____

P wave: _____

PR interval: _____

QRS complex: _____

T wave: _____

QT interval: _____

Other: _____

Junctional tachycardia

In junctional tachycardia, three or more PJCs occur in a row. This supraventricular tachycardia (SVT) generally occurs as a result of enhanced automaticity of the AV junction, which causes the AV junction to override the SA node as the dominant pacemaker.

In junctional tachycardia, the atria depolarize by retrograde conduction. Conduction through the ventricles is normal. If this rhythm starts and stops suddenly, it is referred to as *paroxysmal*. If this rhythm is sustained, it is called *nonparoxysmal*. (See *Identifying junctional tachycardia*.)

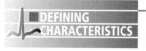

Identifying junctional tachycardia

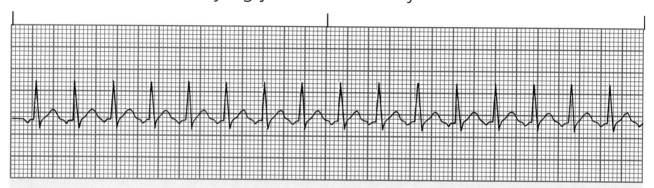

Rhythm

- Atrial: Usually regular but may be difficult to determine if P wave is hidden in QRS complex or precedes T wave
- Ventricular: Usually regular

Rate

- Atrial: Exceeds 100 beats/minute (usually 100 to 200 beats/minute) but may be difficult to determine if P wave is hidden in QRS complex
- Ventricular: Exceeds 100 beats/minute (usually 100 to 200 beats/minute)

P wave

- Usually inverted in leads II, III, and aV$_F$
- May occur before, during, or after QRS complex
- May be hidden in QRS complex

PR interval

- Shortened (less than 0.12 second) if P wave precedes QRS complex
- Unmeasurable if no P wave precedes QRS complex

QRS complex

- Duration: Within normal limits
- Configuration: Usually normal

T wave

- Configuration: Usually normal
- May be abnormal if P wave is hidden in T wave
- May be indiscernible because of fast rate

QT interval

- Usually within normal limits

Other

- May have gradual onset

Junctional tachycardia

Use the 8-step method to interpret the following rhythm strip. Place your answers on the blank lines. See the answer key below.

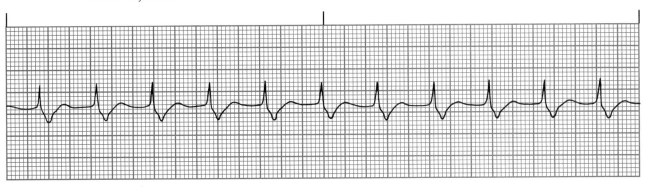

Rhythm: _____

Rate: _____

P wave: _____

PR interval: _____

QRS complex: _____

T wave: _____

QT interval: _____

Other: _____

■ **ANSWER KEY**

Rhythm: **Atrial and ventricular—regular**

Rate: **Atrial and ventricular—115 beats/minute**

P wave: **Inverted; follows QRS complex**

PR interval: **Unmeasurable**

QRS complex: **0.08 second**

T wave: **Normal**

QT interval: **0.36 second**

Other: **None**

AV nodal reentry tachycardia

AV nodal reentry tachycardia is the most common type of narrow complex tachycardia and results from a reentry mechanism. A reentry circuit is set up in the AV node with two pathways: a slow pathway with a shorter refractory period and a fast pathway with a longer refractory period. The rhythm starts and stops suddenly and is usually initiated by a premature atrial contraction (PAC). The PAC finds the fast pathway refractory and is conducted down the slow pathway. There, it travels simultaneously into the ventricles and up the fast pathway to the atria. It establishes a reentry circuit, which causes repeated simultaneous stimulation of the atria and ventricles.

AV nodal reentry tachycardia commonly occurs in young adults without heart disease. It may occur in patients with preexisting heart disease and, if the rate exceeds 200 beats/minute, may cause a decrease in cardiac output. (See *Identifying AV nodal reentry tachycardia*.)

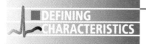

Identifying AV nodal reentry tachycardia

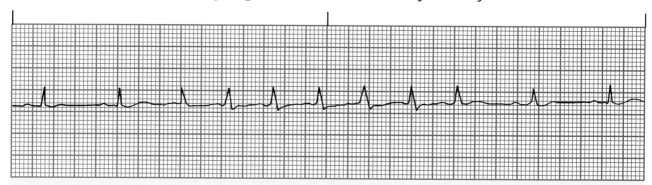

Rhythm
- Atrial: Regular
- Ventricular: Regular

Rate
- Atrial: Can't be determined
- Ventricular: 150 to 250 beats/minute

P wave
- Can't always be identified

PR interval
- Unmeasurable if P wave doesn't precede QRS complex

QRS complex
- Duration: Usually normal
- Configuration: Usually normal

T wave
- Configuration: Usually normal

QT interval
- Usually within normal limits

Other
- May start with a PAC

AV nodal reentry tachycardia

Use the 8-step method to interpret the following rhythm strip. Place your answers on the blank lines. See the answer key below.

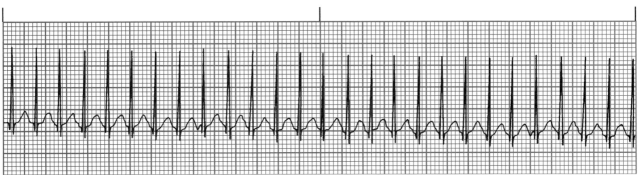

Rhythm: _____

Rate: _____

P wave: _____

PR interval: _____

QRS complex: _____

T wave: _____

QT interval: _____

Other: _____

■ **ANSWER KEY**

Rhythm: **Regular**

Rate: **275 beats/minute**

P wave: **Can't be identified**

PR interval: **Unmeasurable**

QRS complex: **Normal configuration and duration**

T wave: **Normal configuration**

QT interval: **Within normal limits**

Other: **None**

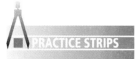

PRACTICE STRIPS

■ PRACTICE 5-1

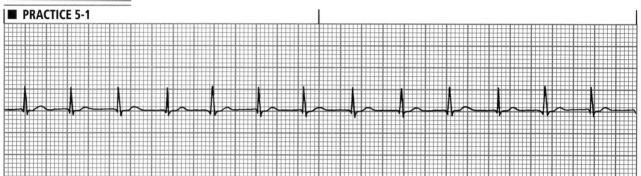

Rhythm: _____   PR interval: _____   QT interval: _____

Rate: _____   QRS complex: _____   Other: _____

P wave: _____   T wave: _____   Interpretation: _____

■ PRACTICE 5-2

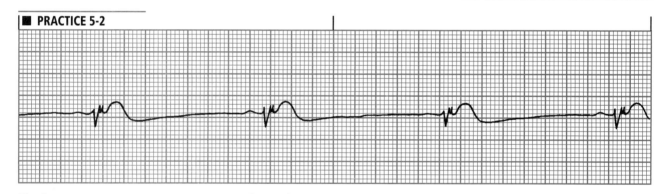

Rhythm: _____   PR interval: _____   QT interval: _____

Rate: _____   QRS complex: _____   Other: _____

P wave: _____   T wave: _____   Interpretation: _____

■ PRACTICE 5-3

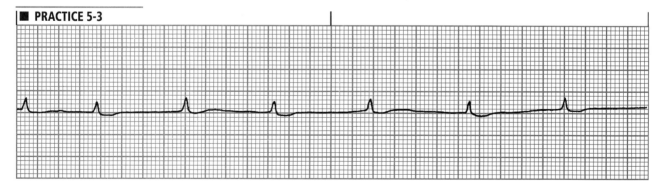

Rhythm: _____   PR interval: _____   QT interval: _____

Rate: _____   QRS complex: _____   Other: _____

P wave: _____   T wave: _____   Interpretation: _____

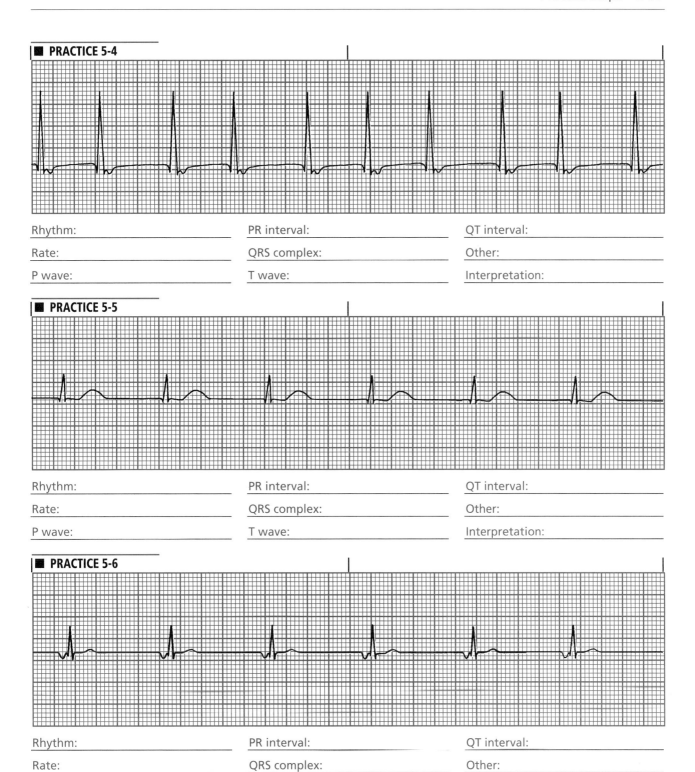

■ PRACTICE 5-4

Rhythm:	PR interval:	QT interval:
Rate:	QRS complex:	Other:
P wave:	T wave:	Interpretation:

■ PRACTICE 5-5

Rhythm:	PR interval:	QT interval:
Rate:	QRS complex:	Other:
P wave:	T wave:	Interpretation:

■ PRACTICE 5-6

Rhythm:	PR interval:	QT interval:
Rate:	QRS complex:	Other:
P wave:	T wave:	Interpretation:

■ **PRACTICE 5-7**

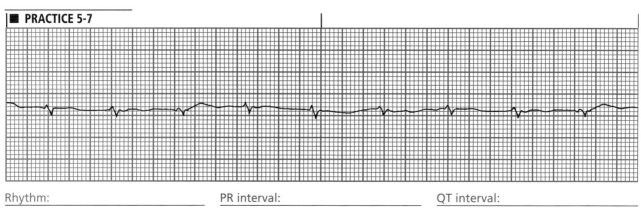

Rhythm: _____

Rate: _____

P wave: _____

PR interval: _____

QRS complex: _____

T wave: _____

QT interval: _____

Other: _____

Interpretation: _____

■ **PRACTICE 5-8**

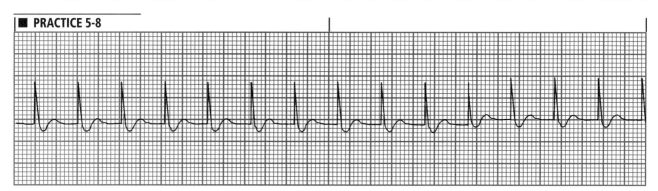

Rhythm: _____

Rate: _____

P wave: _____

PR interval: _____

QRS complex: _____

T wave: _____

QT interval: _____

Other: _____

Interpretation: _____

■ **PRACTICE 5-9**

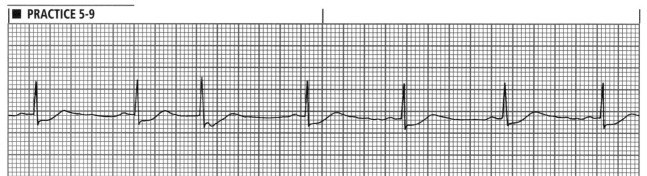

Rhythm: _____

Rate: _____

P wave: _____

PR interval: _____

QRS complex: _____

T wave: _____

QT interval: _____

Other: _____

Interpretation: _____

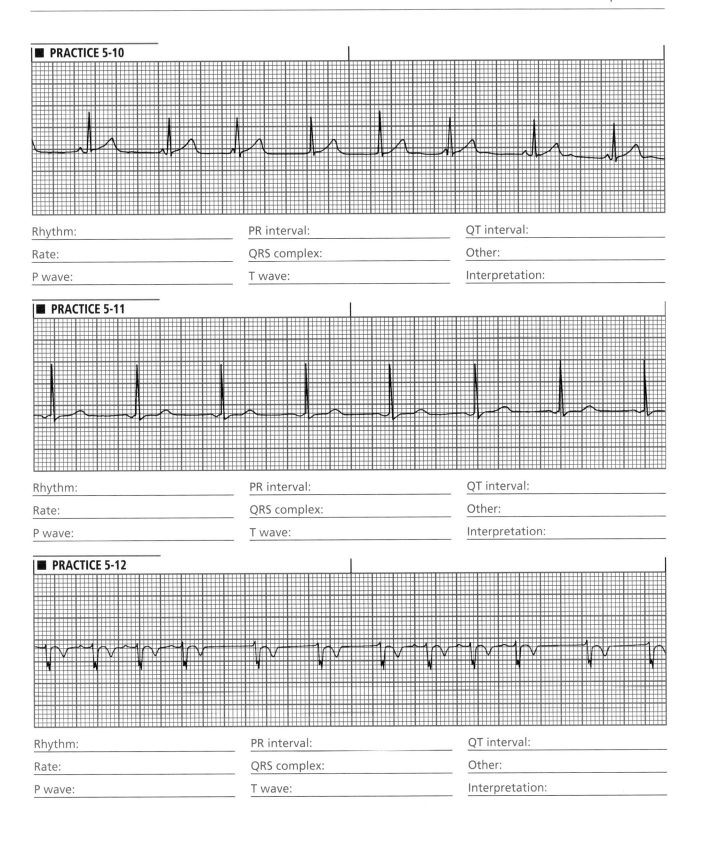

■ PRACTICE 5-10

Rhythm: _____

Rate: _____

P wave: _____

PR interval: _____

QRS complex: _____

T wave: _____

QT interval: _____

Other: _____

Interpretation: _____

■ PRACTICE 5-11

Rhythm: _____

Rate: _____

P wave: _____

PR interval: _____

QRS complex: _____

T wave: _____

QT interval: _____

Other: _____

Interpretation: _____

■ PRACTICE 5-12

Rhythm: _____

Rate: _____

P wave: _____

PR interval: _____

QRS complex: _____

T wave: _____

QT interval: _____

Other: _____

Interpretation: _____

■ **PRACTICE 5-13**

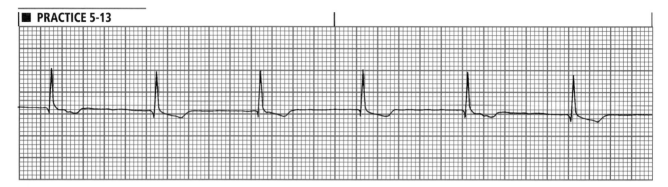

Rhythm: _____   PR interval: _____   QT interval: _____

Rate: _____   QRS complex: _____   Other: _____

P wave: _____   T wave: _____   Interpretation: _____

■ **PRACTICE 5-14**

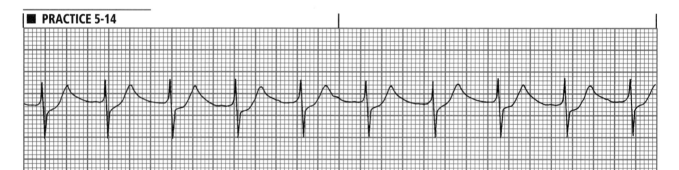

Rhythm: _____   PR interval: _____   QT interval: _____

Rate: _____   QRS complex: _____   Other: _____

P wave: _____   T wave: _____   Interpretation: _____

■ **PRACTICE 5-15**

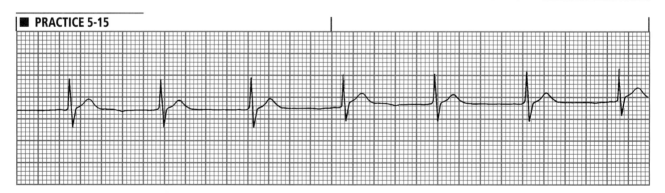

Rhythm: _____   PR interval: _____   QT interval: _____

Rate: _____   QRS complex: _____   Other: _____

P wave: _____   T wave: _____   Interpretation: _____

■ PRACTICE 5-16

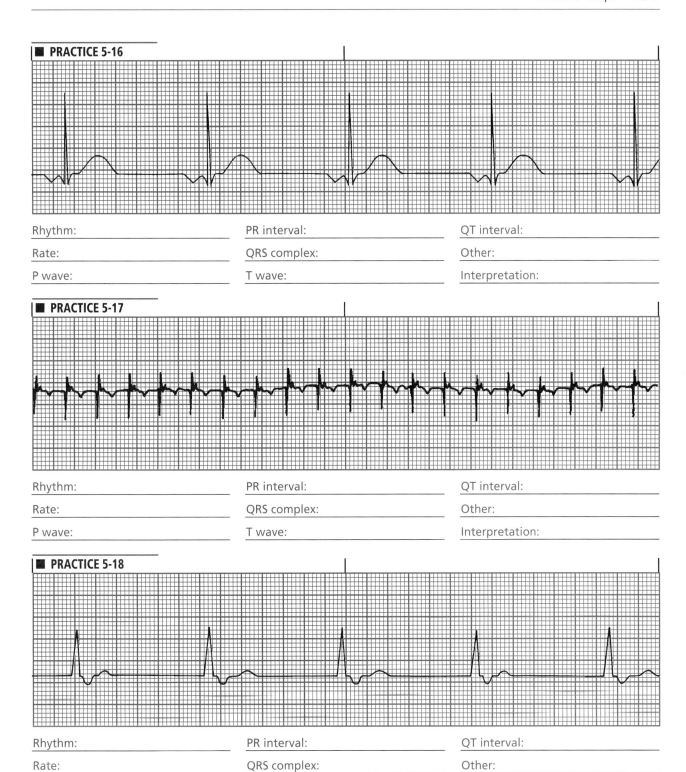

Rhythm: _____   PR interval: _____   QT interval: _____

Rate: _____   QRS complex: _____   Other: _____

P wave: _____   T wave: _____   Interpretation: _____

■ PRACTICE 5-17

Rhythm: _____   PR interval: _____   QT interval: _____

Rate: _____   QRS complex: _____   Other: _____

P wave: _____   T wave: _____   Interpretation: _____

■ PRACTICE 5-18

Rhythm: _____   PR interval: _____   QT interval: _____

Rate: _____   QRS complex: _____   Other: _____

P wave: _____   T wave: _____   Interpretation: _____

■ **PRACTICE 5-19**

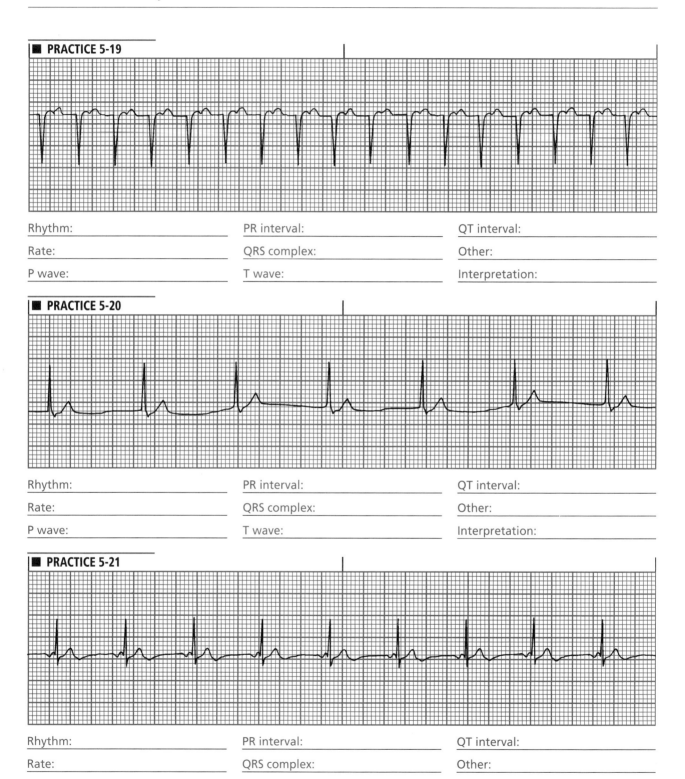

Rhythm: _____

Rate: _____

P wave: _____

PR interval: _____

QRS complex: _____

T wave: _____

QT interval: _____

Other: _____

Interpretation: _____

■ **PRACTICE 5-20**

Rhythm: _____

Rate: _____

P wave: _____

PR interval: _____

QRS complex: _____

T wave: _____

QT interval: _____

Other: _____

Interpretation: _____

■ **PRACTICE 5-21**

Rhythm: _____

Rate: _____

P wave: _____

PR interval: _____

QRS complex: _____

T wave: _____

QT interval: _____

Other: _____

Interpretation: _____

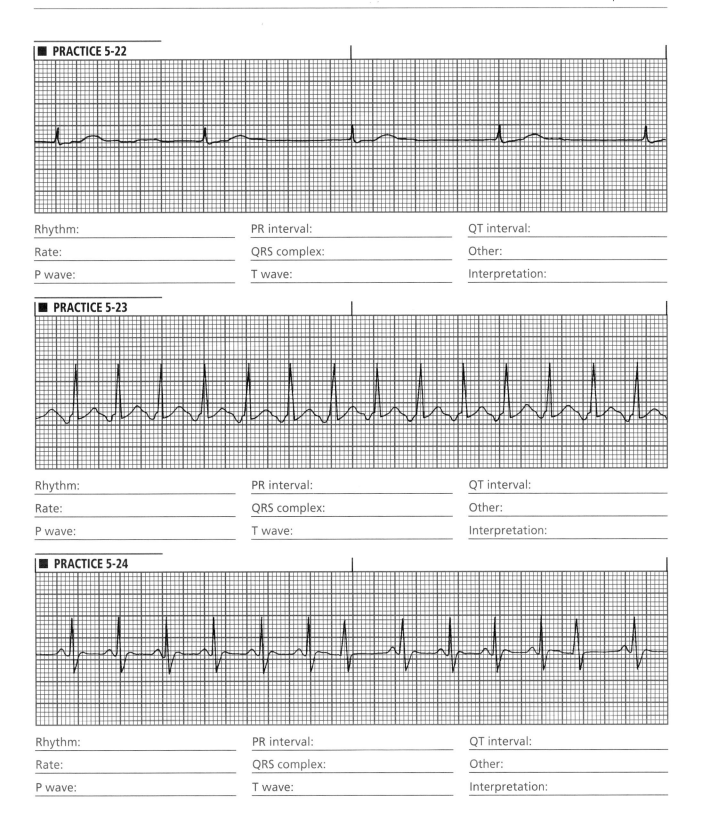

■ **PRACTICE 5-22**

Rhythm: _____   PR interval: _____   QT interval: _____

Rate: _____   QRS complex: _____   Other: _____

P wave: _____   T wave: _____   Interpretation: _____

■ **PRACTICE 5-23**

Rhythm: _____   PR interval: _____   QT interval: _____

Rate: _____   QRS complex: _____   Other: _____

P wave: _____   T wave: _____   Interpretation: _____

■ **PRACTICE 5-24**

Rhythm: _____   PR interval: _____   QT interval: _____

Rate: _____   QRS complex: _____   Other: _____

P wave: _____   T wave: _____   Interpretation: _____

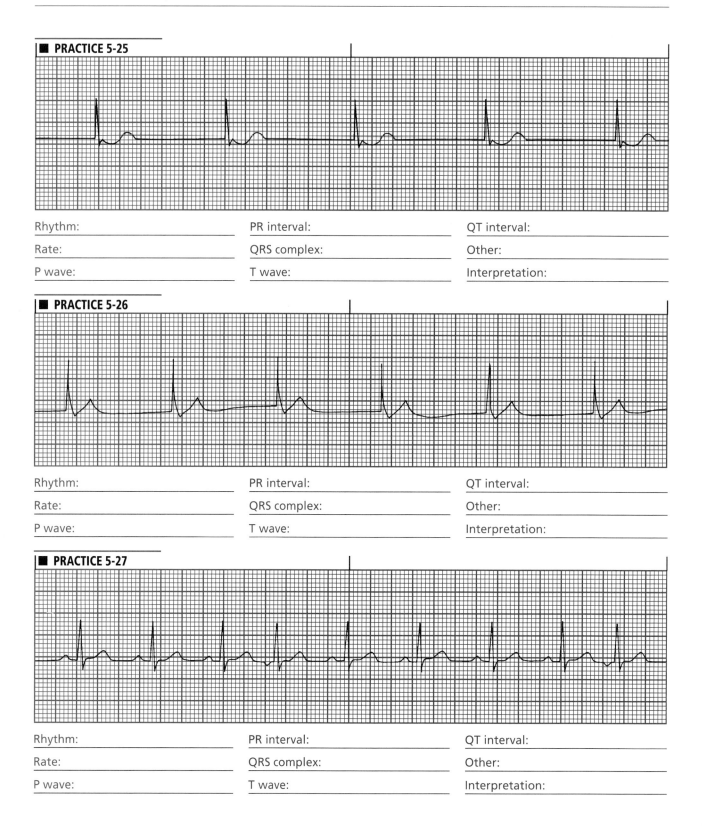

■ **PRACTICE 5-25**

Rhythm:	PR interval:	QT interval:
Rate:	QRS complex:	Other:
P wave:	T wave:	Interpretation:

■ **PRACTICE 5-26**

Rhythm:	PR interval:	QT interval:
Rate:	QRS complex:	Other:
P wave:	T wave:	Interpretation:

■ **PRACTICE 5-27**

Rhythm:	PR interval:	QT interval:
Rate:	QRS complex:	Other:
P wave:	T wave:	Interpretation:

■ PRACTICE 5-28

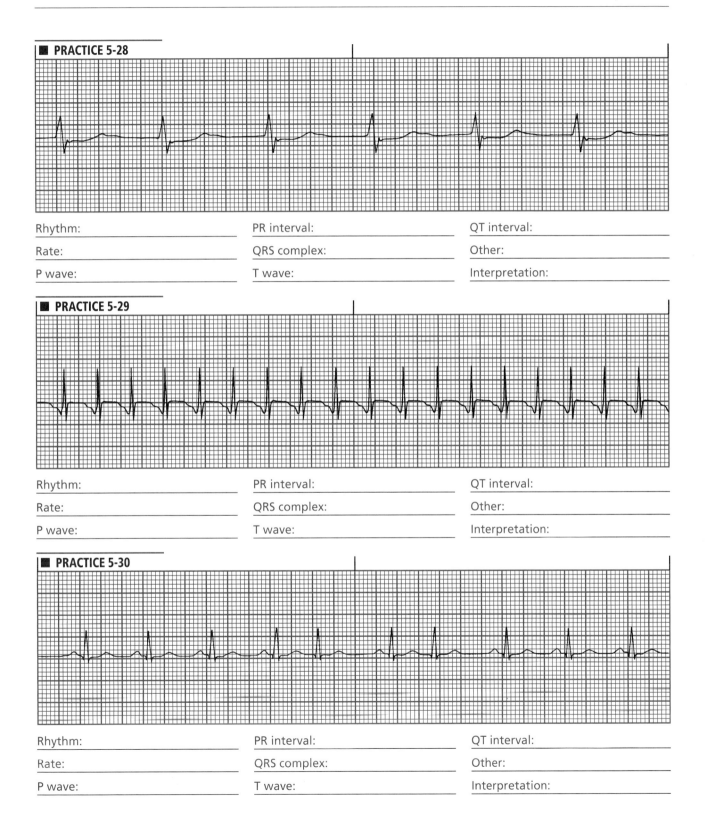

Rhythm: _____   PR interval: _____   QT interval: _____

Rate: _____   QRS complex: _____   Other: _____

P wave: _____   T wave: _____   Interpretation: _____

■ PRACTICE 5-29

Rhythm: _____   PR interval: _____   QT interval: _____

Rate: _____   QRS complex: _____   Other: _____

P wave: _____   T wave: _____   Interpretation: _____

■ PRACTICE 5-30

Rhythm: _____   PR interval: _____   QT interval: _____

Rate: _____   QRS complex: _____   Other: _____

P wave: _____   T wave: _____   Interpretation: _____

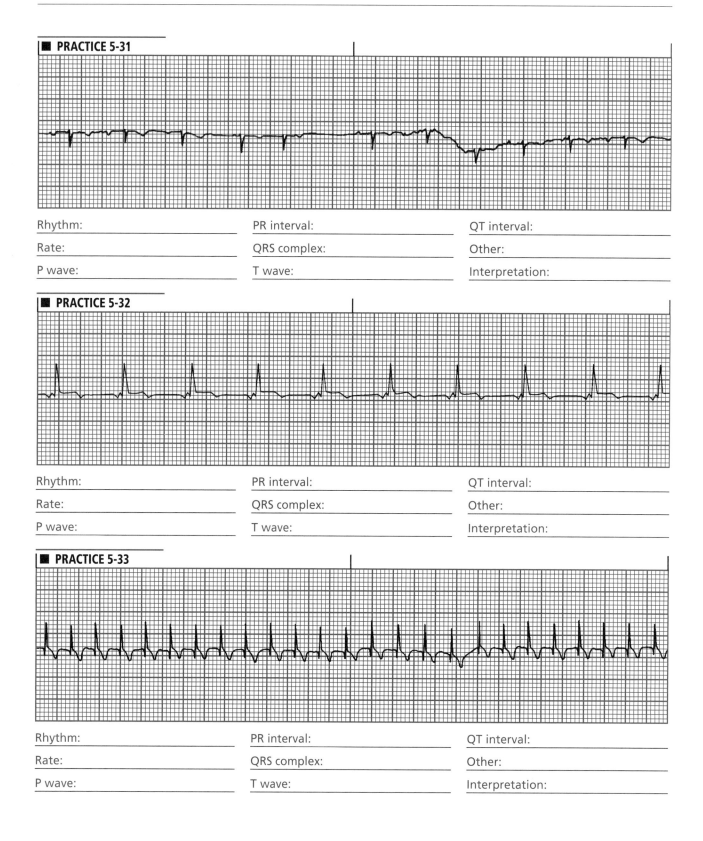

■ PRACTICE 5-31

Rhythm: _____ PR interval: _____ QT interval: _____

Rate: _____ QRS complex: _____ Other: _____

P wave: _____ T wave: _____ Interpretation: _____

■ PRACTICE 5-32

Rhythm: _____ PR interval: _____ QT interval: _____

Rate: _____ QRS complex: _____ Other: _____

P wave: _____ T wave: _____ Interpretation: _____

■ PRACTICE 5-33

Rhythm: _____ PR interval: _____ QT interval: _____

Rate: _____ QRS complex: _____ Other: _____

P wave: _____ T wave: _____ Interpretation: _____

■ **PRACTICE 5-34**

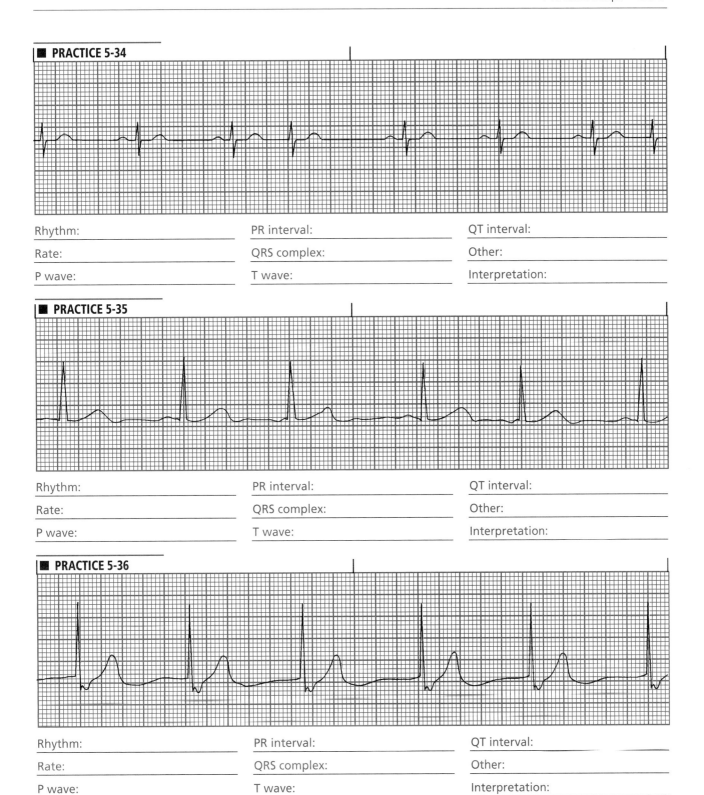

Rhythm: _____   PR interval: _____   QT interval: _____

Rate: _____   QRS complex: _____   Other: _____

P wave: _____   T wave: _____   Interpretation: _____

■ **PRACTICE 5-35**

Rhythm: _____   PR interval: _____   QT interval: _____

Rate: _____   QRS complex: _____   Other: _____

P wave: _____   T wave: _____   Interpretation: _____

■ **PRACTICE 5-36**

Rhythm: _____   PR interval: _____   QT interval: _____

Rate: _____   QRS complex: _____   Other: _____

P wave: _____   T wave: _____   Interpretation: _____

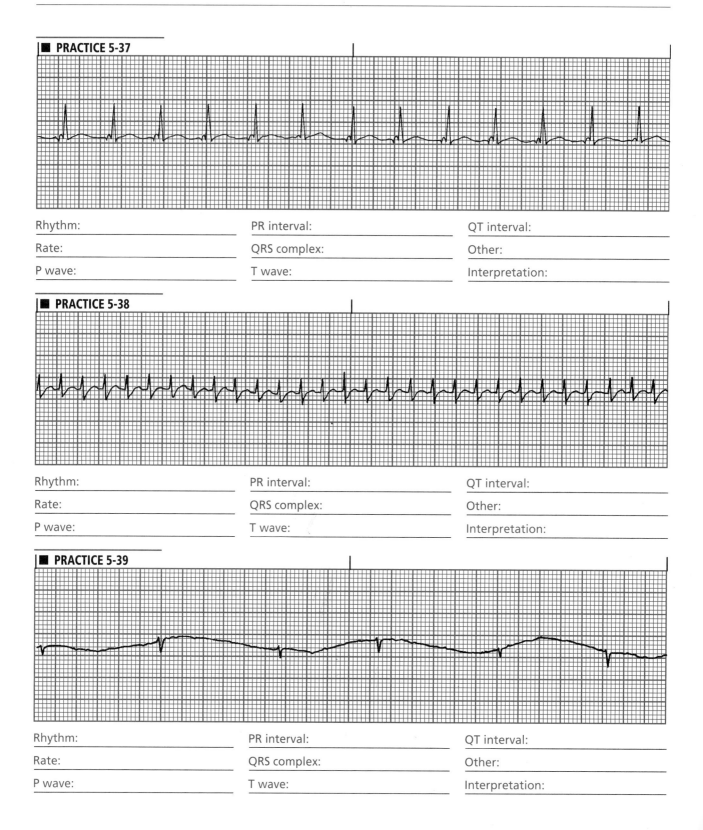

■ **PRACTICE 5-37**

Rhythm: _____   PR interval: _____   QT interval: _____

Rate: _____   QRS complex: _____   Other: _____

P wave: _____   T wave: _____   Interpretation: _____

■ **PRACTICE 5-38**

Rhythm: _____   PR interval: _____   QT interval: _____

Rate: _____   QRS complex: _____   Other: _____

P wave: _____   T wave: _____   Interpretation: _____

■ **PRACTICE 5-39**

Rhythm: _____   PR interval: _____   QT interval: _____

Rate: _____   QRS complex: _____   Other: _____

P wave: _____   T wave: _____   Interpretation: _____

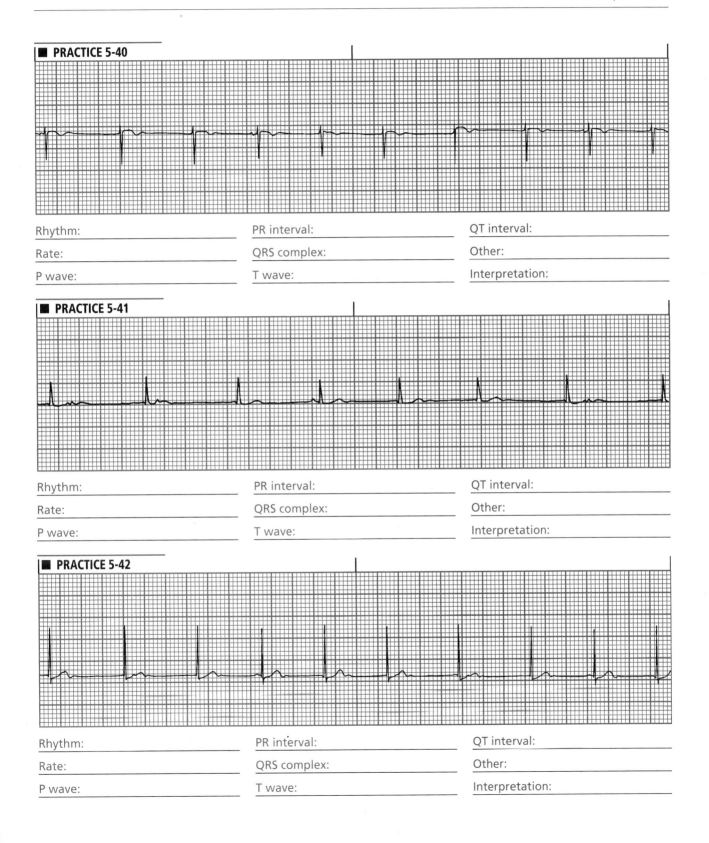

■ PRACTICE 5-40

Rhythm: _____

Rate: _____

P wave: _____

PR interval: _____

QRS complex: _____

T wave: _____

QT interval: _____

Other: _____

Interpretation: _____

■ PRACTICE 5-41

Rhythm: _____

Rate: _____

P wave: _____

PR interval: _____

QRS complex: _____

T wave: _____

QT interval: _____

Other: _____

Interpretation: _____

■ PRACTICE 5-42

Rhythm: _____

Rate: _____

P wave: _____

PR interval: _____

QRS complex: _____

T wave: _____

QT interval: _____

Other: _____

Interpretation: _____

■ PRACTICE 5-43

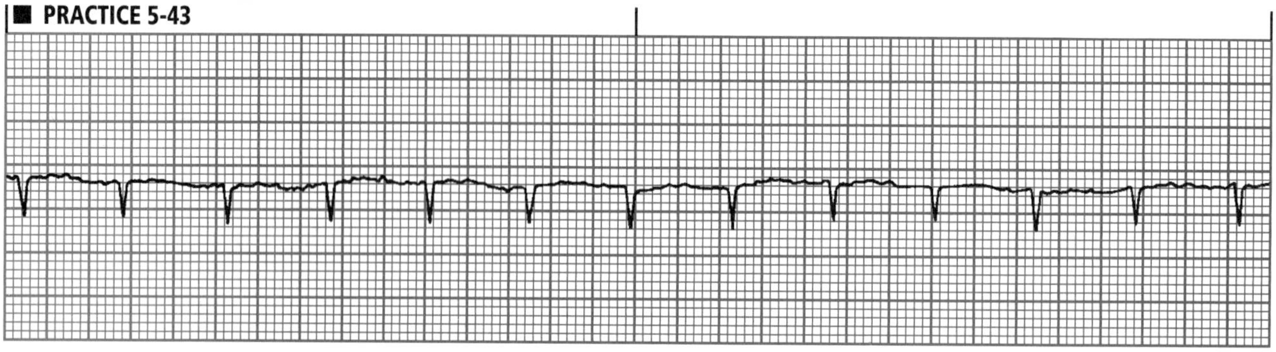

Rhythm: _____   PR interval: _____   QT interval: _____

Rate: _____   QRS complex: _____   Other: _____

P wave: _____   T wave: _____   Interpretation: _____

■ PRACTICE 5-44

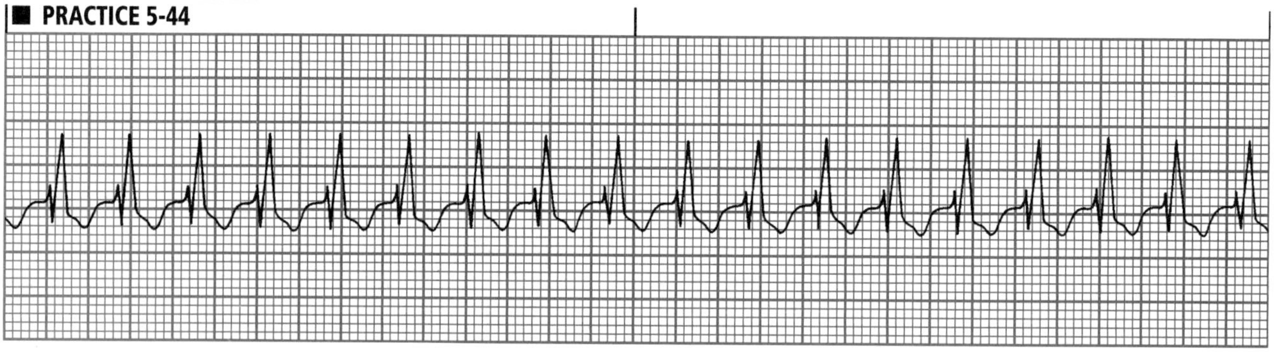

Rhythm: _____   PR interval: _____   QT interval: _____

Rate: _____   QRS complex: _____   Other: _____

P wave: _____   T wave: _____   Interpretation: _____

■ PRACTICE 5-45

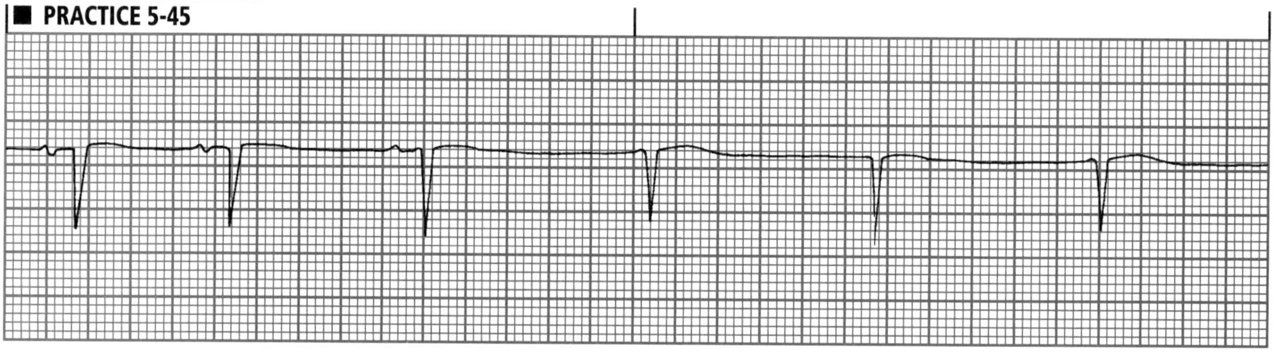

Rhythm: _____   PR interval: _____   QT interval: _____

Rate: _____   QRS complex: _____   Other: _____

P wave: _____   T wave: _____   Interpretation: _____

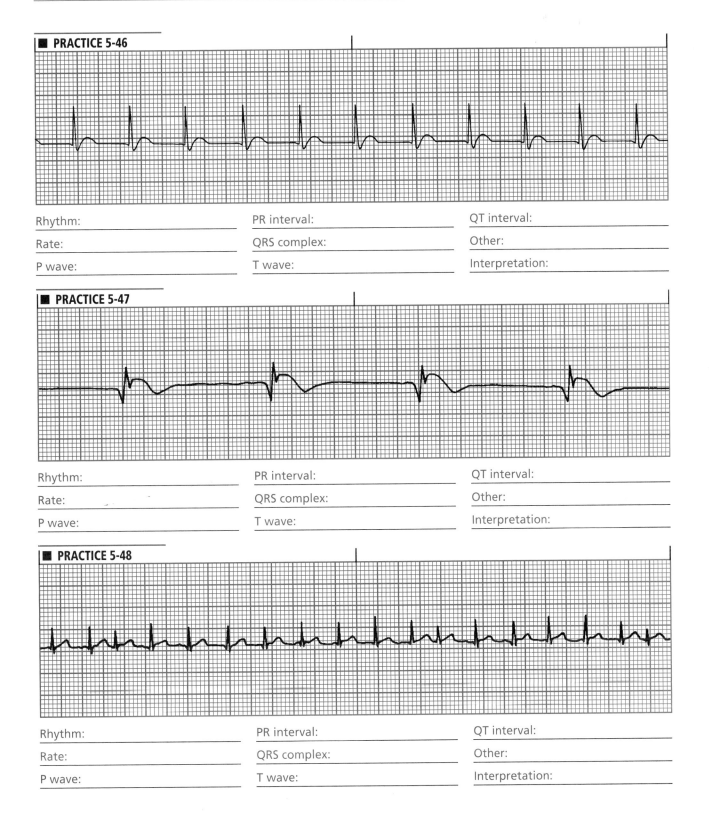

■ **PRACTICE 5-46**

Rhythm: _____

Rate: _____

P wave: _____

PR interval: _____

QRS complex: _____

T wave: _____

QT interval: _____

Other: _____

Interpretation: _____

■ **PRACTICE 5-47**

Rhythm: _____

Rate: _____

P wave: _____

PR interval: _____

QRS complex: _____

T wave: _____

QT interval: _____

Other: _____

Interpretation: _____

■ **PRACTICE 5-48**

Rhythm: _____

Rate: _____

P wave: _____

PR interval: _____

QRS complex: _____

T wave: _____

QT interval: _____

Other: _____

Interpretation: _____

■ **PRACTICE 5-49**

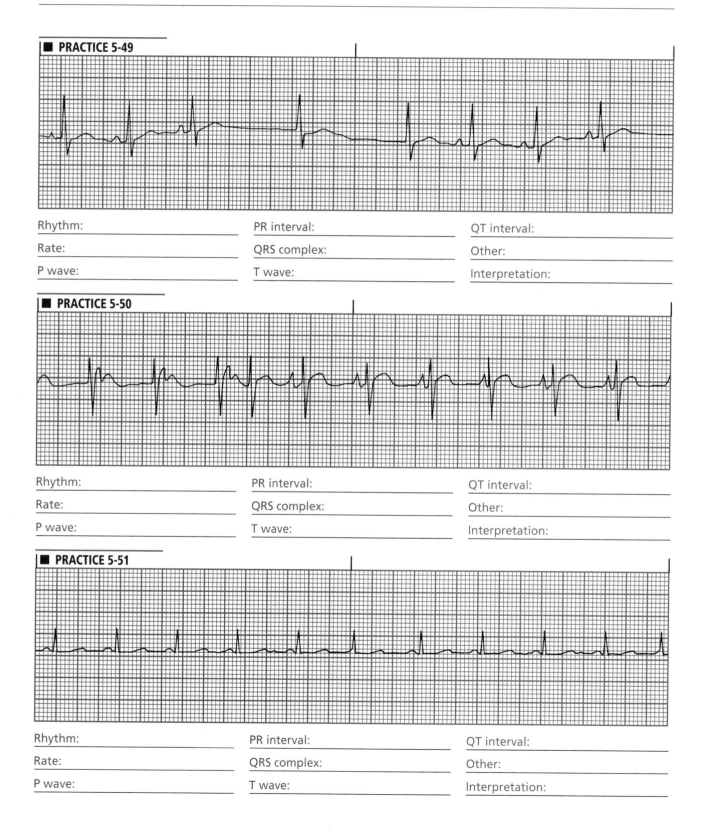

Rhythm: _____   PR interval: _____   QT interval: _____

Rate: _____   QRS complex: _____   Other: _____

P wave: _____   T wave: _____   Interpretation: _____

■ **PRACTICE 5-50**

Rhythm: _____   PR interval: _____   QT interval: _____

Rate: _____   QRS complex: _____   Other: _____

P wave: _____   T wave: _____   Interpretation: _____

■ **PRACTICE 5-51**

Rhythm: _____   PR interval: _____   QT interval: _____

Rate: _____   QRS complex: _____   Other: _____

P wave: _____   T wave: _____   Interpretation: _____

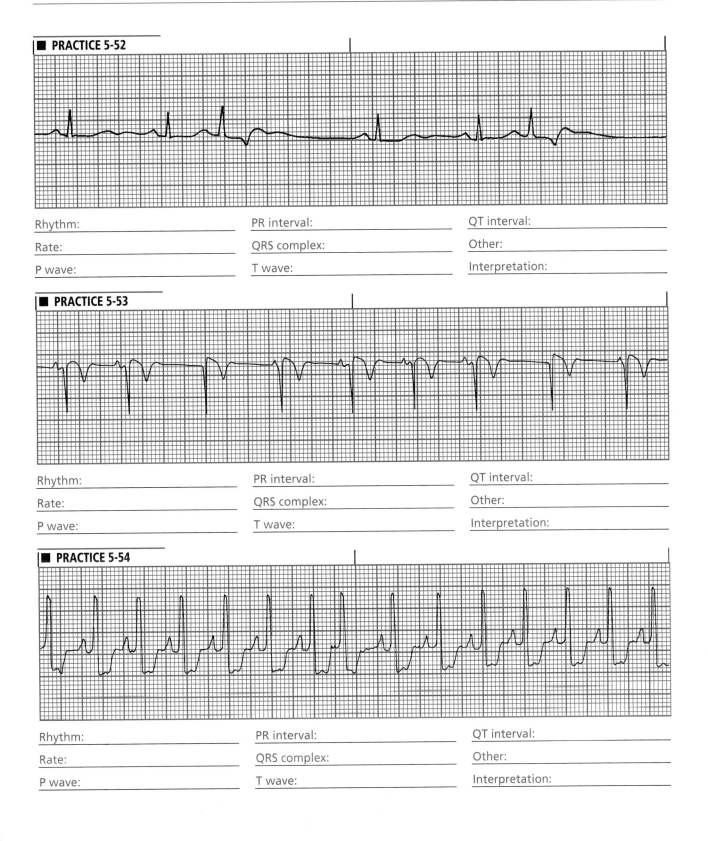

■ PRACTICE 5-52

Rhythm: _____

Rate: _____

P wave: _____

PR interval: _____

QRS complex: _____

T wave: _____

QT interval: _____

Other: _____

Interpretation: _____

■ PRACTICE 5-53

Rhythm: _____

Rate: _____

P wave: _____

PR interval: _____

QRS complex: _____

T wave: _____

QT interval: _____

Other: _____

Interpretation: _____

■ PRACTICE 5-54

Rhythm: _____

Rate: _____

P wave: _____

PR interval: _____

QRS complex: _____

T wave: _____

QT interval: _____

Other: _____

Interpretation: _____

■ **PRACTICE 5-55**

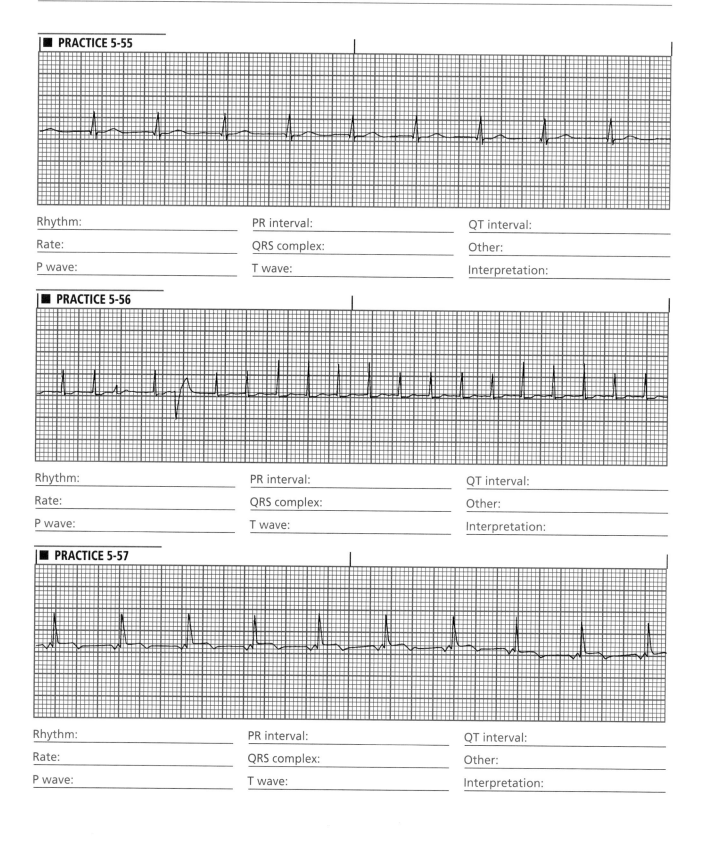

Rhythm: _____ PR interval: _____ QT interval: _____

Rate: _____ QRS complex: _____ Other: _____

P wave: _____ T wave: _____ Interpretation: _____

■ **PRACTICE 5-56**

Rhythm: _____ PR interval: _____ QT interval: _____

Rate: _____ QRS complex: _____ Other: _____

P wave: _____ T wave: _____ Interpretation: _____

■ **PRACTICE 5-57**

Rhythm: _____ PR interval: _____ QT interval: _____

Rate: _____ QRS complex: _____ Other: _____

P wave: _____ T wave: _____ Interpretation: _____

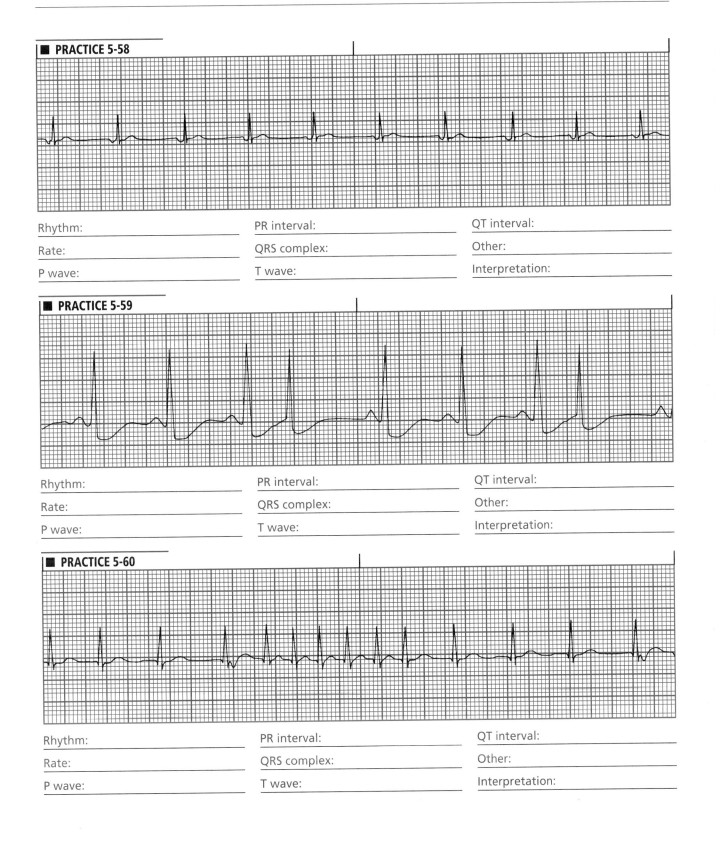

■ PRACTICE 5-58

Rhythm: _____ PR interval: _____ QT interval: _____

Rate: _____ QRS complex: _____ Other: _____

P wave: _____ T wave: _____ Interpretation: _____

■ PRACTICE 5-59

Rhythm: _____ PR interval: _____ QT interval: _____

Rate: _____ QRS complex: _____ Other: _____

P wave: _____ T wave: _____ Interpretation: _____

■ PRACTICE 5-60

Rhythm: _____ PR interval: _____ QT interval: _____

Rate: _____ QRS complex: _____ Other: _____

P wave: _____ T wave: _____ Interpretation: _____

■ PRACTICE STRIP ANSWERS

PRACTICE 5-1
- Rhythm: Regular
- Rate: 125 beats/minute
- P wave: Not present
- PR interval: Unmeasurable
- QRS complex: 0.06 second
- T wave: Normal
- QT interval: 0.24 second
- Other: None
- Interpretation: Junctional tachycardia

PRACTICE 5-2
- Rhythm: Irregular
- Rate: 40 beats/minute
- P wave: Variable; not always present
- PR interval: 0.20 second
- QRS complex: 0.08 second
- T wave: Normal
- QT interval: 0.38 second
- Other: None
- Interpretation: Sinus bradycardia with junctional beat

PRACTICE 5-3
- Rhythm: Mostly regular
- Rate: 70 beats/minute
- P wave: Not present
- PR interval: Unmeasurable
- QRS complex: 0.08 second
- T wave: Almost flat
- QT interval: Unmeasurable
- Other: None
- Interpretation: Accelerated junctional rhythm

PRACTICE 5-4
- Rhythm: Irregular
- Rate: 100 beats/minute
- P wave: Inverted and retrograde
- PR interval: Unmeasurable
- QRS complex: 0.08 second
- T wave: Flattened
- QT interval: Unmeasurable
- Other: Two different R-Rs noted
- Interpretation: Accelerated junctional rhythm

PRACTICE 5-5
- Rhythm: Regular
- Rate: 63 beats/minute
- P wave: Not present
- PR interval: Unmeasurable
- QRS complex: 0.06 second
- T wave: Normal
- QT interval: 0.44 second
- Other: None
- Interpretation: Accelerated junctional rhythm

PRACTICE 5-6
- Rhythm: Regular
- Rate: 63 beats/minute
- P wave: Inverted
- PR interval: 0.10 second
- QRS complex: 0.06 second
- T wave: Normal
- QT interval: 0.28 second
- Other: None
- Interpretation: Accelerated junctional rhythm

PRACTICE 5-7
- Rhythm: Regular
- Rate: 94 beats/minute
- P wave: Not visible
- PR interval: Unmeasurable
- QRS complex: 0.08 second
- T wave: Slightly flattened
- QT interval: 0.32 second
- Other: None
- Interpretation: Accelerated junctional rhythm

PRACTICE 5-8
- Rhythm: Regular
- Rate: 150 beats/minute
- P wave: Not visible
- PR interval: Unmeasurable
- QRS complex: 0.12 second
- T wave: Normal
- QT interval: 0.24 second
- Other: None
- Interpretation: Junctional tachycardia

PRACTICE 5-9
- Rhythm: Irregular
- Rate: 70 beats/minute
- P wave: Normal when present
- PR interval: 0.16 second
- QRS complex: 0.06 second
- T wave: Normal
- QT interval: 0.46 second
- Other: None
- Interpretation: Normal sinus rhythm (NSR) with PJC

PRACTICE 5-10
- Rhythm: Irregular
- Rate: 80 beats/minute
- P wave: Normal when present
- PR interval: Variable
- QRS complex: 0.06 second
- T wave: Normal
- QT interval: 0.28 second
- Other: None
- Interpretation: Wandering pacemaker with junctional beats

PRACTICE 5-11
- Rhythm: Regular
- Rate: 75 beats/minute
- P wave: Inverted
- PR interval: 0.10 second
- QRS complex: 0.04 second
- T wave: Normal
- QT interval: 0.36 second
- Other: None
- Interpretation: Accelerated junctional rhythm

PRACTICE 5-12
- Rhythm: Irregular
- Rate: 120 beats/minute
- P wave: Normal when present
- PR interval: 0.16 second
- QRS complex: 0.08 second
- T wave: Inverted
- QT interval: 0.24 second
- Other: Bundle-branch block
- Interpretation: Sinus tachycardia with period of junctional tachycardia

PRACTICE 5-13
- Rhythm: Regular
- Rate: 60 beats/minute
- P wave: None present
- PR interval: Unmeasurable
- QRS complex: 0.08 second
- T wave: Inverted
- QT interval: 0.32 second
- Other: None
- Interpretation: Accelerated junctional rhythm

PRACTICE 5-14
- Rhythm: Regular
- Rate: 100 beats/minute
- P wave: None present
- PR interval: Unmeasurable
- QRS complex: 0.10 second
- T wave: Normal
- QT interval: 0.44 second
- Other: ST-segment depression
- Interpretation: Accelerated junctional rhythm

PRACTICE 5-15
- Rhythm: Regular
- Rate: 68 beats/minute
- P wave: None present
- PR interval: Unmeasurable
- QRS complex: 0.10 second
- T wave: Normal
- QT interval: 0.32 second
- Other: None
- Interpretation: Accelerated junctional rhythm

PRACTICE 5-16
- Rhythm: Regular
- Rate: 44 beats/minute
- P wave: Inverted
- PR interval: 0.20 second
- QRS complex: 0.10 second
- T wave: Normal
- QT interval: 0.54 second
- Other: None
- Interpretation: Junctional escape rhythm

PRACTICE 5-17
- Rhythm: Regular
- Rate: 188 beats/minute
- P wave: Retrograde
- PR interval: Unmeasurable
- QRS complex: 0.04 second
- T wave: Inverted
- QT interval: 0.20 second
- Other: None
- Interpretation: Junctional tachycardia

PRACTICE 5-18
- Rhythm: Regular
- Rate: 47 beats/minute
- P wave: Inverted and retrograde
- PR interval: Unmeasurable
- QRS complex: 0.12 second
- T wave: Normal
- QT interval: 0.52 second
- Other: None
- Interpretation: Junctional escape rhythm

PRACTICE 5-19
- Rhythm: Regular
- Rate: 167 beats/minute
- P wave: Inverted and retrograde
- PR interval: Unmeasurable
- QRS complex: 0.08 second
- T wave: Normal
- QT interval: 0.24 second
- Other: None
- Interpretation: Junctional tachycardia

PRACTICE 5-20
- Rhythm: Regular
- Rate: 68 beats/minute
- P wave: Not present
- PR interval: Unmeasurable
- QRS complex: 0.06 second
- T wave: Normal
- QT interval: 0.28 second
- Other: None
- Interpretation: Accelerated junctional rhythm

PRACTICE 5-21
- Rhythm: Regular
- Rate: 88 beats/minute
- P wave: Inverted
- PR interval: 0.12 second
- QRS complex: 0.04 second
- T wave: Normal
- QT interval: 0.24 second
- Other: None
- Interpretation: Accelerated junctional rhythm

PRACTICE 5-22
- Rhythm: Regular
- Rate: 43 beats/minute
- P wave: Not present
- PR interval: Unmeasurable
- QRS complex: 0.04 second
- T wave: Normal
- QT interval: 0.44 second
- Other: None
- Interpretation: Junctional escape rhythm

PRACTICE 5-23
- Rhythm: Regular
- Rate: 150 beats/minute
- P wave: Inverted
- PR interval: 0.12 second
- QRS complex: 0.08 second
- T wave: Normal
- QT interval: 0.28 second
- Other: None
- Interpretation: Junctional tachycardia

PRACTICE 5-24
- Rhythm: Irregular
- Rate: 136 beats/minute
- P wave: Normal
- PR interval: 0.12 second
- QRS complex: 0.08 second
- T wave: Normal
- QT interval: 0.20 second
- Other: None
- Interpretation: Sinus tachycardia with PJCs

PRACTICE 5-25
- Rhythm: Regular
- Rate: 48 beats/minute
- P wave: Retrograde
- PR interval: Unmeasurable
- QRS complex: 0.04 second
- T wave: Normal
- QT interval: 0.40 second
- Other: None
- Interpretation: Junctional escape rhythm

PRACTICE 5-26
- Rhythm: Regular
- Rate: 60 beats/minute
- P wave: Not present
- PR interval: Unmeasurable
- QRS complex: 0.06 second
- T wave: Normal
- QT interval: 0.32 second
- Other: None
- Interpretation: Junctional escape rhythm

PRACTICE 5-27
- Rhythm: Irregular
- Rate: 88 beats/minute
- P wave: Mostly normal; inverted with premature beats
- PR interval: 0.16 second
- QRS complex: 0.08 second
- T wave: Normal
- QT interval: 0.32 second
- Other: None
- Interpretation: NSR with PJCs

PRACTICE 5-28
- Rhythm: Regular
- Rate: 60 beats/minute
- P wave: Not present
- PR interval: Unmeasurable
- QRS complex: 0.12 second
- T wave: Normal
- QT interval: 0.60 second
- Other: None
- Interpretation: Accelerated junctional rhythm

PRACTICE 5-29
- Rhythm: Regular
- Rate: 188 beats/minute
- P wave: Inverted
- PR interval: 0.12 second
- QRS complex: 0.06 second
- T wave: Flattened
- QT interval: Unmeasurable
- Other: None
- Interpretation: Junctional tachycardia

PRACTICE 5-30
- Rhythm: Irregular
- Rate: 100 beats/minute
- P wave: Mostly normal; absent with premature beats
- PR interval: 0.14 second
- QRS complex: 0.06 second
- T wave: Normal
- QT interval: 0.28 second
- Other: None
- Interpretation: NSR with PJCs

PRACTICE 5-31
- Rhythm: Irregular
- Rate: 110 beats/minute
- P wave: Mostly inverted; occasionally absent
- PR interval: 0.20 second
- QRS complex: 0.04 second
- T wave: Inverted
- QT interval: 0.26 second
- Other: None
- Interpretation: Junctional tachycardia with PJCs

PRACTICE 5-32
- Rhythm: Regular
- Rate: 94 beats/minute
- P wave: Inverted
- PR interval: 0.08 second
- QRS complex: 0.06 second
- T wave: Inverted
- QT interval: 0.28 second
- Other: Slight ST-segment elevation
- Interpretation: Accelerated junctional rhythm

PRACTICE 5-33
- Rhythm: Regular
- Rate: 250 beats/minute
- P wave: Not present
- PR interval: Unmeasurable
- QRS complex: 0.04 second
- T wave: Inverted
- QT interval: 0.12 second
- Other: Possible SVT
- Interpretation: Junctional tachycardia

PRACTICE 5-34
- Rhythm: Irregular
- Rate: 80 beats/minute
- P wave: Normal; absent with premature beats
- PR interval: 0.16 second
- QRS complex: 0.08 second
- T wave: Normal
- QT interval: 0.32 second
- Other: None
- Interpretation: NSR with PJCs

PRACTICE 5-35
- Rhythm: Irregular
- Rate: 60 beats/minute
- P wave: Mostly normal; inverted with premature beats
- PR interval: 0.20 second
- QRS complex: 0.08 second
- T wave: Normal
- QT interval: 0.48 second
- Other: None
- Interpretation: Sinus bradycardia with PJCs

PRACTICE 5-36
- Rhythm: Regular
- Rate: 56 beats/minute
- P wave: Inverted and retrograde
- PR interval: Unmeasurable
- QRS complex: 0.08 second
- T wave: Normal
- QT interval: 0.44 second
- Other: None
- Interpretation: Junctional escape rhythm

PRACTICE 5-37
- Rhythm: Regular
- Rate: 136 beats/minute
- P wave: Normal
- PR interval: 0.08 second
- QRS complex: 0.06 second
- T wave: Normal
- QT interval: 0.28 second
- Other: None
- Interpretation: Junctional tachycardia

PRACTICE 5-38
- Rhythm: Regular
- Rate: 300 beats/minute
- P wave: Not present
- PR interval: Unmeasurable
- QRS complex: 0.04 second
- T wave: Normal
- QT interval: 0.16 second
- Other: Possible SVT
- Interpretation: Junctional tachycardia

PRACTICE 5-39
- Rhythm: Irregular
- Rate: 60 beats/minute
- P wave: Not present
- PR interval: Unmeasurable
- QRS complex: 0.06 second
- T wave: Flattened
- QT interval: Unmeasurable
- Other: None
- Interpretation: Junctional escape rhythm

PRACTICE 5-40
- Rhythm: Irregular
- Rate: 100 beats/minute
- P wave: Not present
- PR interval: Unmeasurable
- QRS complex: 0.04 second
- T wave: Biphasic
- QT interval: 0.24 second
- Other: One sinus beat noted
- Interpretation: Accelerated junctional rhythm with PJCs

PRACTICE 5-41
- Rhythm: Irregular
- Rate: 80 beats/minute
- P wave: Not present
- PR interval: Unmeasurable
- QRS complex: 0.04 second
- T wave: Normal
- QT interval: 0.24 second
- Other: One sinus beat noted
- Interpretation: Accelerated junctional rhythm with one PAC and one PJC

PRACTICE 5-42
- Rhythm: Irregular
- Rate: 100 beats/minute
- P wave: Not present
- PR interval: Unmeasurable
- QRS complex: 0.04 second
- T wave: Biphasic
- QT interval: 0.24 second
- Other: None
- Interpretation: Accelerated junctional rhythm with one PAC and one PJC

PRACTICE 5-43
- Rhythm: Regular
- Rate: 125 beats/minute
- P wave: Not present
- PR interval: Unmeasurable
- QRS complex: 0.06 second
- T wave: Flattened
- QT interval: Unmeasurable
- Other: None
- Interpretation: Junctional tachycardia

PRACTICE 5-44
- Rhythm: Regular
- Rate: 188 beats/minute
- P wave: Not present
- PR interval: Unmeasurable
- QRS complex: 0.12 second
- T wave: Inverted
- QT interval: 0.24 second
- Other: None
- Interpretation: Junctional tachycardia

PRACTICE 5-45
- Rhythm: Irregular
- Rate: 60 beats/minute
- P wave: Occasionally present
- PR interval: 0.16 second
- QRS complex: 0.08 second
- T wave: Slightly flattened
- QT interval: 0.34 second
- Other: None
- Interpretation: Sinus arrhythmia into junctional escape rhythm

PRACTICE 5-46
- Rhythm: Regular
- Rate: 115 beats/minute
- P wave: Not present
- PR interval: Unmeasurable
- QRS complex: 0.06 second
- T wave: Normal
- QT interval: 0.24 second
- Other: None
- Interpretation: Junctional tachycardia

PRACTICE 5-47
- Rhythm: Regular
- Rate: 43 beats/minute
- P wave: Not present
- PR interval: Unmeasurable
- QRS complex: 0.12 second
- T wave: Normal
- QT interval: 0.40 second
- Other: ST-segment elevation
- Interpretation: Junctional escape rhythm

PRACTICE 5-48
- Rhythm: Irregular
- Rate: 180 beats/minute
- P wave: Not present
- PR interval: Unmeasurable
- QRS complex: 0.06 second
- T wave: Normal
- QT interval: 0.20 second
- Other: None
- Interpretation: Junctional tachycardia with PJCs

PRACTICE 5-49
- Rhythm: Irregular
- Rate: 80 beats/minute
- P wave: Normal when present
- PR interval: 0.16 second
- QRS complex: 0.08 second
- T wave: Normal
- QT interval: 0.32 second
- Other: None
- Interpretation: NSR with junctional escape beats

PRACTICE 5-50
- Rhythm: Irregular
- Rate: 100 beats/minute
- P wave: Some retrograde, some normal
- PR interval: 0.12 second
- QRS complex: 0.08 second
- T wave: Normal
- QT interval: 0.26 second
- Other: Slight ST-segment elevation
- Interpretation: Accelerated junctional changing to sinus tachycardia

PRACTICE 5-51
- Rhythm: Irregular
- Rate: 110 beats/minute
- P wave: Normal except during premature beats
- PR interval: 0.12 second
- QRS complex: 0.04 second
- T wave: Normal
- QT interval: 0.32 second
- Other: None
- Interpretation: Sinus tachycardia with PJC

PRACTICE 5-52
- Rhythm: Irregular
- Rate: 60 beats/minute
- P wave: Normal to retrograde
- PR interval: 0.20 second
- QRS complex: 0.08 second
- T wave: Normal
- QT interval: 0.48 second
- Other: None
- Interpretation: NSR with PJCs

PRACTICE 5-53
- Rhythm: Irregular
- Rate: 90 beats/minute
- P wave: Normal to absent
- PR interval: 0.12 second
- QRS complex: 0.04 second
- T wave: Inverted
- QT interval: 0.28 second
- Other: ST-segment elevation
- Interpretation: NSR with junctional escape beats

PRACTICE 5-54
- Rhythm: Irregular
- Rate: 150 beats/minute
- P wave: Normal except during premature beats
- PR interval: 0.12 second
- QRS complex: 0.08 second
- T wave: Inverted
- QT interval: 0.24 second
- Other: None
- Interpretation: Sinus tachycardia with PJC

PRACTICE 5-55
- Rhythm: Regular
- Rate: 94 beats/minute
- P wave: Not present
- PR interval: Unmeasurable
- QRS complex: 0.06 second
- T wave: Normal
- QT interval: 0.32 second
- Other: None
- Interpretation: Accelerated junctional rhythm

PRACTICE 5-56
- Rhythm: Irregular
- Rate: 200 beats/minute
- P wave: Not present
- PR interval: Unmeasurable
- QRS complex: 0.04 second
- T wave: Normal
- QT interval: 0.20 second
- Other: None
- Interpretation: Junctional tachycardia with PVCs

PRACTICE 5-57
- Rhythm: Regular
- Rate: 94 beats/minute
- P wave: Inverted
- PR interval: 0.12 second
- QRS complex: 0.08 second
- T wave: Inverted
- QT interval: 0.30 second
- Other: None
- Interpretation: Accelerated junctional rhythm

PRACTICE 5-58
- Rhythm: Regular
- Rate: 94 beats/minute
- P wave: Inverted
- PR interval: 0.08 second
- QRS complex: 0.06 second
- T wave: Normal
- QT interval: 0.24 second
- Other: None
- Interpretation: Accelerated junctional rhythm

PRACTICE 5-59
- Rhythm: Irregular
- Rate: 80 beats/minute
- P wave: Normal but absent in premature beats
- PR interval: 0.20 second
- QRS complex: 0.08 second
- T wave: Flattened
- QT interval: Unmeasurable
- Other: None
- Interpretation: NSR with PJCs

PRACTICE 5-60
- Rhythm: Irregular
- Rate: 140 beats/minute
- P wave: Not present
- PR interval: Unmeasurable
- QRS complex: 0.08 second
- T wave: Normal
- QT interval: Variable
- Other: None
- Interpretation: Junctional tachycardia

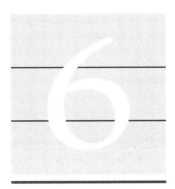

Ventricular arrhythmias

Ventricular arrhythmias originate in the ventricles below the bifurcation of the bundle of His. These arrhythmias occur when electrical impulses depolarize the myocardium using a different pathway from normal impulse conduction.

Ventricular arrhythmias appear on an electrocardiogram (ECG) in characteristic ways. The QRS complex in most of these arrhythmias is wider than normal because of the prolonged conduction time through, and abnormal depolarization of, the ventricles. The deflections of the T wave and the QRS complex are in opposite directions because ventricular repolarization, as well as ventricular depolarization, is abnormal. The P wave in many ventricular arrhythmias is absent because atrial depolarization doesn't occur.

When electrical impulses come from the ventricles instead of the atria, atrial kick is lost and cardiac output can decrease by as much as 30%. This is one reason patients with ventricular arrhythmias may show signs and symptoms of heart failure, including hypotension, angina, syncope, and respiratory distress.

Although ventricular arrhythmias may be benign, they're generally considered the most serious arrhythmias, because the ventricles are ultimately responsible for cardiac output. Rapid recognition and treatment of ventricular arrhythmias increases the chances of successful resuscitation.

Ventricular arrhythmias

In ventricular arrhythmias, impulses originate in the ventricles below the bifurcation of the bundle of His.

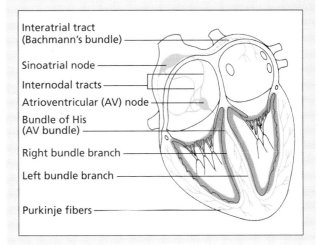

- Interatrial tract (Bachmann's bundle)
- Sinoatrial node
- Internodal tracts
- Atrioventricular (AV) node
- Bundle of His (AV bundle)
- Right bundle branch
- Left bundle branch
- Purkinje fibers

Premature ventricular contractions

Premature ventricular contractions (PVCs) are ectopic beats that originate in the ventricles and occur earlier than expected. PVCs may occur in healthy people without being clinically significant. When PVCs occur in patients with underlying heart disease, however, they may herald the development of lethal ventricular arrhythmias, including ventricular tachycardia and ventricular fibrillation.

In many cases, PVCs are followed by a compensatory pause. PVCs may be uniform in appearance, arising from a single ectopic ventricular pacemaker site, or multiform, originating from different sites or originating from a single pacemaker site but having QRS complexes that differ in size, shape, and direction. (See *Identifying premature ventricular contractions.*)

PVCs may also be described as *unifocal* or *multifocal.* Unifocal PVCs originate from the same ventricular ectopic pacemaker site, whereas multifocal PVCs originate from different ectopic pacemaker sites in the ventricles.

PVCs may occur singly, in pairs (couplets), or in clusters. PVCs may also appear in patterns, such as bigeminy or trigeminy. (See *Patterns of potentially dangerous PVCs.*)

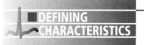

Identifying premature ventricular contractions

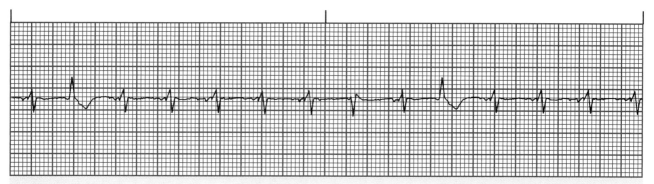

Rhythm
- Atrial: Irregular during PVCs
- Ventricular: Irregular during PVCs
- Underlying rhythm possibly regular

Rate
- Atrial: Reflects underlying rhythm
- Ventricular: Reflects underlying rhythm

P wave
- Usually absent in ectopic beat
- May appear after QRS complex with retrograde conduction to atria
- Usually normal if present in underlying rhythm

PR interval
- Unmeasurable except in underlying rhythm

QRS complex
- Occurs earlier than expected
- Duration: Exceeds 0.12 second
- Configuration: Bizarre and wide with PVC
- Usually normal in underlying rhythm

T wave
- Opposite direction to QRS complex
- May trigger more serious rhythm disturbances when PVC occurs on the downslope of the preceding normal T wave (R-on-T phenomenon)

QT interval
- Not usually measured except in underlying rhythm

Other
- PVC may be followed by a full or occasionally an incomplete compensatory pause
- Full compensatory pause existing if the P-P interval encompassing the PVC has twice the duration of a normal sinus beat's P-P interval
- Incomplete compensatory pause existing if the P-P interval encompassing the PVC is less than twice the duration of a normal sinus beat's P-P interval
- Interpolated PVC: Occurs between two normally conducted QRS complexes without great disturbance to underlying rhythm
- Full compensatory pause absent with interpolated PVCs
- May be difficult to distinguish PVCs from aberrant ventricular conduction

Patterns of potentially dangerous PVCs

Some premature ventricular contractions (PVCs) are more dangerous than others. Here are examples of patterns of potentially dangerous PVCs.

Paired PVCs

Two PVCs in a row, called *paired PVCs* or a *ventricular couplet* (see shaded areas below), can produce ventricular tachycardia (VT). That's because the second contraction usually meets refractory tissue. A burst, or *salvo*, of three or more PVCs in a row is considered a run of VT.

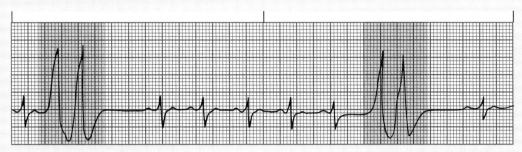

Multiform PVCs

Multiform PVCs, which look different from one another, arise from different sites or from the same site with abnormal conduction (see shaded areas below). Multiform PVCs may indicate severe heart disease or digoxin toxicity.

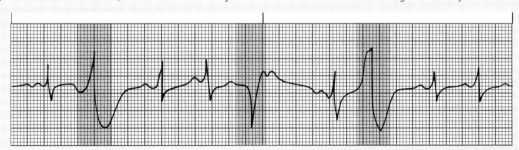

Bigeminy and trigeminy

PVCs that occur every other beat (*bigeminy*) (see shaded areas below) or every third beat (*trigeminy*) may indicate increased ventricular irritability, which can result in VT or ventricular fibrillation. The rhythm strip shown below illustrates ventricular bigeminy.

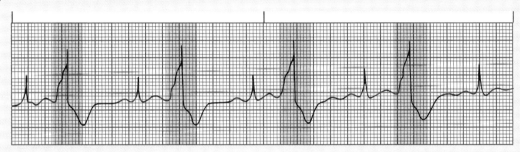

(continued)

Patterns of potentially dangerous PVCs *(continued)*

R-on-T phenomenon

In R-on-T phenomenon, a PVC occurs so early that it falls on the T wave of the preceding beat (see shaded area below). Because the cells haven't fully repolarized, VT or ventricular fibrillation can result.

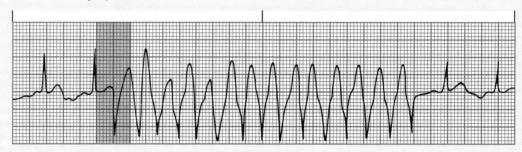

PRACTICE # Premature ventricular contractions

Use the 8-step method to interpret the following rhythm strip. Place your answers on the blank lines. See the answer key below.

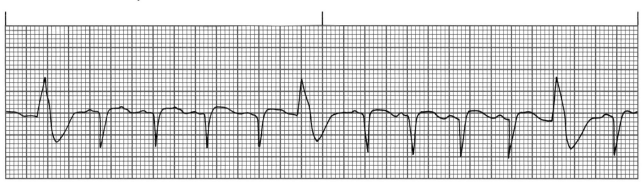

Rhythm: _____

Rate: _____

P wave: _____

PR interval: _____

QRS complex: _____

T wave: _____

QT interval: _____

Other: _____

Idioventricular rhythm

Idioventricular rhythm, also referred to as *ventricular escape rhythm*, originates in an escape pacemaker site in the ventricles. The inherent firing rate of this ectopic pacemaker is usually 20 to 40 beats/minute. The rhythm acts as a safety mechanism by preventing ventricular standstill, or *asystole*—the absence of electrical activity in the ventricles. Although idioventricular rhythms act to protect the heart from ventricular standstill, a continuous idioventricular rhythm presents a clinically serious situation. If not rapidly identified and appropriately managed, idioventricular arrhythmias can cause death.

When fewer than three QRS complexes arising from the escape pacemaker occur, they're called *ventricular escape beats* or *complexes*. Idioventricular rhythms occur when all of the heart's higher pacemakers fail to function or when supraventricular impulses can't reach the ventricles because of a block in the conduction system. Idioventricular rhythms may accompany third-degree heart block. (See *Identifying idioventricular rhythm.*)

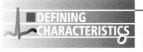

DEFINING CHARACTERISTICS

Identifying idioventricular rhythm

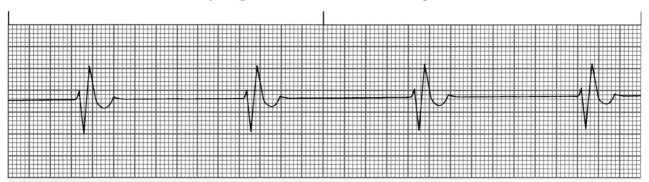

Rhythm
- Atrial: Usually can't be determined
- Ventricular: Usually regular

Rate
- Atrial: Usually can't be determined
- Ventricular: 20 to 40 beats/minute

P wave
- Usually absent

PR interval
- Unmeasurable because of absent P wave

QRS complex
- Duration: Exceeds 0.12 second because of abnormal ventricular depolarization
- Configuration: Wide and bizarre

T wave
- Abnormal
- Usually deflects in opposite direction from QRS complex

QT interval
- Usually prolonged

Other
- Commonly occurs with third-degree atrioventricular (AV) block
- If any P waves present, not associated with QRS complex

Identifying idioventricular rhythm

Use the 8-step method to interpret the following rhythm strip. Place your answers on the blank lines. See the answer key below.

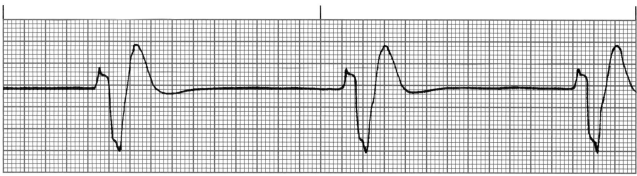

Rhythm:

Rate:

P wave:

PR interval:

QRS complex:

T wave:

QT interval:

Other:

Accelerated idioventricular rhythm

When the rate of an ectopic pacemaker site in the ventricles is under 100 beats/minute but exceeds the inherent ventricular escape rate of 20 to 40 beats/minute, it's called *accelerated idioventricular rhythm* (AIVR). The rate of AIVR isn't fast enough to be considered ventricular tachycardia. The rhythm is usually related to enhanced automaticity of the ventricular tissue. AIVR and idioven-tricular rhythm share the same ECG characteristics, differing only in heart rate. (See *Identifying accelerated idioventricular rhythm.*)

Accelerated idioventricular rhythm can sometimes be difficult to distinguish from accelerated junctional rhythm. (See *Distinguishing AIVR from accelerated junctional rhythm.*)

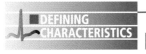

Identifying accelerated idioventricular rhythm

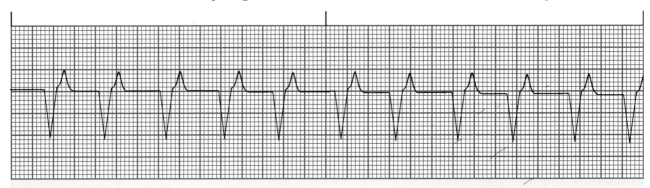

Rhythm
- Atrial: Can't be determined
- Ventricular: Usually regular

Rate
- Atrial: Usually can't be determined
- Ventricular: 40 to 100 beats/minute

P wave
- Usually absent

PR interval
- Unmeasurable

QRS complex
- Duration: Exceeds 0.12 second
- Configuration: Wide and bizarre

T wave
- Abnormal
- Usually deflects in opposite direction from QRS complex

QT interval
- Usually prolonged

Other
- If any P waves present, not associated with QRS complex

Distinguishing AIVR from accelerated junctional rhythm

Accelerated idioventricular rhythm (AIVR) and accelerated junctional rhythm appear similar but have different causes. To distinguish between the two, closely examine the duration of the QRS complex and then look for P waves.

AIVR

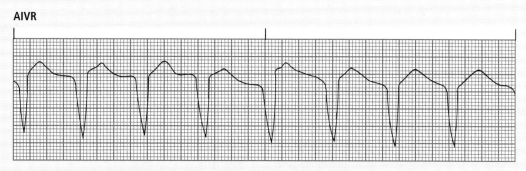

- The QRS duration will be greater than 0.12 second.
- The QRS will have a wide and bizarre configuration.

- P waves are usually absent.
- The ventricular rate is generally between 40 and 100 beats/minute.

Accelerated junctional rhythm

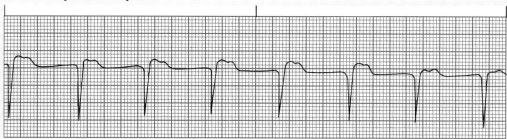

- The QRS duration and configuration are usually normal.
- Inverted P waves generally occur before or after the QRS complex. However, remember

that the P waves may also appear absent when hidden within the QRS complex.
- The ventricular rate is typically between 60 and 100 beats/minute.

Accelerated idioventricular rhythm

Use the 8-step method to interpret the following rhythm strip. Place your answers on the blank lines. See the answer key below.

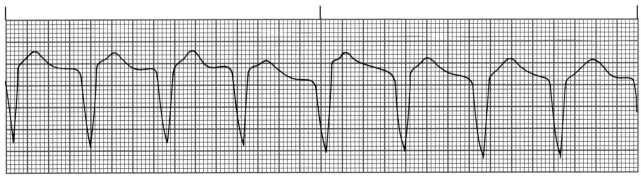

Rhythm: _____

Rate: _____

P wave: _____

PR interval: _____

QRS complex: _____

T wave: _____

QT interval: _____

Other: _____

■ **ANSWER KEY**

Rhythm: Regular

Rate: Ventricular—80 beats/minute

P wave: Absent; sometimes, inverted P wave follows QRS complex

PR interval: Unmeasurable

QRS complex: 0.18 second; wide and bizarre

T wave: Directly opposite last part of QRS complex

QT interval: 0.52 second; prolonged

Other: None

Ventricular tachycardia

Ventricular tachycardia, also called *V-tach* or VT, occurs when three or more PVCs occur in a row and the ventricular rate exceeds 100 beats/minute. VT may produce a palpable pulse, indicating a perfusing rhythm. Pulseless VT is a life-threatening arrhythmia that may precede ventricular fibrillation and sudden cardiac death.

VT is an unstable rhythm and may be sustained or nonsustained. When it occurs in short, paroxysmal bursts lasting less than 30 seconds and causing few or no symptoms, it's called *nonsustained*. When the rhythm is sustained, however, it requires immediate treatment to prevent death, even in patients initially able to maintain adequate cardiac output. (See *Identifying ventricular tachycardia.*)

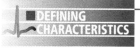
DEFINING CHARACTERISTICS

Identifying ventricular tachycardia

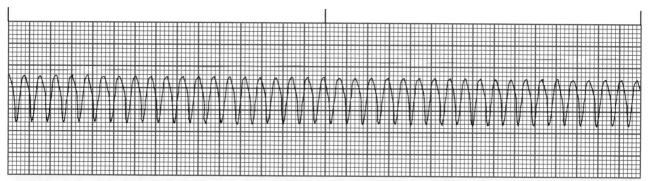

Rhythm

- Atrial: Can't be determined
- Ventricular: Usually regular but may be slightly irregular

Rate

- Atrial: Can't be determined
- Ventricular: Usually rapid (100 to 250 beats/minute)

P wave

- Usually absent
- If present, not associated with QRS complex

PR interval

- Unmeasurable

QRS complex

- Duration: Exceeds 0.12 second
- Configuration: Usually bizarre, with increased amplitude
- Uniform in monomorphic VT
- Constantly changes shape in polymorphic VT

T wave

- If visible, occurs opposite the QRS complex

QT interval

- Unmeasurable

Other

- Ventricular flutter: A variation of VT
- Torsades de pointes: A variation of polymorphic VT that's sometimes difficult to distinguish from ventricular flutter

■ PRACTICE Ventricular tachycardia

Use the 8-step method to interpret the following rhythm strip. Place your answers on the blank lines. See the answer key below.

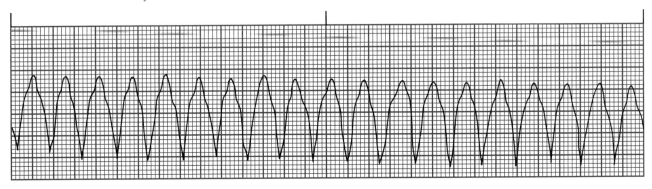

Rhythm:

Rate:

P wave:

PR interval:

QRS complex:

T wave:

QT interval:

Other:

Torsades de pointes

Torsades de pointes is a special variation of polymorphic VT. Polymorphic VT is a form of VT in which the QRS complex morphology is unstable and continually varies because the site of origin changes. A life-threatening arrhythmia, torsades de pointes is characterized by a prolonged QT interval and QRS polarity that seems to spiral around the isoelectric line. Any condition that causes a prolonged QT interval can also cause torsades de pointes. (See *Identifying torsades de pointes*.)

Torsades de pointes at an early age is usually caused by congenital long QT syndrome. Ask parents about a family history of sudden cardiac death or sudden infant death syndrome.

It may be difficult to distinguish torsades de pointes from ventricular flutter (See *Distinguishing torsades de pointes from ventricular flutter,* page 184.)

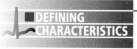

DEFINING CHARACTERISTICS

Identifying torsades de pointes

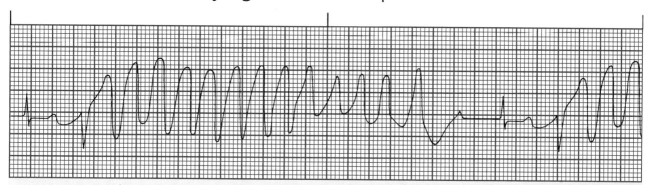

Rhythm
- Atrial: Can't be determined
- Ventricular: May be regular or irregular

Rate
- Atrial: Can't be determined
- Ventricular: 150 to 300 beats/minute

P wave
- Indiscernible

PR interval
- Unmeasurable

QRS complex
- Usually wide
- Usually a phasic variation of electrical polarity, with complexes that point downward for several beats and then upward for several beats

T wave
- Indiscernible

QT interval
- Prolonged

Other
- May be paroxysmal, starting and stopping suddenly

Distinguishing torsades de pointes from ventricular flutter

Ventricular flutter, although rarely recognized, results from the rapid, regular, repetitive beating of the ventricles. It's produced by a single ventricular focus firing at a rapid rate of 250 to 350 beats/minute. The hallmark of this arrhythmia is its smooth sine-wave appearance.

Torsades de pointes is a variant form of ventricular tachycardia, with a rapid ventricular rate that varies between 150 and 300 beats/minute. It's characterized by QRS complexes that gradually change back and forth, with the amplitude of each successive complex gradually increasing and decreasing. This results in an overall outline of the rhythm commonly described as *spindle shaped*.

The illustrations shown here highlight key differences in the two arrhythmias.

Ventricular flutter

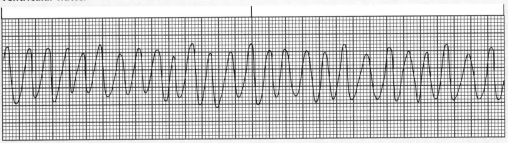

■ Smooth, sine-wave appearance

Torsades de pointes

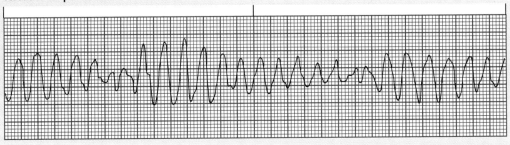

■ Spindle-shaped appearance

PRACTICE # Torsades de pointes

Use the 8-step method to interpret the following rhythm strip. Place your answers on the blank lines. See the answer key below.

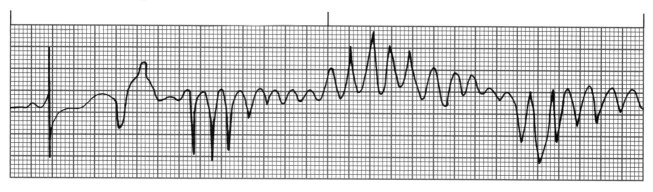

Rhythm:

Rate:

P wave:

PR interval:

QRS complex:

T wave:

QT interval:

Other:

■ **ANSWER KEY**

Rhythm: Atrial rhythm—can't be determined; ventricular rhythm—irregular

Rate: Atrial rate—can't be determined; ventricular rate—150 to 250 beats/minute

P wave: Not identifiable because it's buried in the QRS complex

PR interval: Not applicable because P wave can't be identified

QRS complex: Usually wide with a phasic variation in its electrical polarity, shown by complexes that point downward for several beats, and vice versa

T wave: Indiscernible

QT interval: Prolonged in underlying rhythm

Other: Started suddenly

Ventricular fibrillation

Ventricular fibrillation, commonly called *V-fib* or VF, is characterized by a chaotic, disorganized pattern of electrical activity. The pattern arises from electrical impulses coming from multiple ectopic pacemakers in the ventricles.

The arrhythmia produces no effective ventricular mechanical activity or contractions and no cardiac output. The patient in VF is in full cardiac arrest, unresponsive, and without a detectable blood pressure or central pulses. Whenever you see an ECG pattern resembling VF, check the patient immediately and initiate definitive emergency treatment.

Untreated VF is the most common cause of sudden cardiac death in people outside of a health care facility. (See *Identifying ventricular fibrillation.*)

Identifying ventricular fibrillation

Coarse fibrillatory waves

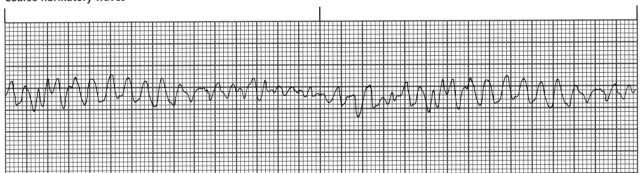

Fine fibrillatory waves

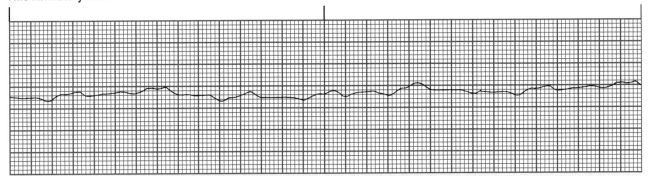

Rhythm
- Atrial: Can't be determined
- Ventricular: No pattern or regularity, just fibrillatory waves

Rate
- Atrial: Can't be determined
- Ventricular: Can't be determined

P wave
- Can't be determined

PR interval
- Can't be determined

QRS complex
- Can't be determined

T wave
- Can't be determined

QT interval
- Unmeasurable

Other
- Electrical defibrillation more successful with coarse fibrillatory waves than with fine waves, which indicate more advanced hypoxemia and acidosis

Ventricular fibrillation

Use the 8-step method to interpret the following rhythm strips. Place your answers on the blank lines. See the answer key below.

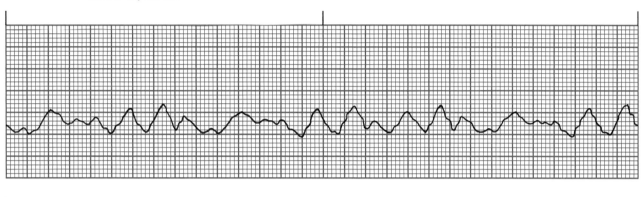

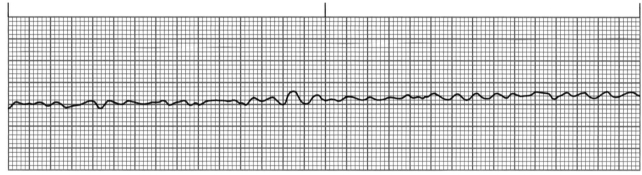

Rhythm: _____

Rate: _____

P wave: _____

PR interval: _____

QRS complex: _____

T wave: _____

QT interval: _____

Other: _____

■ **ANSWER KEY**

Rhythm: **Chaotic**

Rate: **Can't be determined**

P wave: **Absent**

PR interval: **Unmeasurable**

QRS complex: **Indiscernible**

T wave: **Indiscernible**

QT interval: **Not applicable**

Other: The presence of large fibrillatory waves indicates coarse VF (as shown in the top ECG strip); the presence of small fibrillatory waves indicates fine VF (as shown in the bottom ECG strip)

Asystole

Ventricular asystole, also called *asystole* and *ventricular standstill*, is the absence of discernible electrical activity in the ventricles. Although some electrical activity may be evident in the atria, these impulses aren't conducted to the ventricles. Asystole usually results from a prolonged period of cardiac arrest without effective resuscitation. It's important to distinguish asystole from fine ventricular fibrillation, which is managed differently. Therefore, asystole must be confirmed in more than one ECG lead. (See *Identifying asystole*.)

Identifying asystole

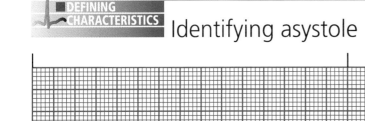

Rhythm
■ Atrial: Usually indiscernible
■ Ventricular: Not present

Rate
■ Atrial: Usually indiscernible
■ Ventricular: Not present

P wave
■ May be present

PR interval
■ Unmeasurable

QRS complex
■ Absent or occasional escape beats

T wave
■ Absent

QT interval
■ Unmeasurable

Other
■ Looks like a nearly flat line on a rhythm strip except during chest compressions with cardiopulmonary resuscitation
■ If the patient has a pacemaker, pacer spikes may show on the strip but no P wave or QRS complex occurs in response

■ PRACTICE # Asystole

Use the 8-step method to interpret the following rhythm strip. Place your answers on the blank lines. See the answer key below.

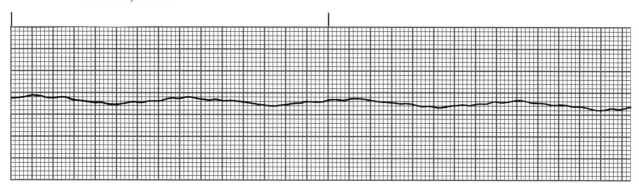

Rhythm:

Rate:

P wave:

PR interval:

QRS complex:

T wave:

QT interval:

Other:

■ **ANSWER KEY**

Rhythm: Atrial—indiscernible; ventricular—none

Rate: Atrial—indiscernible; ventricular—none

P wave: Not present

PR interval: Unmeasurable

QRS complex: Absent

T wave: Absent

QT interval: Unmeasurable

Other: Absence of electrical activity in the ventricles results in a nearly flat line

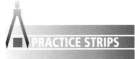

■ PRACTICE 6-1

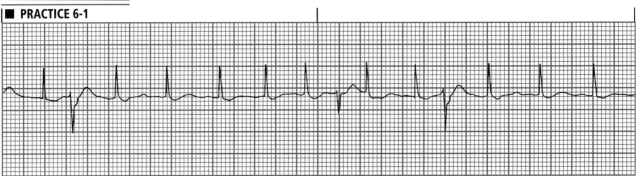

Rhythm: _____

PR interval: _____

QT interval: _____

Rate: _____

QRS complex: _____

Other: _____

P wave: _____

T wave: _____

Interpretation: _____

■ PRACTICE 6-2

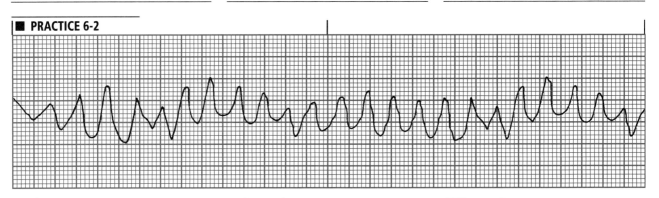

Rhythm: _____

PR interval: _____

QT interval: _____

Rate: _____

QRS complex: _____

Other: _____

P wave: _____

T wave: _____

Interpretation: _____

■ PRACTICE 6-3

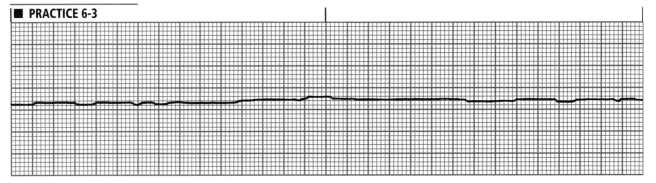

Rhythm: _____

PR interval: _____

QT interval: _____

Rate: _____

QRS complex: _____

Other: _____

P wave: _____

T wave: _____

Interpretation: _____

■ PRACTICE 6-4

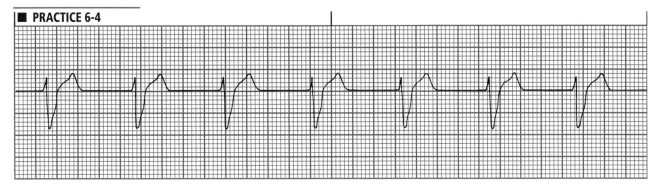

Rhythm: _____   PR interval: _____   QT interval: _____

Rate: _____   QRS complex: _____   Other: _____

P wave: _____   T wave: _____   Interpretation: _____

■ PRACTICE 6-5

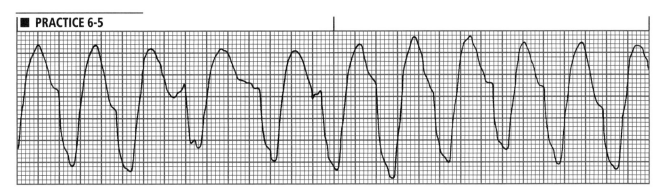

Rhythm: _____   PR interval: _____   QT interval: _____

Rate: _____   QRS complex: _____   Other: _____

P wave: _____   T wave: _____   Interpretation: _____

■ PRACTICE 6-6

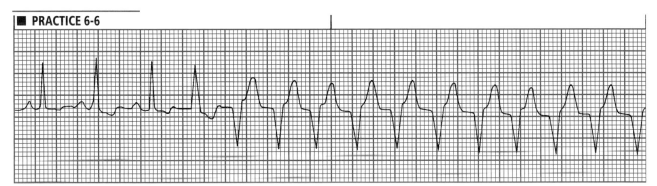

Rhythm: _____   PR interval: _____   QT interval: _____

Rate: _____   QRS complex: _____   Other: _____

P wave: _____   T wave: _____   Interpretation: _____

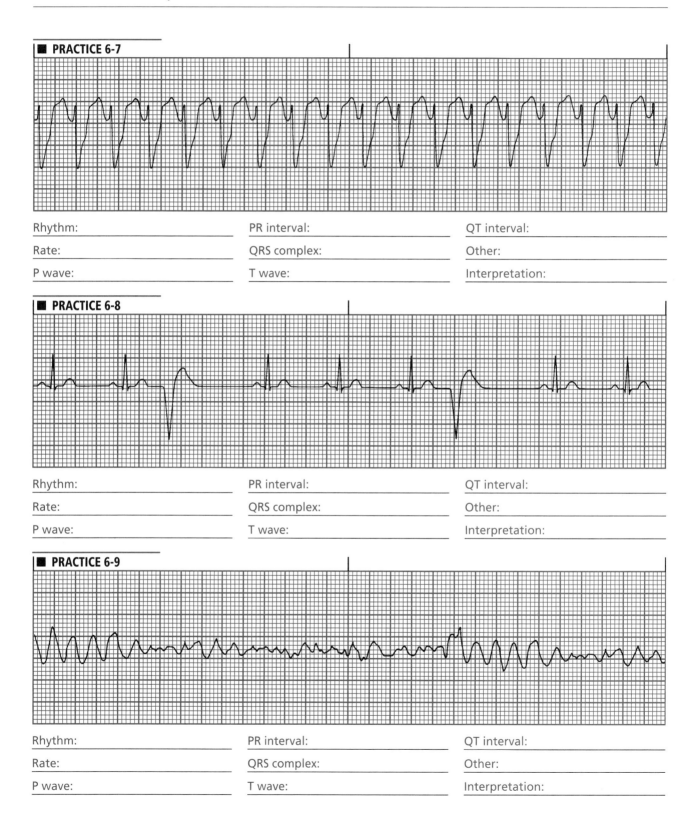

■ **PRACTICE 6-7**

Rhythm: _____ PR interval: _____ QT interval: _____

Rate: _____ QRS complex: _____ Other: _____

P wave: _____ T wave: _____ Interpretation: _____

■ **PRACTICE 6-8**

Rhythm: _____ PR interval: _____ QT interval: _____

Rate: _____ QRS complex: _____ Other: _____

P wave: _____ T wave: _____ Interpretation: _____

■ **PRACTICE 6-9**

Rhythm: _____ PR interval: _____ QT interval: _____

Rate: _____ QRS complex: _____ Other: _____

P wave: _____ T wave: _____ Interpretation: _____

■ **PRACTICE 6-10**

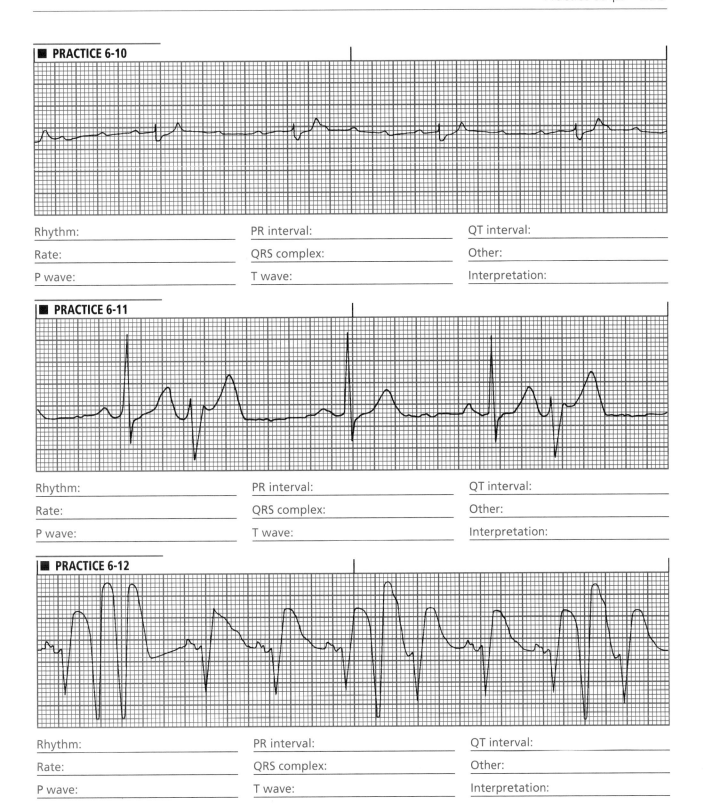

Rhythm: _____   PR interval: _____   QT interval: _____

Rate: _____   QRS complex: _____   Other: _____

P wave: _____   T wave: _____   Interpretation: _____

■ **PRACTICE 6-11**

Rhythm: _____   PR interval: _____   QT interval: _____

Rate: _____   QRS complex: _____   Other: _____

P wave: _____   T wave: _____   Interpretation: _____

■ **PRACTICE 6-12**

Rhythm: _____   PR interval: _____   QT interval: _____

Rate: _____   QRS complex: _____   Other: _____

P wave: _____   T wave: _____   Interpretation: _____

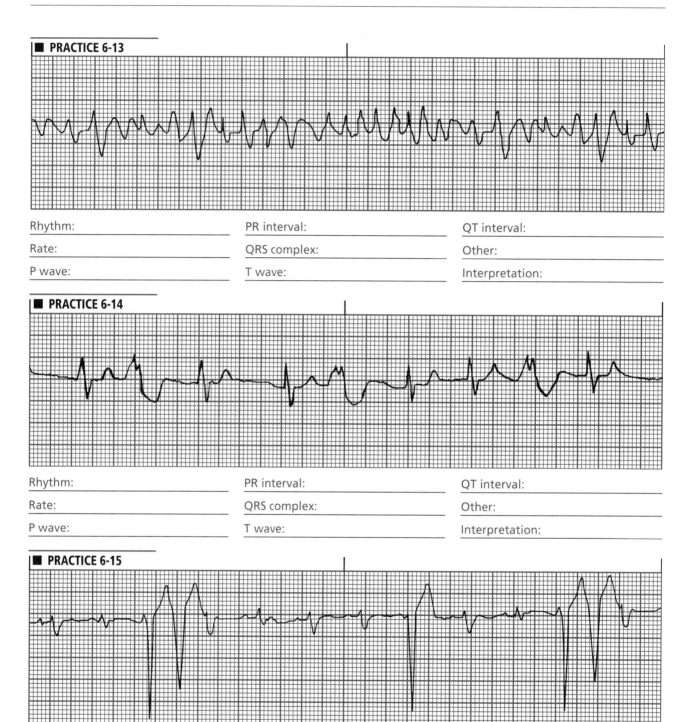

■ PRACTICE 6-13

Rhythm: _____   PR interval: _____   QT interval: _____

Rate: _____   QRS complex: _____   Other: _____

P wave: _____   T wave: _____   Interpretation: _____

■ PRACTICE 6-14

Rhythm: _____   PR interval: _____   QT interval: _____

Rate: _____   QRS complex: _____   Other: _____

P wave: _____   T wave: _____   Interpretation: _____

■ PRACTICE 6-15

Rhythm: _____   PR interval: _____   QT interval: _____

Rate: _____   QRS complex: _____   Other: _____

P wave: _____   T wave: _____   Interpretation: _____

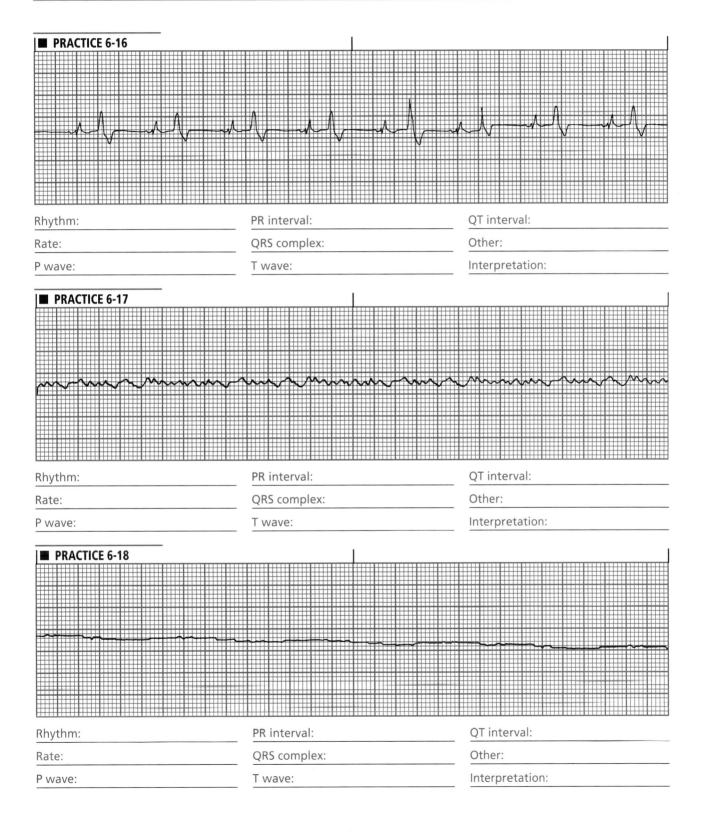

PRACTICE 6-16

Rhythm:	PR interval:	QT interval:
Rate:	QRS complex:	Other:
P wave:	T wave:	Interpretation:

PRACTICE 6-17

Rhythm:	PR interval:	QT interval:
Rate:	QRS complex:	Other:
P wave:	T wave:	Interpretation:

PRACTICE 6-18

Rhythm:	PR interval:	QT interval:
Rate:	QRS complex:	Other:
P wave:	T wave:	Interpretation:

■ PRACTICE 6-19

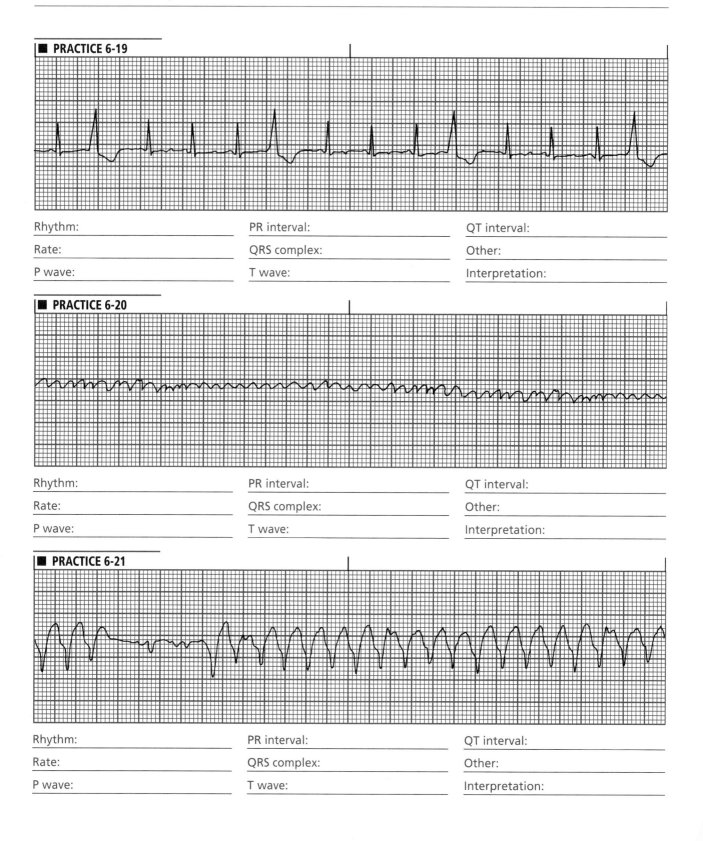

Rhythm: _____   PR interval: _____   QT interval: _____

Rate: _____   QRS complex: _____   Other: _____

P wave: _____   T wave: _____   Interpretation: _____

■ PRACTICE 6-20

Rhythm: _____   PR interval: _____   QT interval: _____

Rate: _____   QRS complex: _____   Other: _____

P wave: _____   T wave: _____   Interpretation: _____

■ PRACTICE 6-21

Rhythm: _____   PR interval: _____   QT interval: _____

Rate: _____   QRS complex: _____   Other: _____

P wave: _____   T wave: _____   Interpretation: _____

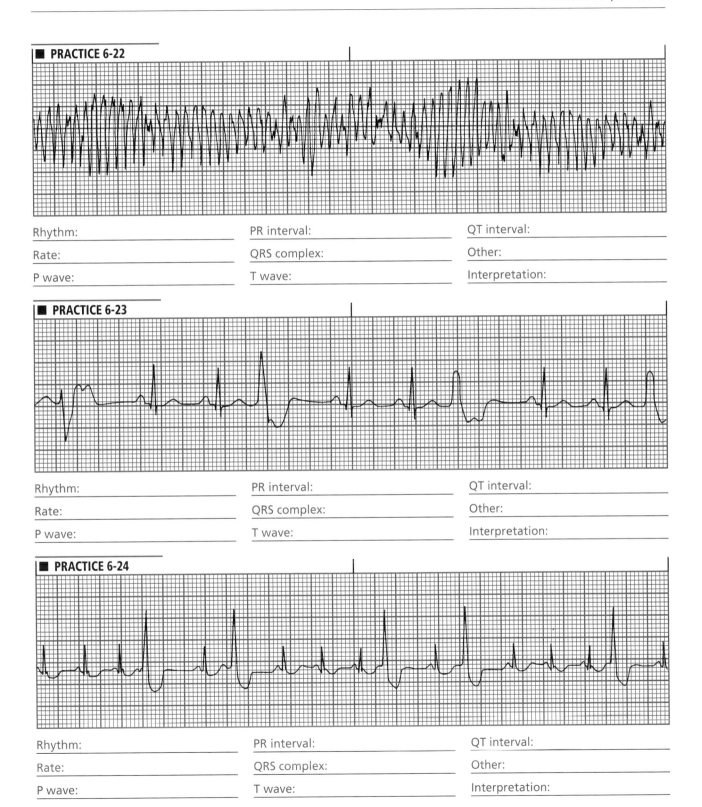

PRACTICE 6-22

Rhythm: _____   PR interval: _____   QT interval: _____

Rate: _____   QRS complex: _____   Other: _____

P wave: _____   T wave: _____   Interpretation: _____

PRACTICE 6-23

Rhythm: _____   PR interval: _____   QT interval: _____

Rate: _____   QRS complex: _____   Other: _____

P wave: _____   T wave: _____   Interpretation: _____

PRACTICE 6-24

Rhythm: _____   PR interval: _____   QT interval: _____

Rate: _____   QRS complex: _____   Other: _____

P wave: _____   T wave: _____   Interpretation: _____

■ PRACTICE 6-25

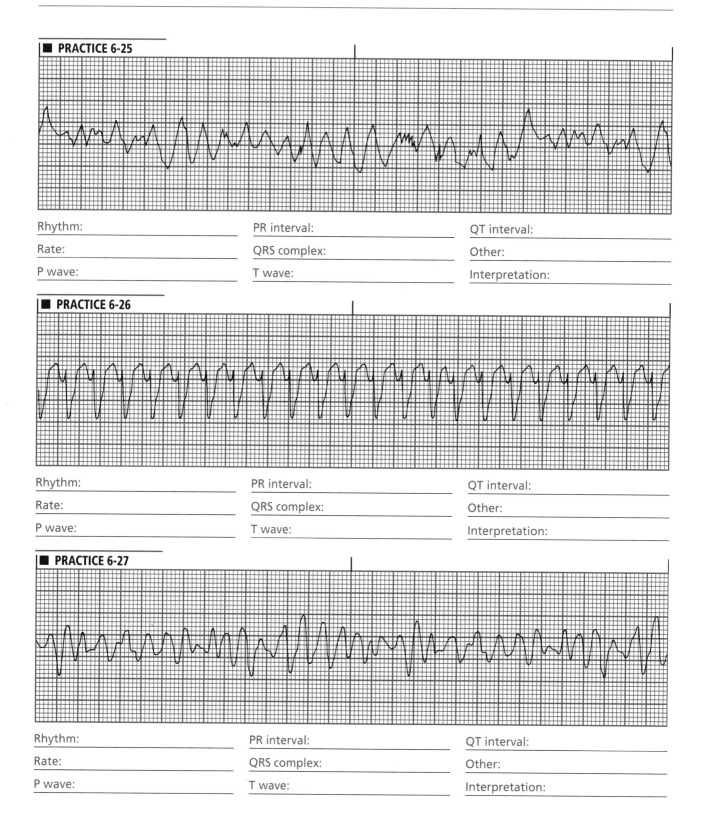

Rhythm: _____   PR interval: _____   QT interval: _____

Rate: _____   QRS complex: _____   Other: _____

P wave: _____   T wave: _____   Interpretation: _____

■ PRACTICE 6-26

Rhythm: _____   PR interval: _____   QT interval: _____

Rate: _____   QRS complex: _____   Other: _____

P wave: _____   T wave: _____   Interpretation: _____

■ PRACTICE 6-27

Rhythm: _____   PR interval: _____   QT interval: _____

Rate: _____   QRS complex: _____   Other: _____

P wave: _____   T wave: _____   Interpretation: _____

■ PRACTICE 6-28

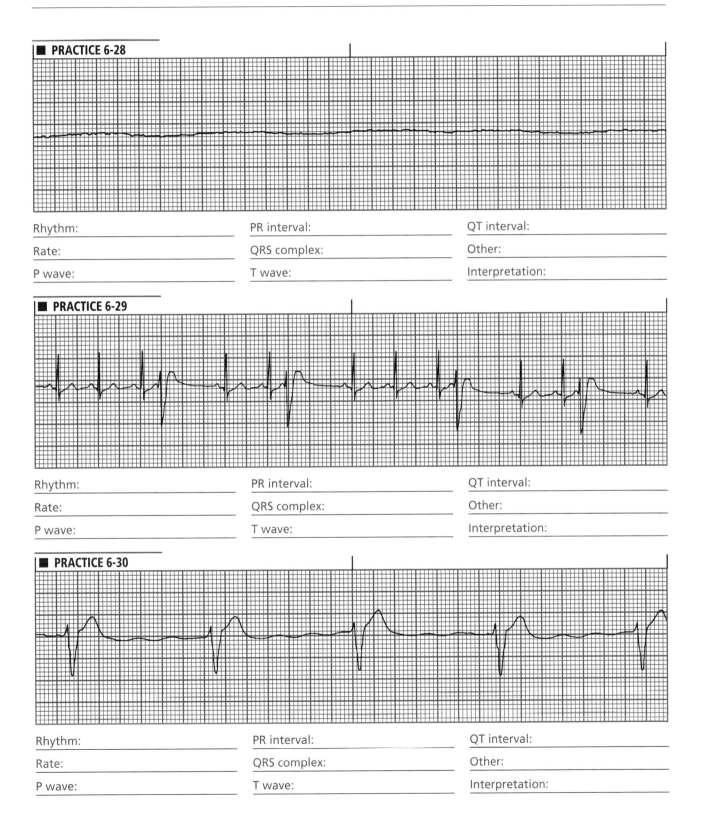

Rhythm: _____

Rate: _____

P wave: _____

PR interval: _____

QRS complex: _____

T wave: _____

QT interval: _____

Other: _____

Interpretation: _____

■ PRACTICE 6-29

Rhythm: _____

Rate: _____

P wave: _____

PR interval: _____

QRS complex: _____

T wave: _____

QT interval: _____

Other: _____

Interpretation: _____

■ PRACTICE 6-30

Rhythm: _____

Rate: _____

P wave: _____

PR interval: _____

QRS complex: _____

T wave: _____

QT interval: _____

Other: _____

Interpretation: _____

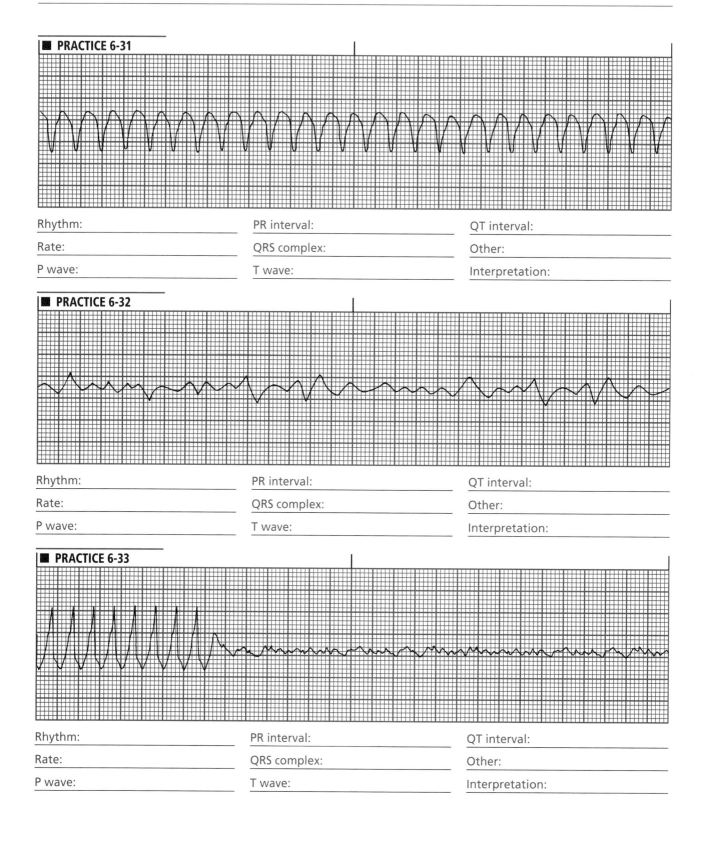

■ PRACTICE 6-31

Rhythm: _____   PR interval: _____   QT interval: _____

Rate: _____   QRS complex: _____   Other: _____

P wave: _____   T wave: _____   Interpretation: _____

■ PRACTICE 6-32

Rhythm: _____   PR interval: _____   QT interval: _____

Rate: _____   QRS complex: _____   Other: _____

P wave: _____   T wave: _____   Interpretation: _____

■ PRACTICE 6-33

Rhythm: _____   PR interval: _____   QT interval: _____

Rate: _____   QRS complex: _____   Other: _____

P wave: _____   T wave: _____   Interpretation: _____

■ PRACTICE 6-34

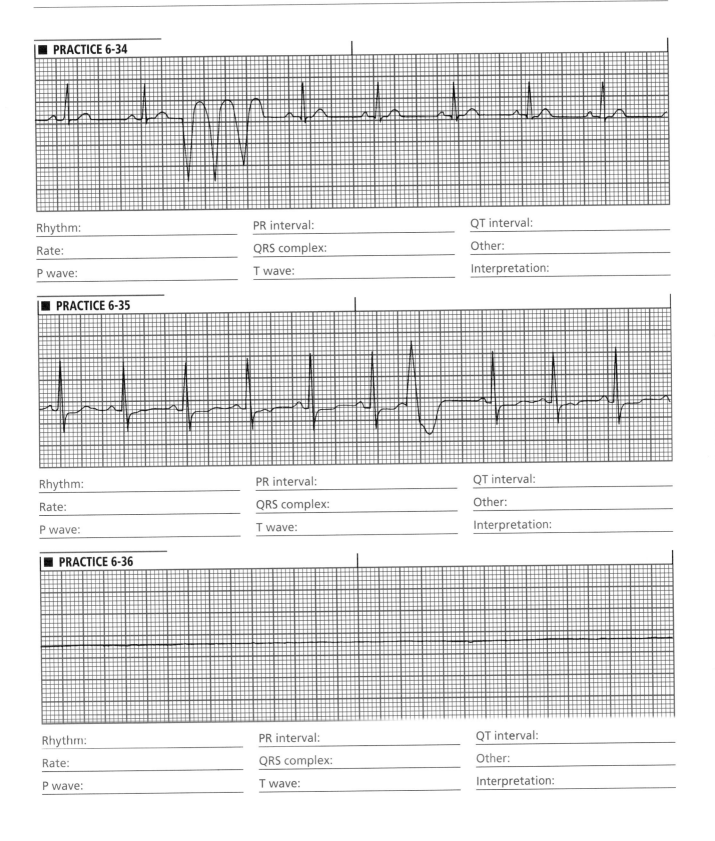

Rhythm: _____

Rate: _____

P wave: _____

PR interval: _____

QRS complex: _____

T wave: _____

QT interval: _____

Other: _____

Interpretation: _____

■ PRACTICE 6-35

Rhythm: _____

Rate: _____

P wave: _____

PR interval: _____

QRS complex: _____

T wave: _____

QT interval: _____

Other: _____

Interpretation: _____

■ PRACTICE 6-36

Rhythm: _____

Rate: _____

P wave: _____

PR interval: _____

QRS complex: _____

T wave: _____

QT interval: _____

Other: _____

Interpretation: _____

■ **PRACTICE 6-37**

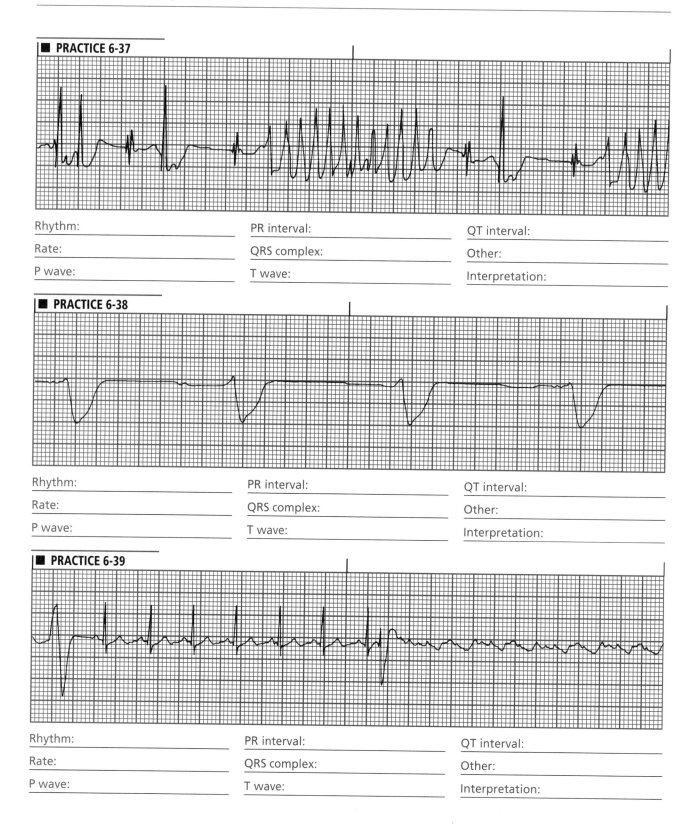

Rhythm: _____

Rate: _____

P wave: _____

PR interval: _____

QRS complex: _____

T wave: _____

QT interval: _____

Other: _____

Interpretation: _____

■ **PRACTICE 6-38**

Rhythm: _____

Rate: _____

P wave: _____

PR interval: _____

QRS complex: _____

T wave: _____

QT interval: _____

Other: _____

Interpretation: _____

■ **PRACTICE 6-39**

Rhythm: _____

Rate: _____

P wave: _____

PR interval: _____

QRS complex: _____

T wave: _____

QT interval: _____

Other: _____

Interpretation: _____

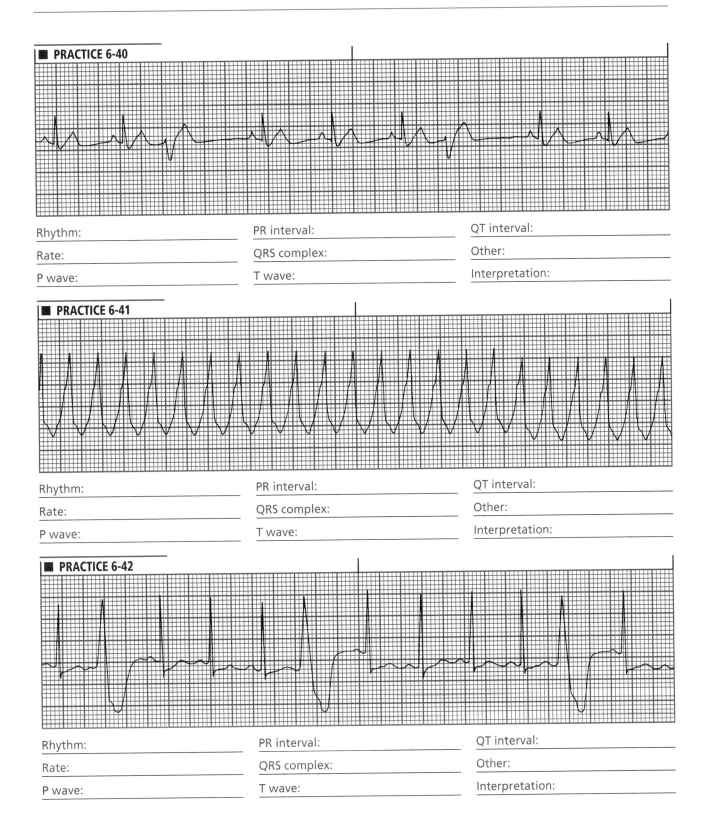

■ PRACTICE 6-40

Rhythm: _____   PR interval: _____   QT interval: _____

Rate: _____   QRS complex: _____   Other: _____

P wave: _____   T wave: _____   Interpretation: _____

■ PRACTICE 6-41

Rhythm: _____   PR interval: _____   QT interval: _____

Rate: _____   QRS complex: _____   Other: _____

P wave: _____   T wave: _____   Interpretation: _____

■ PRACTICE 6-42

Rhythm: _____   PR interval: _____   QT interval: _____

Rate: _____   QRS complex: _____   Other: _____

P wave: _____   T wave: _____   Interpretation: _____

■ PRACTICE 6-43

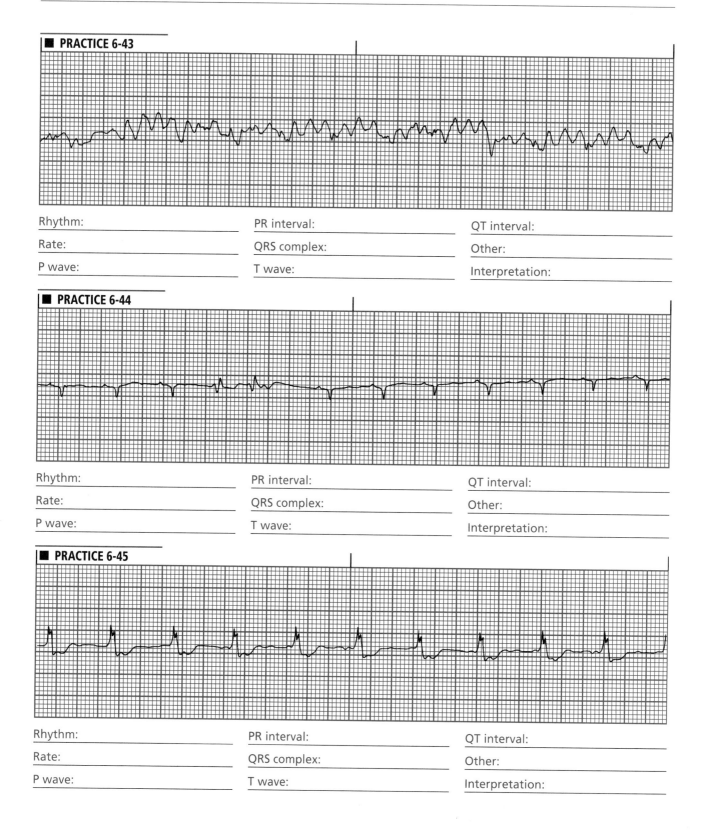

Rhythm: _____   PR interval: _____   QT interval: _____

Rate: _____   QRS complex: _____   Other: _____

P wave: _____   T wave: _____   Interpretation: _____

■ PRACTICE 6-44

Rhythm: _____   PR interval: _____   QT interval: _____

Rate: _____   QRS complex: _____   Other: _____

P wave: _____   T wave: _____   Interpretation: _____

■ PRACTICE 6-45

Rhythm: _____   PR interval: _____   QT interval: _____

Rate: _____   QRS complex: _____   Other: _____

P wave: _____   T wave: _____   Interpretation: _____

■ **PRACTICE 6-46**

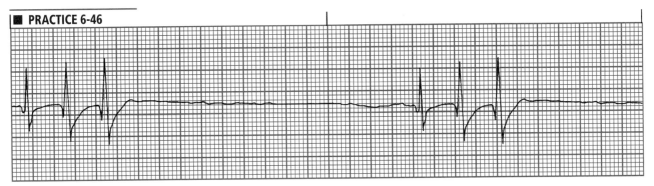

Rhythm: _____

Rate: _____

P wave: _____

PR interval: _____

QRS complex: _____

T wave: _____

QT interval: _____

Other: _____

Interpretation: _____

■ **PRACTICE 6-47**

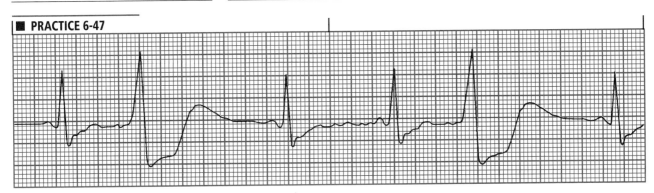

Rhythm: _____

Rate: _____

P wave: _____

PR interval: _____

QRS complex: _____

T wave: _____

QT interval: _____

Other: _____

Interpretation: _____

■ **PRACTICE 6-48**

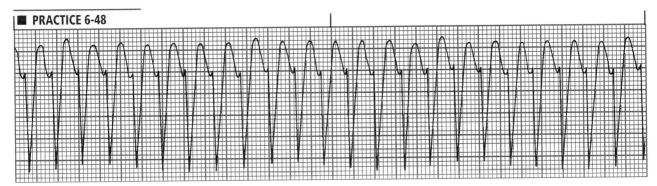

Rhythm: _____

Rate: _____

P wave: _____

PR interval: _____

QRS complex: _____

T wave: _____

QT interval: _____

Other: _____

Interpretation: _____

■ PRACTICE 6-49

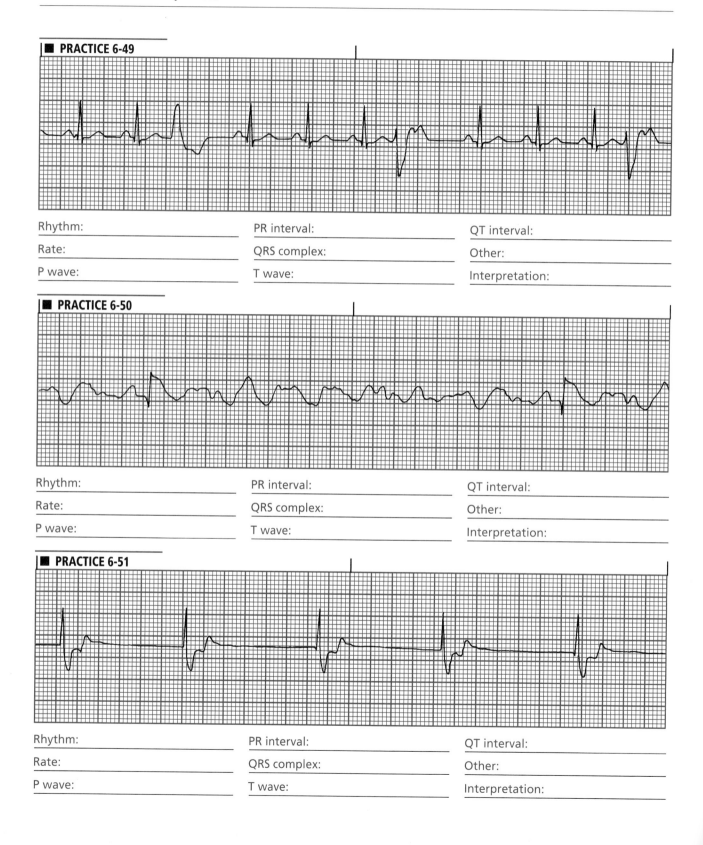

Rhythm: _____

Rate: _____

P wave: _____

PR interval: _____

QRS complex: _____

T wave: _____

QT interval: _____

Other: _____

Interpretation: _____

■ PRACTICE 6-50

Rhythm: _____

Rate: _____

P wave: _____

PR interval: _____

QRS complex: _____

T wave: _____

QT interval: _____

Other: _____

Interpretation: _____

■ PRACTICE 6-51

Rhythm: _____

Rate: _____

P wave: _____

PR interval: _____

QRS complex: _____

T wave: _____

QT interval: _____

Other: _____

Interpretation: _____

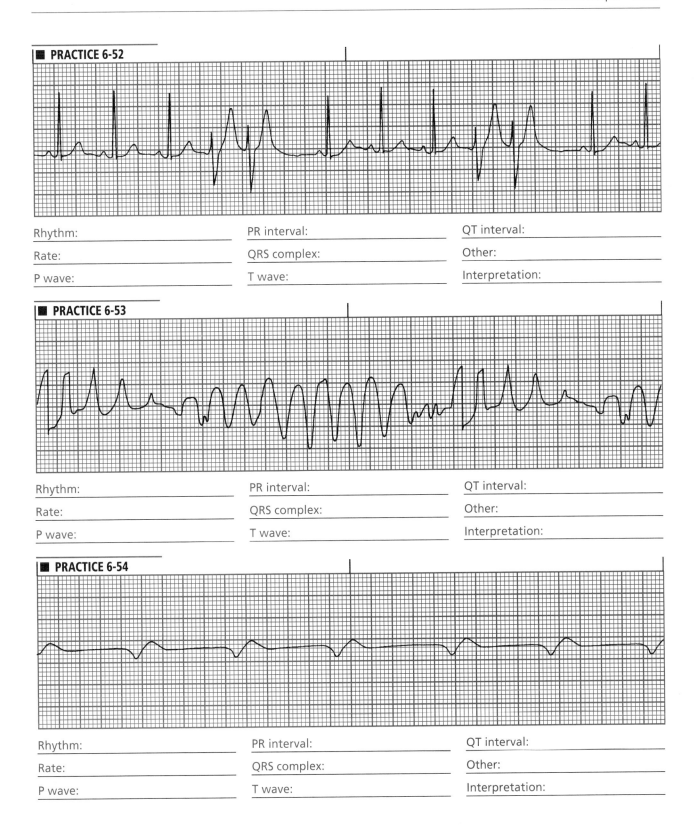

■ **PRACTICE 6-52**

Rhythm: _____

Rate: _____

P wave: _____

PR interval: _____

QRS complex: _____

T wave: _____

QT interval: _____

Other: _____

Interpretation: _____

■ **PRACTICE 6-53**

Rhythm: _____

Rate: _____

P wave: _____

PR interval: _____

QRS complex: _____

T wave: _____

QT interval: _____

Other: _____

Interpretation: _____

■ **PRACTICE 6-54**

Rhythm: _____

Rate: _____

P wave: _____

PR interval: _____

QRS complex: _____

T wave: _____

QT interval: _____

Other: _____

Interpretation: _____

■ **PRACTICE 6-55**

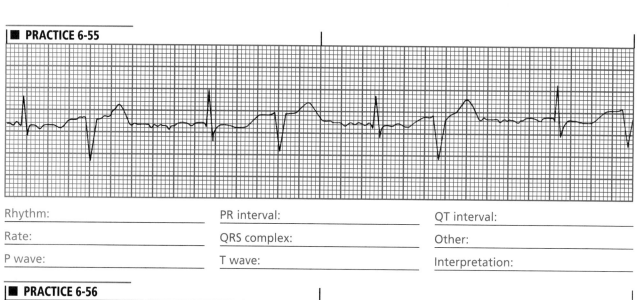

Rhythm: _____ PR interval: _____ QT interval: _____

Rate: _____ QRS complex: _____ Other: _____

P wave: _____ T wave: _____ Interpretation: _____

■ **PRACTICE 6-56**

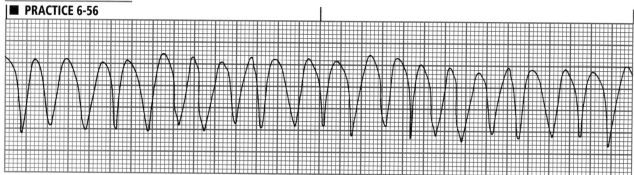

Rhythm: _____ PR interval: _____ QT interval: _____

Rate: _____ QRS complex: _____ Other: _____

P wave: _____ T wave: _____ Interpretation: _____

■ **PRACTICE 6-57**

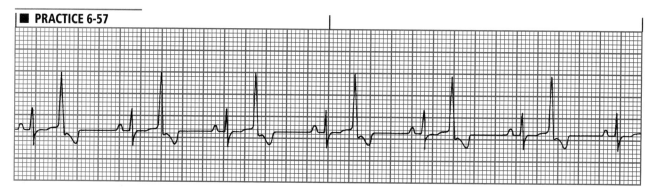

Rhythm: _____ PR interval: _____ QT interval: _____

Rate: _____ QRS complex: _____ Other: _____

P wave: _____ T wave: _____ Interpretation: _____

■ PRACTICE 6-58

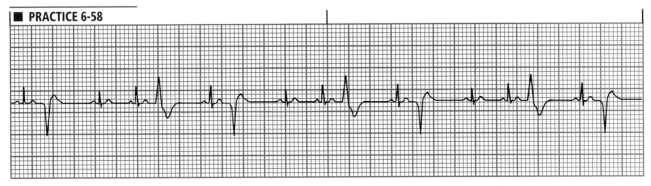

Rhythm:	PR interval:	QT interval:
Rate:	QRS complex:	Other:
P wave:	T wave:	Interpretation:

■ PRACTICE 6-59

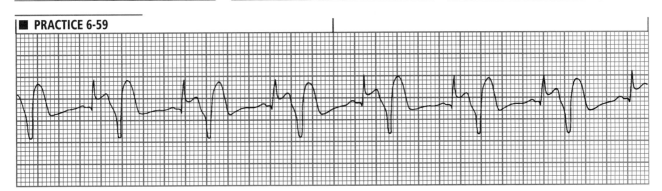

Rhythm:	PR interval:	QT interval:
Rate:	QRS complex:	Other:
P wave:	T wave:	Interpretation:

■ PRACTICE 6-60

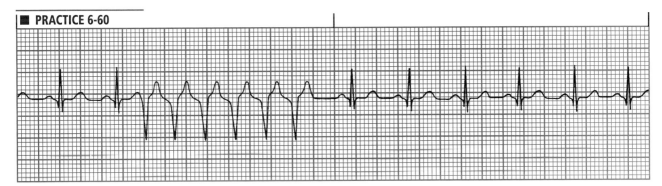

Rhythm:	PR interval:	QT interval:
Rate:	QRS complex:	Other:
P wave:	T wave:	Interpretation:

■ PRACTICE 6-61

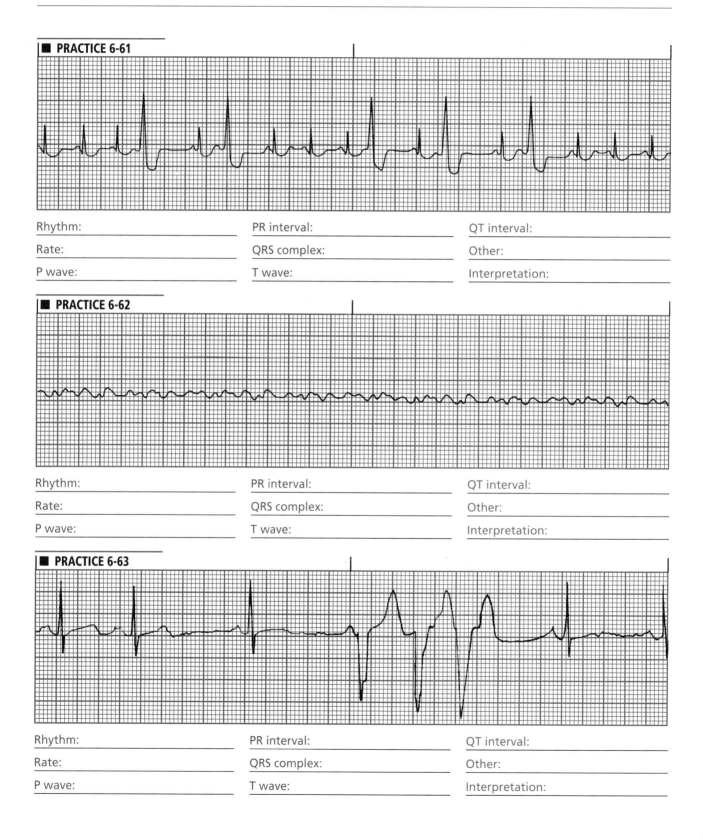

Rhythm: _____

Rate: _____

P wave: _____

PR interval: _____

QRS complex: _____

T wave: _____

QT interval: _____

Other: _____

Interpretation: _____

■ PRACTICE 6-62

Rhythm: _____

Rate: _____

P wave: _____

PR interval: _____

QRS complex: _____

T wave: _____

QT interval: _____

Other: _____

Interpretation: _____

■ PRACTICE 6-63

Rhythm: _____

Rate: _____

P wave: _____

PR interval: _____

QRS complex: _____

T wave: _____

QT interval: _____

Other: _____

Interpretation: _____

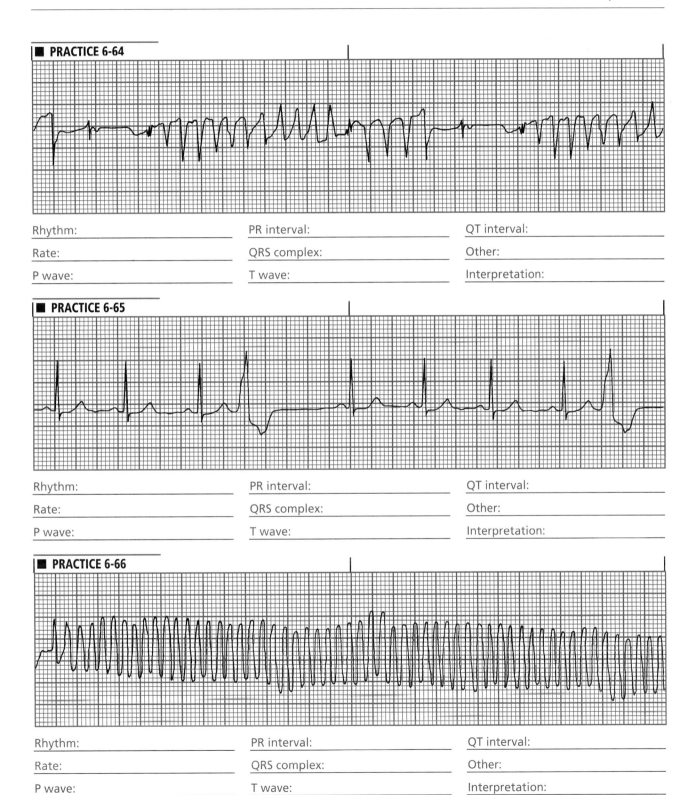

■ **PRACTICE 6-64**

Rhythm: _____   PR interval: _____   QT interval: _____

Rate: _____   QRS complex: _____   Other: _____

P wave: _____   T wave: _____   Interpretation: _____

■ **PRACTICE 6-65**

Rhythm: _____   PR interval: _____   QT interval: _____

Rate: _____   QRS complex: _____   Other: _____

P wave: _____   T wave: _____   Interpretation: _____

■ **PRACTICE 6-66**

Rhythm: _____   PR interval: _____   QT interval: _____

Rate: _____   QRS complex: _____   Other: _____

P wave: _____   T wave: _____   Interpretation: _____

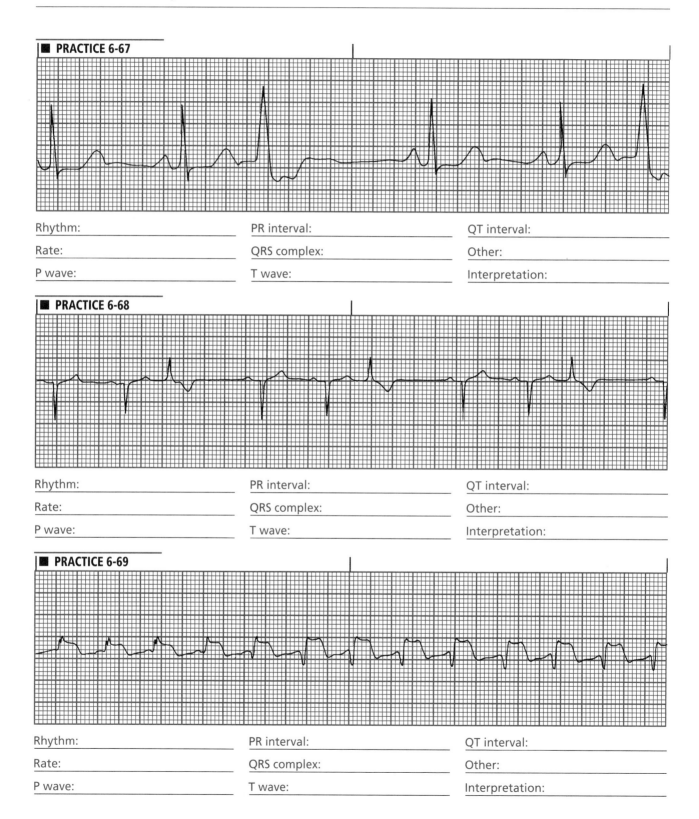

■ PRACTICE 6-67

Rhythm:	PR interval:	QT interval:
Rate:	QRS complex:	Other:
P wave:	T wave:	Interpretation:

■ PRACTICE 6-68

Rhythm:	PR interval:	QT interval:
Rate:	QRS complex:	Other:
P wave:	T wave:	Interpretation:

■ PRACTICE 6-69

Rhythm:	PR interval:	QT interval:
Rate:	QRS complex:	Other:
P wave:	T wave:	Interpretation:

■ PRACTICE 6-70

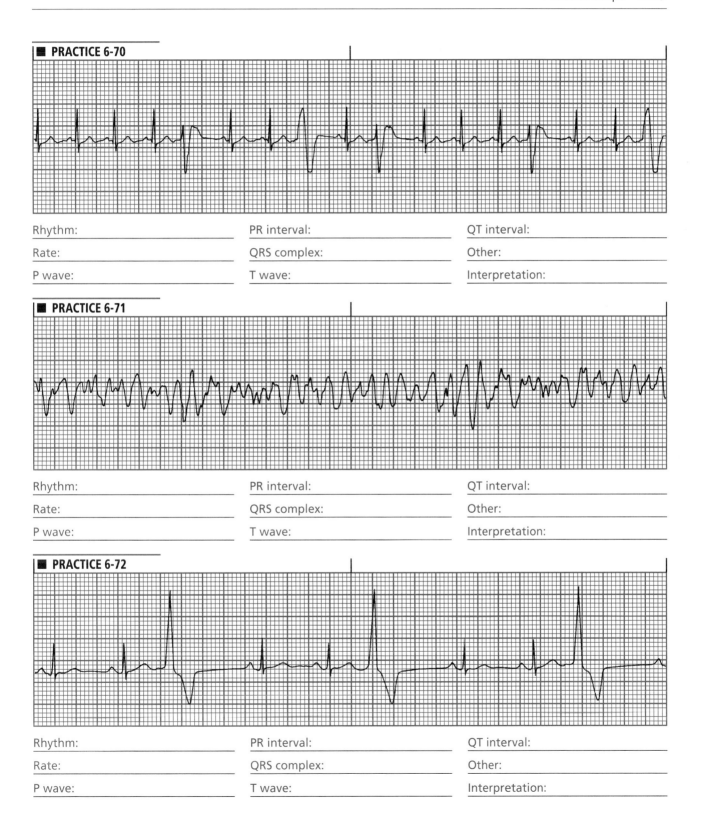

Rhythm: _____

Rate: _____

P wave: _____

PR interval: _____

QRS complex: _____

T wave: _____

QT interval: _____

Other: _____

Interpretation: _____

■ PRACTICE 6-71

Rhythm: _____

Rate: _____

P wave: _____

PR interval: _____

QRS complex: _____

T wave: _____

QT interval: _____

Other: _____

Interpretation: _____

■ PRACTICE 6-72

Rhythm: _____

Rate: _____

P wave: _____

PR interval: _____

QRS complex: _____

T wave: _____

QT interval: _____

Other: _____

Interpretation: _____

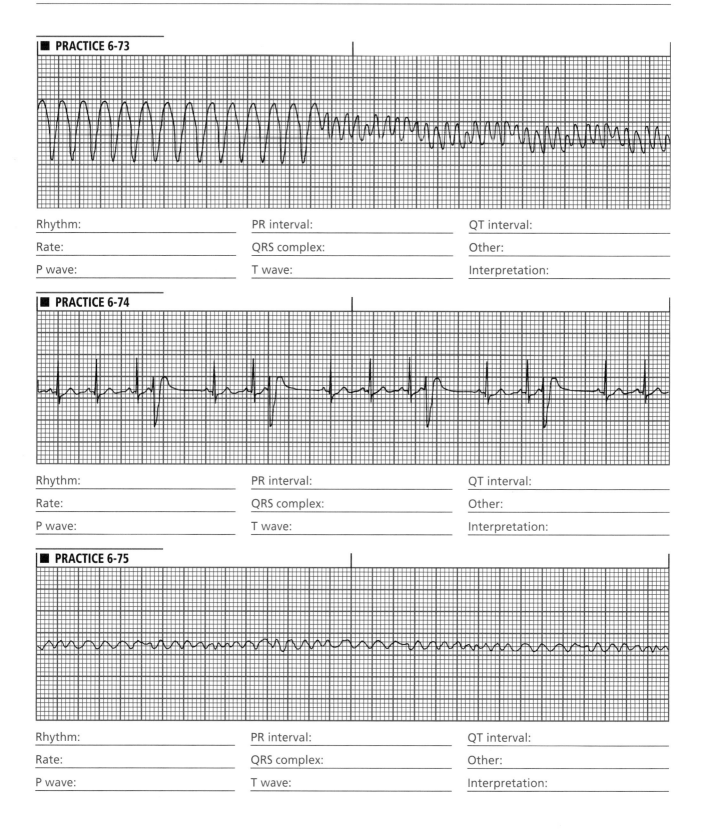

PRACTICE 6-73

Rhythm: _____ PR interval: _____ QT interval: _____

Rate: _____ QRS complex: _____ Other: _____

P wave: _____ T wave: _____ Interpretation: _____

PRACTICE 6-74

Rhythm: _____ PR interval: _____ QT interval: _____

Rate: _____ QRS complex: _____ Other: _____

P wave: _____ T wave: _____ Interpretation: _____

PRACTICE 6-75

Rhythm: _____ PR interval: _____ QT interval: _____

Rate: _____ QRS complex: _____ Other: _____

P wave: _____ T wave: _____ Interpretation: _____

■ **PRACTICE 6-76**

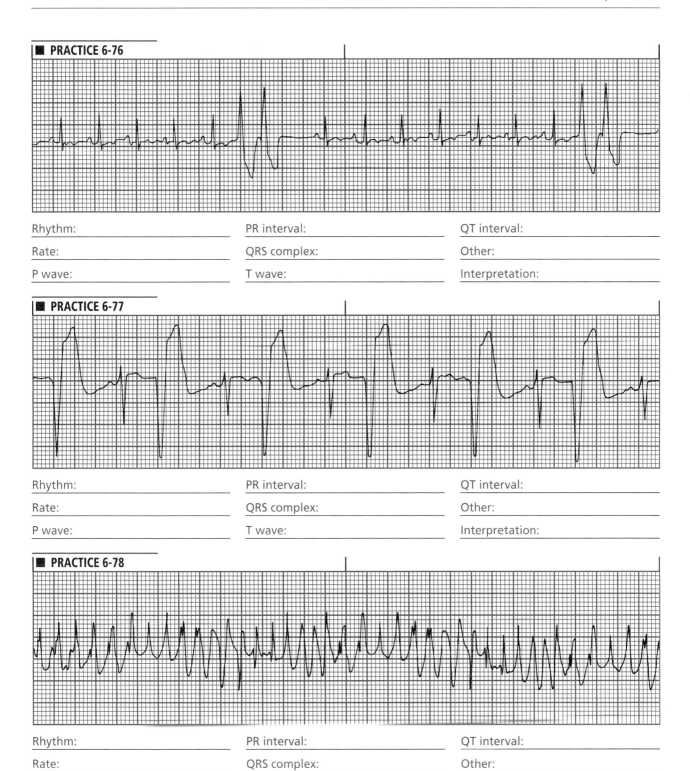

Rhythm: _____   PR interval: _____   QT interval: _____

Rate: _____   QRS complex: _____   Other: _____

P wave: _____   T wave: _____   Interpretation: _____

■ **PRACTICE 6-77**

Rhythm: _____   PR interval: _____   QT interval: _____

Rate: _____   QRS complex: _____   Other: _____

P wave: _____   T wave: _____   Interpretation: _____

■ **PRACTICE 6-78**

Rhythm: _____   PR interval: _____   QT interval: _____

Rate: _____   QRS complex: _____   Other: _____

P wave: _____   T wave: _____   Interpretation: _____

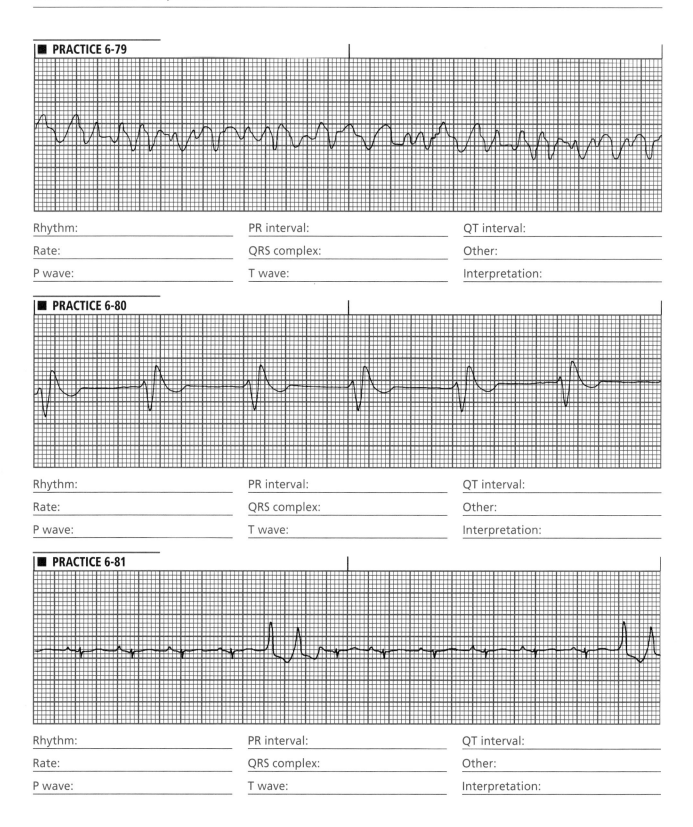

■ **PRACTICE 6-79**

Rhythm: _____   PR interval: _____   QT interval: _____

Rate: _____   QRS complex: _____   Other: _____

P wave: _____   T wave: _____   Interpretation: _____

■ **PRACTICE 6-80**

Rhythm: _____   PR interval: _____   QT interval: _____

Rate: _____   QRS complex: _____   Other: _____

P wave: _____   T wave: _____   Interpretation: _____

■ **PRACTICE 6-81**

Rhythm: _____   PR interval: _____   QT interval: _____

Rate: _____   QRS complex: _____   Other: _____

P wave: _____   T wave: _____   Interpretation: _____

■ **PRACTICE 6-82**

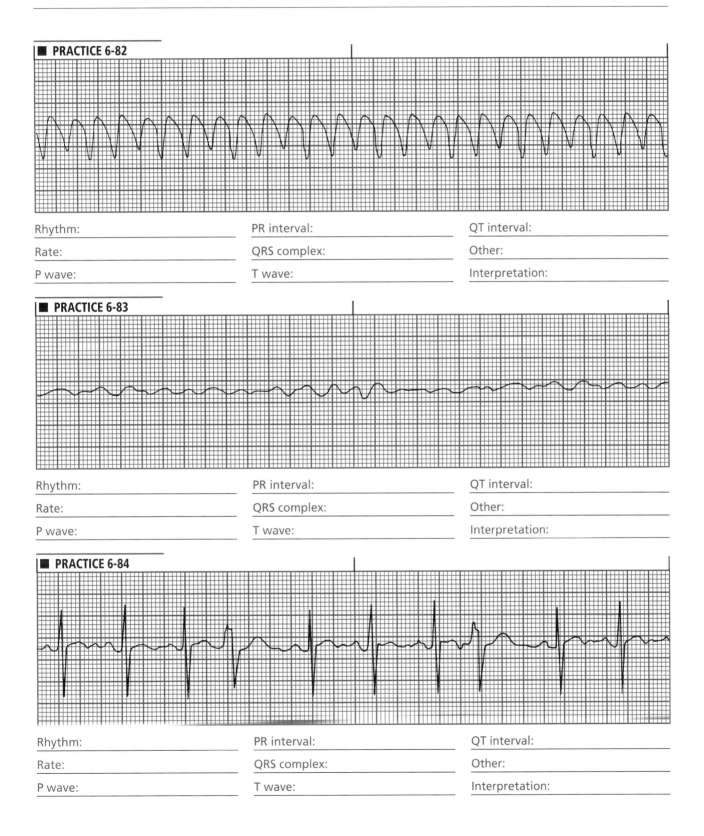

Rhythm: _____

Rate: _____

P wave: _____

PR interval: _____

QRS complex: _____

T wave: _____

QT interval: _____

Other: _____

Interpretation: _____

■ **PRACTICE 6-83**

Rhythm: _____

Rate: _____

P wave: _____

PR interval: _____

QRS complex: _____

T wave: _____

QT interval: _____

Other: _____

Interpretation: _____

■ **PRACTICE 6-84**

Rhythm: _____

Rate: _____

P wave: _____

PR interval: _____

QRS complex: _____

T wave: _____

QT interval: _____

Other: _____

Interpretation: _____

■ PRACTICE 6-85

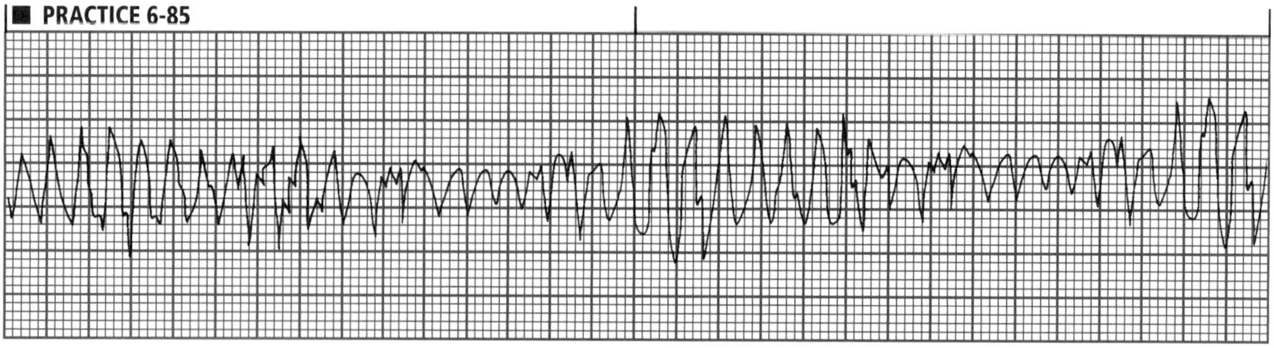

Rhythm: _____   PR interval: _____   QT interval: _____

Rate: _____   QRS complex: _____   Other: _____

P wave: _____   T wave: _____   Interpretation: _____

■ PRACTICE 6-86

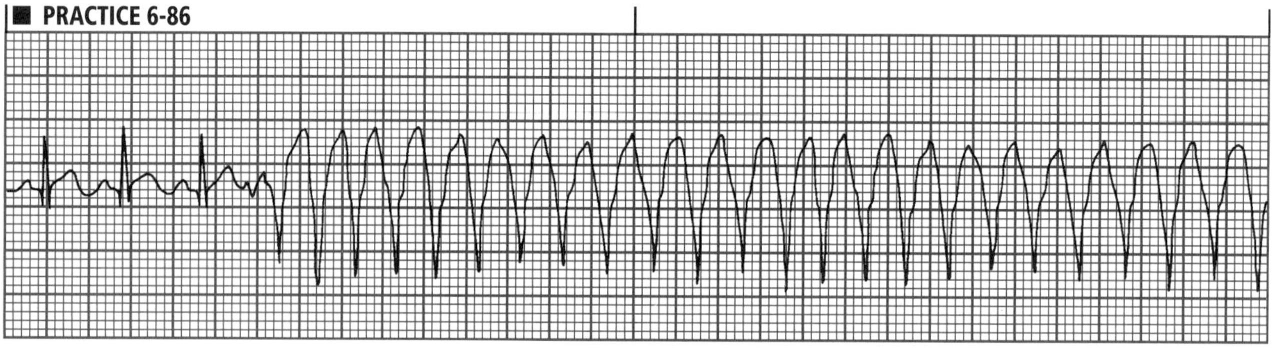

Rhythm: _____   PR interval: _____   QT interval: _____

Rate: _____   QRS complex: _____   Other: _____

P wave: _____   T wave: _____   Interpretation: _____

■ PRACTICE 6-87

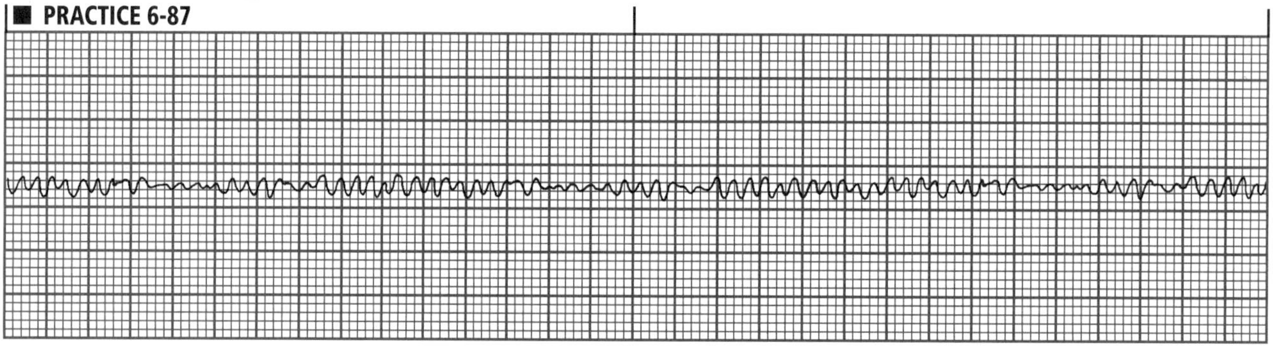

Rhythm: _____   PR interval: _____   QT interval: _____

Rate: _____   QRS complex: _____   Other: _____

P wave: _____   T wave: _____   Interpretation: _____

■ **PRACTICE 6-88**

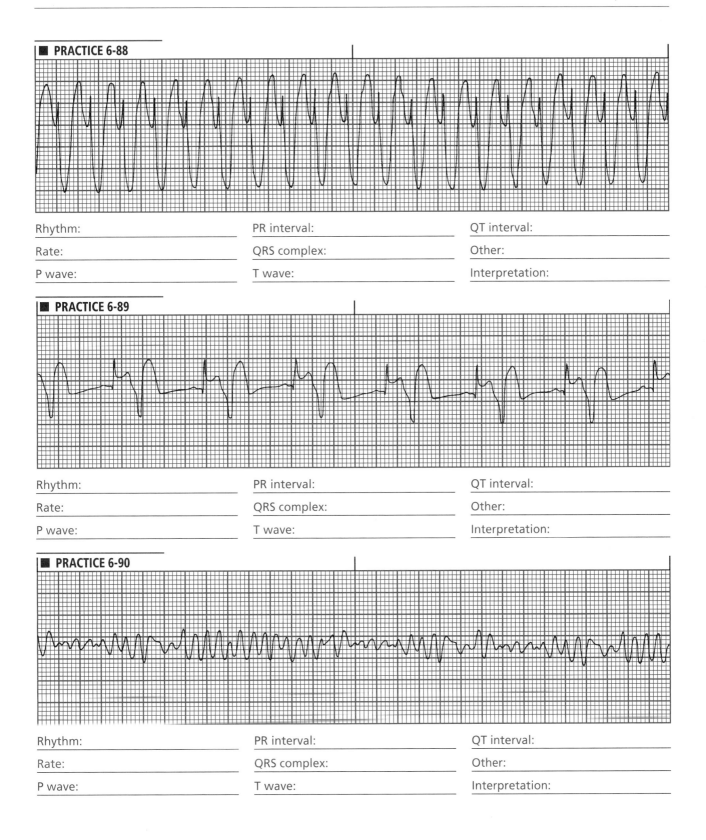

Rhythm: _____

Rate: _____

P wave: _____

PR interval: _____

QRS complex: _____

T wave: _____

QT interval: _____

Other: _____

Interpretation: _____

■ **PRACTICE 6-89**

Rhythm: _____

Rate: _____

P wave: _____

PR interval: _____

QRS complex: _____

T wave: _____

QT interval: _____

Other: _____

Interpretation: _____

■ **PRACTICE 6-90**

Rhythm: _____

Rate: _____

P wave: _____

PR interval: _____

QRS complex: _____

T wave: _____

QT interval: _____

Other: _____

Interpretation: _____

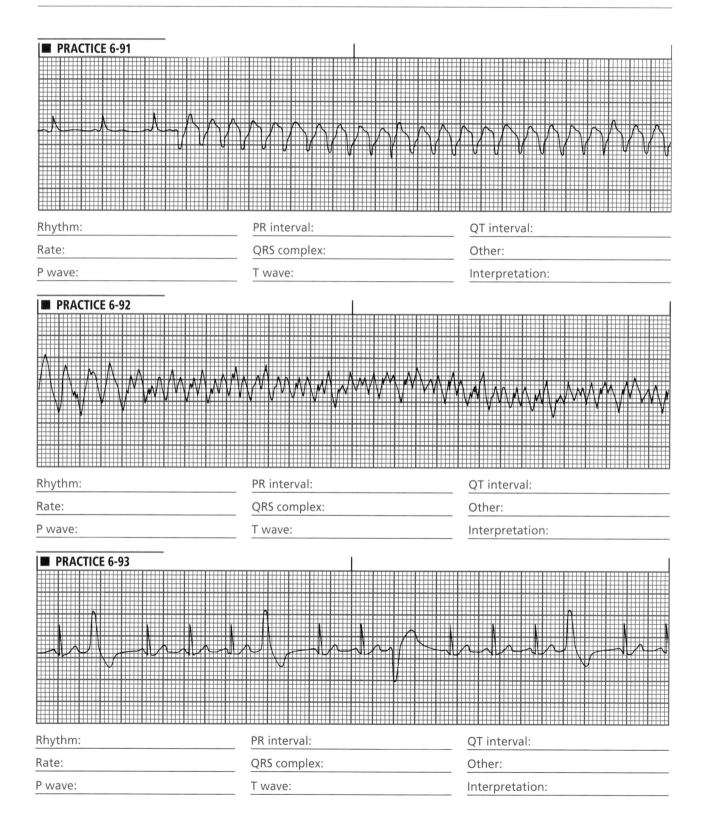

■ PRACTICE 6-91

Rhythm: _____   PR interval: _____   QT interval: _____

Rate: _____   QRS complex: _____   Other: _____

P wave: _____   T wave: _____   Interpretation: _____

■ PRACTICE 6-92

Rhythm: _____   PR interval: _____   QT interval: _____

Rate: _____   QRS complex: _____   Other: _____

P wave: _____   T wave: _____   Interpretation: _____

■ PRACTICE 6-93

Rhythm: _____   PR interval: _____   QT interval: _____

Rate: _____   QRS complex: _____   Other: _____

P wave: _____   T wave: _____   Interpretation: _____

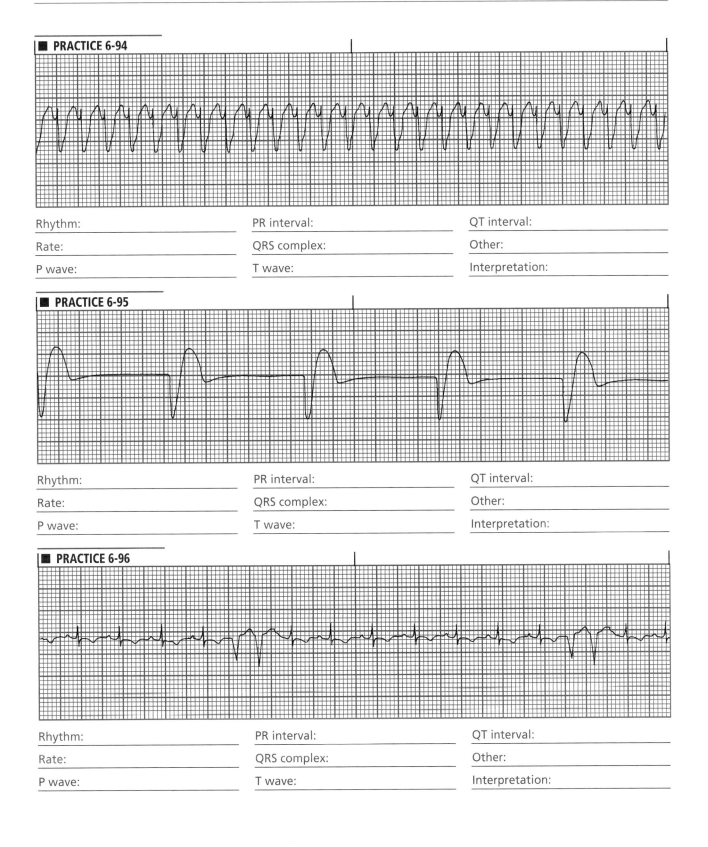

■ PRACTICE 6-94

Rhythm: _____   PR interval: _____   QT interval: _____

Rate: _____   QRS complex: _____   Other: _____

P wave: _____   T wave: _____   Interpretation: _____

■ PRACTICE 6-95

Rhythm: _____   PR interval: _____   QT interval: _____

Rate: _____   QRS complex: _____   Other: _____

P wave: _____   T wave: _____   Interpretation: _____

■ PRACTICE 6-96

Rhythm: _____   PR interval: _____   QT interval: _____

Rate: _____   QRS complex: _____   Other: _____

P wave: _____   T wave: _____   Interpretation: _____

■ PRACTICE 6-97

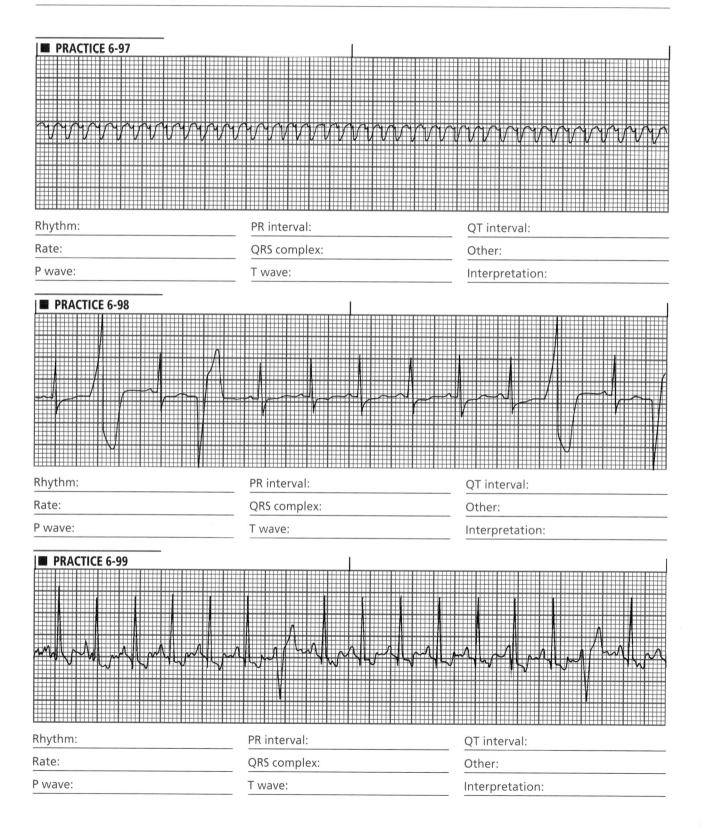

Rhythm: _____

PR interval: _____

QT interval: _____

Rate: _____

QRS complex: _____

Other: _____

P wave: _____

T wave: _____

Interpretation: _____

■ PRACTICE 6-98

Rhythm: _____

PR interval: _____

QT interval: _____

Rate: _____

QRS complex: _____

Other: _____

P wave: _____

T wave: _____

Interpretation: _____

■ PRACTICE 6-99

Rhythm: _____

PR interval: _____

QT interval: _____

Rate: _____

QRS complex: _____

Other: _____

P wave: _____

T wave: _____

Interpretation: _____

■ **PRACTICE 6-100**

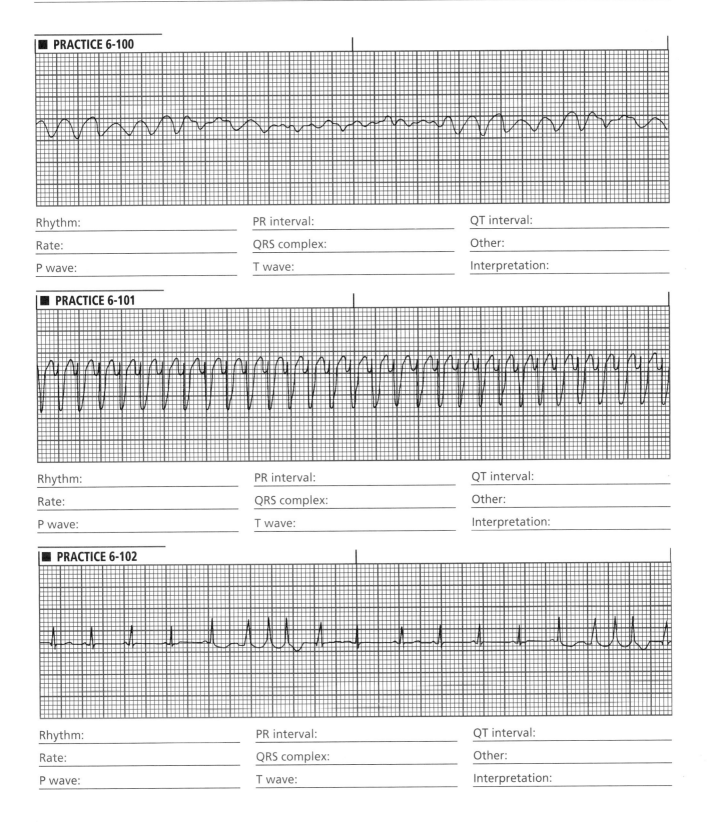

Rhythm: _____

Rate: _____

P wave: _____

PR interval: _____

QRS complex: _____

T wave: _____

QT interval: _____

Other: _____

Interpretation: _____

■ **PRACTICE 6-101**

Rhythm: _____

Rate: _____

P wave: _____

PR interval: _____

QRS complex: _____

T wave: _____

QT interval: _____

Other: _____

Interpretation: _____

■ **PRACTICE 6-102**

Rhythm: _____

Rate: _____

P wave: _____

PR interval: _____

QRS complex: _____

T wave: _____

QT interval: _____

Other: _____

Interpretation: _____

■ **PRACTICE 6-103**

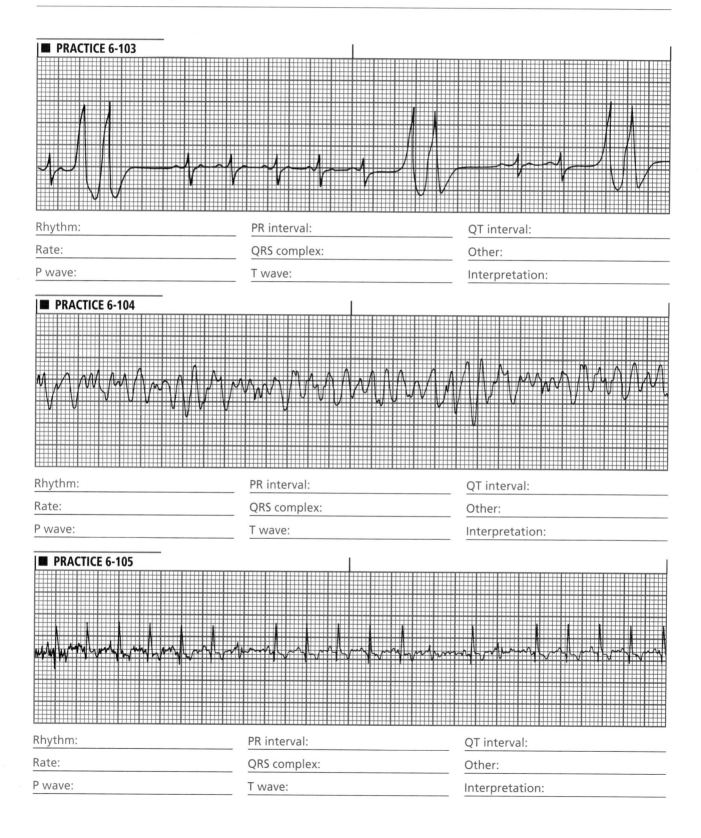

Rhythm: _____   PR interval: _____   QT interval: _____

Rate: _____   QRS complex: _____   Other: _____

P wave: _____   T wave: _____   Interpretation: _____

■ **PRACTICE 6-104**

Rhythm: _____   PR interval: _____   QT interval: _____

Rate: _____   QRS complex: _____   Other: _____

P wave: _____   T wave: _____   Interpretation: _____

■ **PRACTICE 6-105**

Rhythm: _____   PR interval: _____   QT interval: _____

Rate: _____   QRS complex: _____   Other: _____

P wave: _____   T wave: _____   Interpretation: _____

■ PRACTICE 6-106

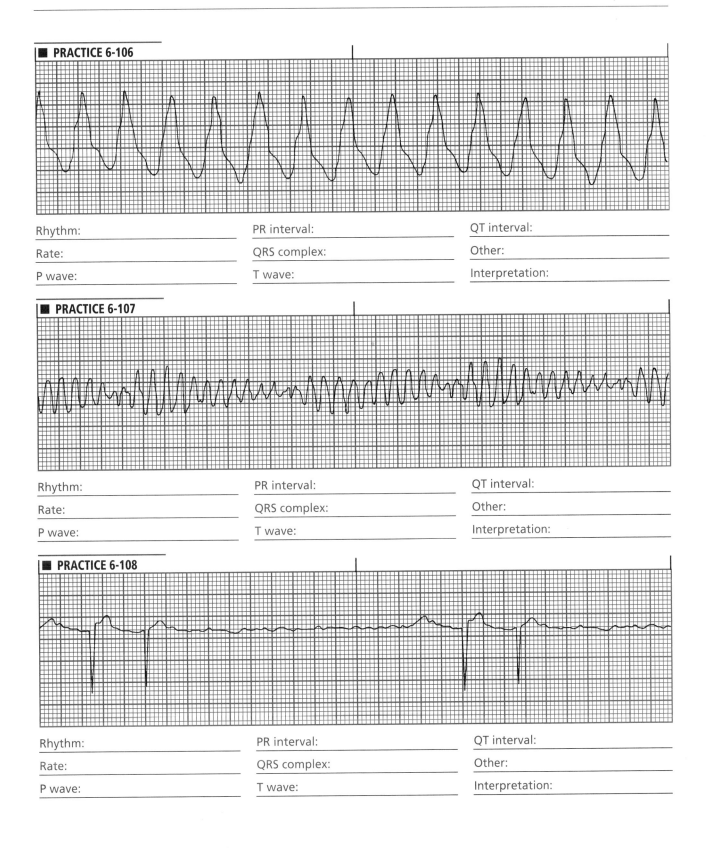

Rhythm: _____

Rate: _____

P wave: _____

PR interval: _____

QRS complex: _____

T wave: _____

QT interval: _____

Other: _____

Interpretation: _____

■ PRACTICE 6-107

Rhythm: _____

Rate: _____

P wave: _____

PR interval: _____

QRS complex: _____

T wave: _____

QT interval: _____

Other: _____

Interpretation: _____

■ PRACTICE 6-108

Rhythm: _____

Rate: _____

P wave: _____

PR interval: _____

QRS complex: _____

T wave: _____

QT interval: _____

Other: _____

Interpretation: _____

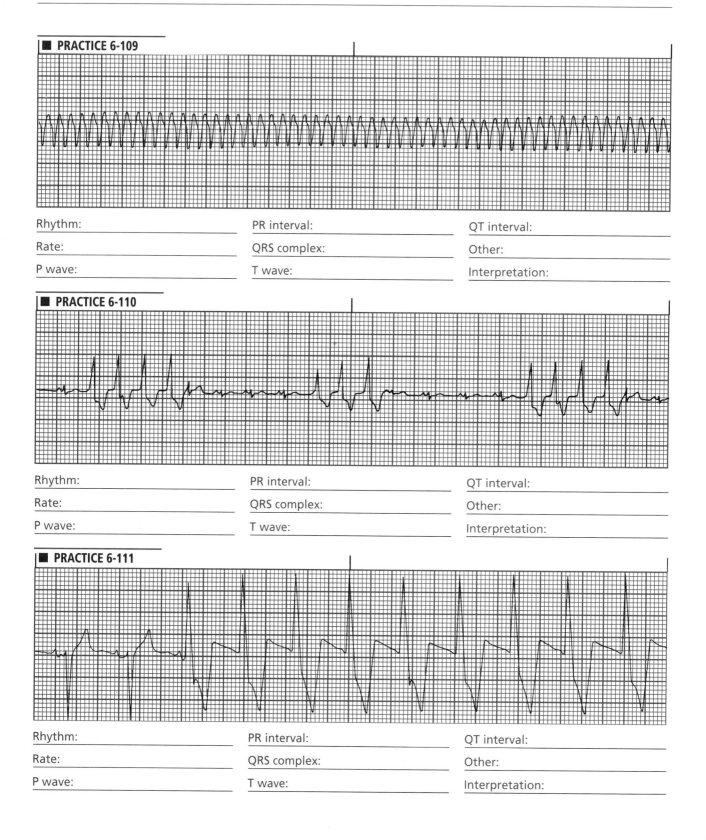

■ PRACTICE 6-109

Rhythm: _____ PR interval: _____ QT interval: _____

Rate: _____ QRS complex: _____ Other: _____

P wave: _____ T wave: _____ Interpretation: _____

■ PRACTICE 6-110

Rhythm: _____ PR interval: _____ QT interval: _____

Rate: _____ QRS complex: _____ Other: _____

P wave: _____ T wave: _____ Interpretation: _____

■ PRACTICE 6-111

Rhythm: _____ PR interval: _____ QT interval: _____

Rate: _____ QRS complex: _____ Other: _____

P wave: _____ T wave: _____ Interpretation: _____

■ **PRACTICE 6-112**

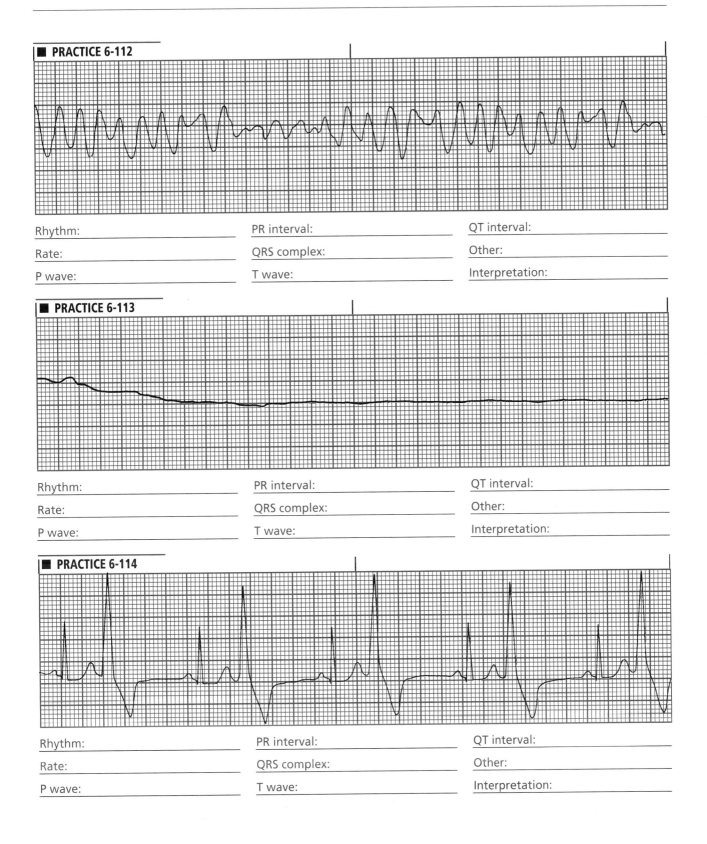

Rhythm: _____

Rate: _____

P wave: _____

PR interval: _____

QRS complex: _____

T wave: _____

QT interval: _____

Other: _____

Interpretation: _____

■ **PRACTICE 6-113**

Rhythm: _____

Rate: _____

P wave: _____

PR interval: _____

QRS complex: _____

T wave: _____

QT interval: _____

Other: _____

Interpretation: _____

■ **PRACTICE 6-114**

Rhythm: _____

Rate: _____

P wave: _____

PR interval: _____

QRS complex: _____

T wave: _____

QT interval: _____

Other: _____

Interpretation: _____

■ PRACTICE 6-115

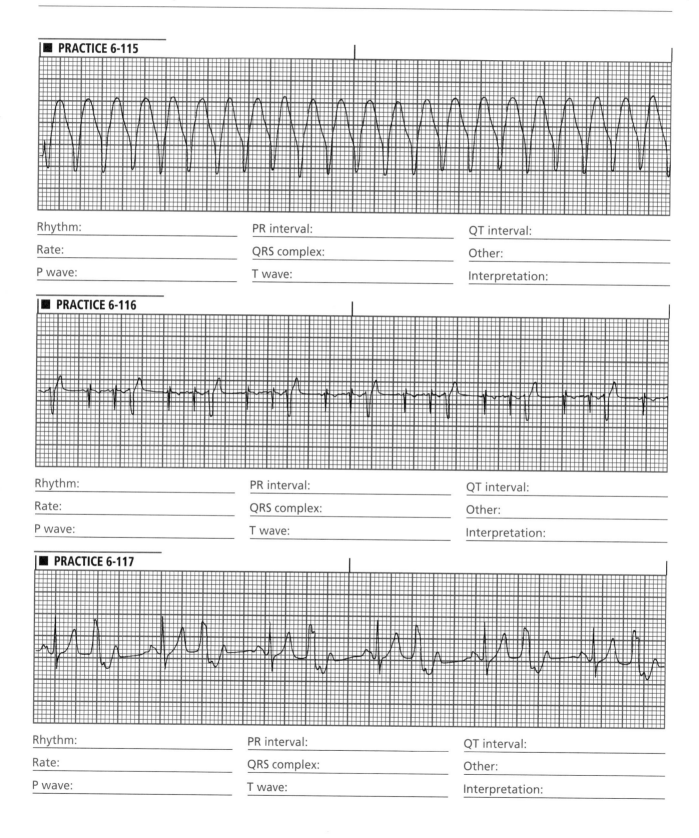

Rhythm: _____   PR interval: _____   QT interval: _____

Rate: _____   QRS complex: _____   Other: _____

P wave: _____   T wave: _____   Interpretation: _____

■ PRACTICE 6-116

Rhythm: _____   PR interval: _____   QT interval: _____

Rate: _____   QRS complex: _____   Other: _____

P wave: _____   T wave: _____   Interpretation: _____

■ PRACTICE 6-117

Rhythm: _____   PR interval: _____   QT interval: _____

Rate: _____   QRS complex: _____   Other: _____

P wave: _____   T wave: _____   Interpretation: _____

■ **PRACTICE 6-118**

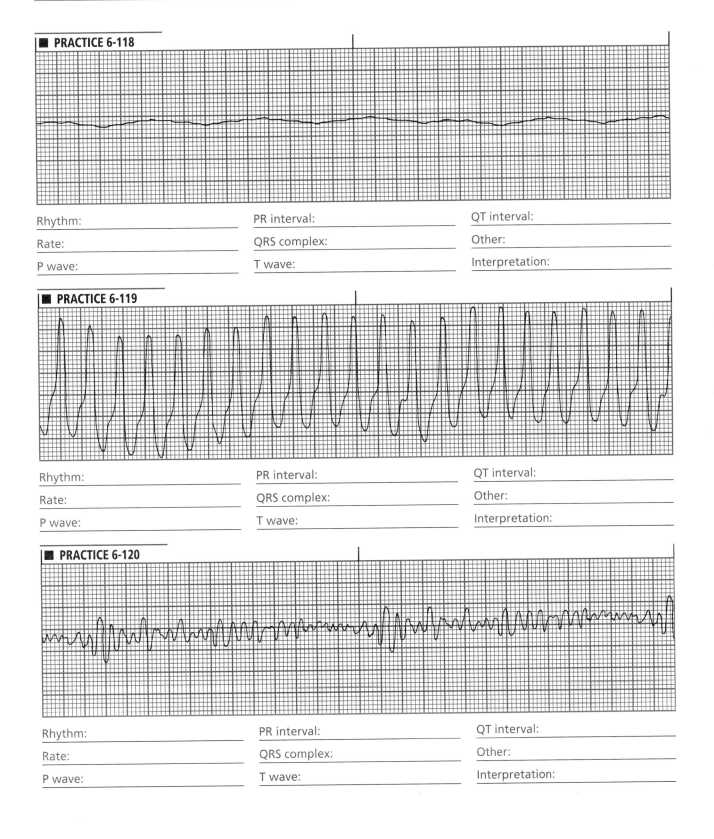

Rhythm: _____

Rate: _____

P wave: _____

PR interval: _____

QRS complex: _____

T wave: _____

QT interval: _____

Other: _____

Interpretation: _____

■ **PRACTICE 6-119**

Rhythm: _____

Rate: _____

P wave: _____

PR interval: _____

QRS complex: _____

T wave: _____

QT interval: _____

Other: _____

Interpretation: _____

■ **PRACTICE 6-120**

Rhythm: _____

Rate: _____

P wave: _____

PR interval: _____

QRS complex: _____

T wave: _____

QT interval: _____

Other: _____

Interpretation: _____

PRACTICE 6-1
▩ Rhythm: Irregular
▩ Rate: 140 beats/minute
▩ P wave: Fibrillatory
▩ PR interval: Unmeasurable
▩ QRS complex: 0.06 second
▩ T wave: Flattened
▩ QT interval: 0.32 second
▩ Other: None
▩ Interpretation: Uncontrolled atrial fibrillation with PVCs

PRACTICE 6-2
▩ Rhythm: Irregular
▩ Rate: 230 beats/minute
▩ P wave: None
▩ PR interval: Unmeasurable
▩ QRS complex: Abnormal
▩ T wave: None
▩ QT interval: Unmeasurable
▩ Other: None
▩ Interpretation: VF

PRACTICE 6-3
▩ Rhythm: Absent
▩ Rate: None
▩ P wave: None
▩ PR interval: Unmeasurable
▩ QRS complex: None
▩ T wave: None
▩ QT interval: Unmeasurable
▩ Other: None
▩ Interpretation: Asystole

PRACTICE 6-4
▩ Rhythm: Regular
▩ Rate: 72 beats/minute
▩ P wave: Indiscernible
▩ PR interval: Unmeasurable
▩ QRS complex: 0.12 second
▩ T wave: Normal
▩ QT interval: 0.36 second
▩ Other: None
▩ Interpretation: AIVR

PRACTICE 6-5
▩ Rhythm: Irregular
▩ Rate: 100 beats/minute
▩ P wave: Indiscernible
▩ PR interval: Unmeasurable
▩ QRS complex: Abnormal
▩ T wave: Indiscernible
▩ QT interval: Unmeasurable
▩ Other: None
▩ Interpretation: VT

PRACTICE 6-6
▩ Rhythm: Irregular
▩ Rate:150 beats/minute
▩ P wave: Normal when present
▩ PR interval: 0.18 second
▩ QRS complex: 0.08 second
▩ T wave: Inverted with sinus beats
▩ QT interval: 0.24 second
▩ Other: None
▩ Interpretation: Normal sinus rhythm (NSR) leading to VT

PRACTICE 6-7
▩ Rhythm: Regular
▩ Rate: 167 beats/minute
▩ P wave: Indiscernible
▩ PR interval: Unmeasurable
▩ QRS complex: 0.12 second
▩ T wave: Indiscernible
▩ QT interval: Unmeasurable
▩ Other: None
▩ Interpretation: VT

PRACTICE 6-8
▩ Rhythm: Irregular
▩ Rate: 90 beats/minute
▩ P wave: Normal when present
▩ PR interval: 0.12 second
▩ QRS complex: 0.06 second
▩ T wave: Normal with sinus beats
▩ QT interval: 0.26 second
▩ Other: None
▩ Interpretation: NSR with PVCs

PRACTICE 6-9
▩ Rhythm: Chaotic
▩ Rate: Greater than 300 beats/minute
▩ P wave: None
▩ PR interval: Unmeasurable
▩ QRS complex: Abnormal
▩ T wave: Indiscernible
▩ QT interval: Unmeasurable
▩ Other: None
▩ Interpretation: VF

PRACTICE 6-10
▩ Rhythm: Irregular
▩ Rate: 45 beats/minute
▩ P wave: Normal
▩ PR interval: Unmeasurable
▩ QRS complex: 0.10 second
▩ T wave: Normal
▩ QT interval: 0.32 second
▩ Other: P wave not related to QRS complex
▩ Interpretation: Idioventricular rhythm

PRACTICE 6-11
▩ Rhythm: Irregular
▩ Rate: 50 beats/minute
▩ P wave: Normal when present
▩ PR interval: 0.24 second
▩ QRS complex: 0.12 second
▩ T wave: Normal
▩ QT interval: 0.52 second
▩ Other: None
▩ Interpretation: Sinus bradycardia first-degree AV block and PVC

PRACTICE 6-12
▩ Rhythm: Irregular
▩ Rate: 120 beats/minute
▩ P wave: Biphasic when present
▩ PR interval: 0.16 second
▩ QRS complex: 0.10 second
▩ T wave: Elevated
▩ QT interval: 0.40 second when measurable
▩ Other: None
▩ Interpretation: NSR with PVCs

PRACTICE 6-13
▩ Rhythm: Chaotic
▩ Rate: Greater than 300 beats/minute
▩ P wave: None
▩ PR interval: Unmeasurable
▩ QRS complex: Unmeasurable
▩ T wave: None
▩ QT interval: Unmeasurable
▩ Other: None
▩ Interpretation: VF

PRACTICE 6-14
- Rhythm: Irregular
- Rate: 90 beats/minute
- P wave: Indiscernible
- PR interval: Unmeasurable
- QRS complex: 0.08 second
- T wave: Abnormal
- QT interval: 0.32 second
- Other: None
- Interpretation: Atrial fibrillation with PVCs

PRACTICE 6-15
- Rhythm: Irregular
- Rate: 125 beats/minute
- P wave: Normal with sinus beats
- PR interval: 0.12 second
- QRS complex: 0.12 second
- T wave: Flattened
- QT interval: 0.26 second
- Other: None
- Interpretation: NSR with PVCs (pair and single)

PRACTICE 6-16
- Rhythm: Irregular
- Rate: 160 beats/minute
- P wave: Normal with sinus beats
- PR interval: 0.08 second; shortened
- QRS complex: 0.08 second
- T wave: Flattened
- QT interval: 0.14 second
- Other: None
- Interpretation: Junctional escape rhythm with PVCs (bigeminy)

PRACTICE 6-17
- Rhythm: Absent
- Rate: Unmeasurable
- P wave: Indiscernible
- PR interval: Unmeasurable
- QRS complex: Indiscernible
- T wave: Indiscernible
- QT interval: Unmeasurable
- Other: None
- Interpretation: VF

PRACTICE 6-18
- Rhythm: Absent
- Rate: None
- P wave: None
- PR interval: None
- QRS complex: None
- T wave: None
- QT interval: None
- Other: None
- Interpretation: Asystole

PRACTICE 6-19
- Rhythm: Irregular
- Rate: 140 beats/minute
- P wave: Normal with sinus beats
- PR interval: 0.12 second
- QRS complex: 0.08 second
- I wave: Flattened
- QT interval: 0.20 second
- Other: None
- Interpretation: Sinus tachycardia with PVCs (quadrigeminy)

PRACTICE 6-20
- Rhythm: Chaotic
- Rate: Unmeasurable
- P wave: Indiscernible
- PR interval: Unmeasurable
- QRS complex: Unmeasurable
- T wave: Indiscernible
- QT interval: Unmeasurable
- Other: None
- Interpretation: VF

PRACTICE 6-21
- Rhythm: Irregular
- Rate: 240 beats/minute
- P wave: Indiscernible
- PR interval: Unmeasurable
- QRS complex: Abnormal
- T wave: Indiscernible
- QT interval: Unmeasurable
- Other: None
- Interpretation: VT

PRACTICE 6-22
- Rhythm: Chaotic
- Rate: Greater than 300 beats/minute
- P wave: Indiscernible
- PR interval: Unmeasurable
- QRS complex: Abnormal
- T wave: Indiscernible
- QT interval: Unmeasurable
- Other: Complex size increases and decreases
- Interpretation: Torsades de pointes

PRACTICE 6-23
- Rhythm: Irregular
- Rate: 100 beats/minute
- P wave: Normal with sinus beats
- PR interval: 0.16 second
- QRS complex: 0.08 second
- T wave: Normal
- QT interval: 0.30 second
- Other: None
- Interpretation: NSR with multifocal PVCs (trigeminy)

PRACTICE 6-24
- Rhythm: Irregular
- Rate: 170 beats/minute
- P wave: Normal with sinus beats
- PR interval: 0.12 second
- QRS complex: 0.04 second
- T wave: Flattened
- QT interval: Unmeasurable
- Other: ST-segment depression
- Interpretation: Sinus tachycardia with PVCs

PRACTICE 6-25
- Rhythm: Chaotic
- Rate: Unmeasurable
- P wave: Indiscernible
- PR interval: Unmeasurable
- QRS complex: Indiscernible
- T wave: Indiscernible
- QT interval: Unmeasurable
- Other: None
- Interpretation: VF

PRACTICE 6-26
- Rhythm: Regular
- Rate: 214 beats/minute
- P wave: Indiscernible
- PR interval: Unmeasurable
- QRS complex: 0.12 second
- T wave: Indiscernible
- QT interval: Unmeasurable
- Other: None
- Interpretation: VT

PRACTICE 6-27
- Rhythm: Chaotic
- Rate: Unmeasurable
- P wave: Indiscernible
- PR interval: Unmeasurable
- QRS complex: Indiscernible
- T wave: Indiscernible
- QT interval: Unmeasurable
- Other: None
- Interpretation: VF

PRACTICE 6-28
- Rhythm: Absent
- Rate: None
- P wave: None
- PR interval: Unmeasurable
- QRS complex: Unmeasurable
- T wave: None
- QT interval: Unmeasurable
- Other: None
- Interpretation: Asystole

PRACTICE 6-29
- Rhythm: Irregular
- Rate: 150 beats/minute
- P wave: Normal with sinus beats
- PR interval: 0.12 second
- QRS complex: 0.04 second
- T wave: Normal
- QT interval: 0.22 second
- Other: None
- Interpretation: Sinus tachycardia with PVCs

PRACTICE 6-30
- Rhythm: Regular
- Rate: 44 beats/minute
- P wave: Indiscernible
- PR interval: Unmeasurable
- QRS complex: 0.12 second
- T wave: Normal
- QT interval: 0.36 second
- Other: None
- Interpretation: AIVR

PRACTICE 6-31
- Rhythm: Regular
- Rate: 250 beats/minute
- P wave: Indiscernible
- PR interval: Unmeasurable
- QRS complex: 0.12 second
- T wave: Indiscernible
- QT interval: Unmeasurable
- Other: None
- Interpretation: VT

PRACTICE 6-32
- Rhythm: Chaotic
- Rate: Unmeasurable
- P wave: Indiscernible
- PR interval: Unmeasurable
- QRS complex: Indiscernible
- T wave: Indiscernible
- QT interval: Unmeasurable
- Other: None
- Interpretation: VF

PRACTICE 6-33
- Rhythm: Irregular
- Rate: 300 beats/minute initially
- P wave: Indiscernible
- PR interval: Unmeasurable
- QRS complex: 0.10 second initially
- T wave: Indiscernible
- QT interval: Unmeasurable
- Other: None
- Interpretation: VT leading to VF

PRACTICE 6-34
- Rhythm: Irregular
- Rate: 83 beats/minute
- P wave: Normal with sinus beats
- PR interval: 0.14 second
- QRS complex: 0.06 second
- T wave: Normal
- QT interval: 0.28 second
- Other: None
- Interpretation: NSR with PVCs (triplet)

PRACTICE 6-35
- Rhythm: Irregular
- Rate: 100 beats/minute
- P wave: Normal with sinus beats
- PR interval: 0.16 second
- QRS complex: 0.08 second
- T wave: Flattened
- QT interval: 0.36 second
- Other: None
- Interpretation: Sinus tachycardia with PVC

PRACTICE 6-36
- Rhythm: Absent
- Rate: None
- P wave: None
- PR interval: Unmeasurable
- QRS complex: Unmeasurable
- T wave: None
- QT interval: Unmeasurable
- Other: None
- Interpretation: Asystole

PRACTICE 6-37
- Rhythm: Irregular
- Rate: 240 beats/minute
- P wave: Indiscernible
- PR interval: Unmeasurable
- QRS complex: Abnormal
- T wave: Indiscernible
- QT interval: Unmeasurable
- Other: Complex size increases and decreases
- Interpretation: Torsades de pointes

PRACTICE 6-38
- Rhythm: Regular
- Rate: 38 beats/minute
- P wave: Indiscernible
- PR interval: Unmeasurable
- QRS complex: 0.36 second
- T wave: Indiscernible
- QT interval: Unmeasurable
- Other: None
- Interpretation: Idioventricular rhythm

PRACTICE 6-39
- Rhythm: Irregular
- Rate: 150 beats/minute
- P wave: Normal with sinus beats
- PR interval: 0.12 second
- QRS complex: 0.06 second
- T wave: Normal with sinus beats
- QT interval: 0.22 second
- Other: None
- Interpretation: Sinus tachycardia with PVC leading to VF

PRACTICE 6-40
- Rhythm: Irregular
- Rate: 90 beats/minute
- P wave: Normal with sinus beats
- PR interval: 0.12 second
- QRS complex: 0.08 second
- T wave: Peaked
- QT interval: 0.24 second
- Other: None
- Interpretation: NSR with PVCs

PRACTICE 6-41
- Rhythm: Regular
- Rate: 214 beats/minute
- P wave: Indiscernible
- PR interval: Unmeasurable
- QRS complex: 0.20 second
- T wave: Indiscernible
- QT interval: Unmeasurable
- Other: None
- Interpretation: VT

PRACTICE 6-42
- Rhythm: Irregular
- Rate: 125 beats/minute
- P wave: Normal with sinus beats
- PR interval: 0.12 second
- QRS complex: 0.08 second
- T wave: Normal
- QT interval: 0.28 second
- Other: None
- Interpretation: Sinus tachycardia with PVCs

PRACTICE 6-43
- Rhythm: Chaotic
- Rate: Unmeasurable
- P wave: Indiscernible
- PR interval: Unmeasurable
- QRS complex: Abnormal
- T wave: Indiscernible
- QT interval: Unmeasurable
- Other: None
- Interpretation: VF

PRACTICE 6-44
- Rhythm: Irregular
- Rate: 120 beats/minute
- P wave: Normal with sinus beats
- PR interval: 0.12 second
- QRS complex: 0.06 second
- T wave: Flattened
- QT interval: Unmeasurable
- Other: None
- Interpretation: Sinus tachycardia with PVCs (pair)

PRACTICE 6-45
- Rhythm: Regular
- Rate: 100 beats/minute
- P wave: Indiscernible
- PR interval: Unmeasurable
- QRS complex: 0.08 second
- T wave: Inverted
- QT interval: 0.24 second
- Other: None
- Interpretation: AIVR

PRACTICE 6-46
- Rhythm: Irregular
- Rate: 60 beats/minute
- P wave: Indiscernible
- PR interval: Unmeasurable
- QRS complex: 0.10 second
- T wave: Indiscernible
- QT interval: Unmeasurable
- Other: None
- Interpretation: AIVR with periods of asystole

PRACTICE 6-47
- Rhythm: Irregular
- Rate: 60 beats/minute
- P wave: Variable when present
- PR interval: 0.16 second
- QRS complex: 0.14 second
- T wave: Flattened
- QT interval: 0.40 second
- Other: None
- Interpretation: Wandering pacemaker with PVCs

PRACTICE 6-48
- Rhythm: Regular
- Rate: 250 beats/minute
- P wave: Indiscernible
- PR interval: Unmeasurable
- QRS complex: 0.12 second
- T wave: Indiscernible
- QT interval: Unmeasurable
- Other: None
- Interpretation: VT

PRACTICE 6-49
- Rhythm: Irregular
- Rate: 107 beats/minute
- P wave: Normal with sinus beats
- PR interval: 0.14 second
- QRS complex: 0.06 second
- T wave: Normal
- QT interval: 0.28 second
- Other: None
- Interpretation: Sinus tachycardia with multifocal PVCs

PRACTICE 6-50
- Rhythm: Chaotic
- Rate: Unmeasurable
- P wave: Indiscernible
- PR interval: Unmeasurable
- QRS complex: Indiscernible
- T wave: Indiscernible
- QT interval: Unmeasurable
- Other: None
- Interpretation: VF

PRACTICE 6-51
- Rhythm: Irregular
- Rate: 50 beats/minute
- P wave: Indiscernible
- PR interval: Unmeasurable
- QRS complex: 0.14 second
- T wave: Abnormal
- QT interval: 0.36 second
- Other: None
- Interpretation: AIVR

PRACTICE 6-52
- Rhythm: Irregular
- Rate: 115 beats/minute
- P wave: Normal with sinus beats
- PR interval: 0.12 second
- QRS complex: 0.06 second
- T wave: Normal
- QT interval: 0.28 second
- Other: None
- Interpretation: Sinus tachycardia with PVCs (couplet)

PRACTICE 6-53
- Rhythm: Chaotic
- Rate: Unmeasurable
- P wave: Indiscernible
- PR interval: Unmeasurable
- QRS complex: Abnormal
- T wave: Indiscernible
- QT interval: Unmeasurable
- Other: Complex size increases and decreases
- Interpretation: Torsades de pointes

PRACTICE 6-54
- Rhythm: Irregular
- Rate: 60 beats/minute
- P wave: Indiscernible
- PR interval: Unmeasurable
- QRS complex: 0.18 second
- T wave: Indiscernible
- QT interval: Unmeasurable
- Other: None
- Interpretation: AIVR

PRACTICE 6-55
- Rhythm: Irregular
- Rate: 70 beats/minute
- P wave: Indiscernible
- PR interval: Unmeasurable
- QRS complex: 0.10 second
- T wave: Indiscernible
- QT interval: Unmeasurable
- Other: None
- Interpretation: Atrial fibrillation with PVCs

PRACTICE 6-56
- Rhythm: Irregular
- Rate: 210 beats/minute
- P wave: Indiscernible
- PR interval: Unmeasurable
- QRS complex: Abnormal
- T wave: Indiscernible
- QT interval: Unmeasurable
- Other: None
- Interpretation: VT

PRACTICE 6-57
- Rhythm: Irregular
- Rate: 130 beats/minute
- P wave: Normal with sinus beats
- PR interval: 0.12 second
- QRS complex: 0.06 second
- T wave: Flattened
- QT interval: 0.18 second
- Other: None
- Interpretation: NSR with PVCs (bigeminy)

PRACTICE 6-58
- Rhythm: Irregular
- Rate: 170 beats/minute
- P wave: Normal with sinus beats
- PR interval: 0.08 second
- QRS complex: 0.04 second
- T wave: Normal
- QT interval: 0.16 second
- Other: None
- Interpretation: Sinus tachycardia with PVCs

PRACTICE 6-59
- Rhythm: Irregular
- Rate: 140 beats/minute
- P wave: Normal with sinus beats
- PR interval: 0.14 second
- QRS complex: 0.08 second
- T wave: Distorted
- QT interval: Unmeasurable
- Other: None
- Interpretation: NSR with PVCs (bigeminy)

PRACTICE 6-60
- Rhythm: Irregular
- Rate: 140 beats/minute
- P wave: Normal with sinus beats
- PR interval: 0.16 second
- QRS complex: 0.06 second
- T wave: Normal
- QT interval: 0.28 second
- Other: None
- Interpretation: Sinus tachycardia with a run of VT

PRACTICE 6-61
- Rhythm: Irregular
- Rate: 170 beats/minute
- P wave: Normal with sinus beats
- PR interval: 0.12 second
- QRS complex: 0.04 second
- T wave: Inverted
- QT interval: 0.16 second
- Other: None
- Interpretation: Sinus tachycardia with PVCs

PRACTICE 6-62
- Rhythm: Chaotic
- Rate: Unmeasurable
- P wave: Indiscernible
- PR interval: Unmeasurable
- QRS complex: Indiscernible
- T wave: Indiscernible
- QT interval: Unmeasurable
- Other: None
- Interpretation: VF

PRACTICE 6-63
- Rhythm: Irregular
- Rate: 80 beats/minute
- P wave: Variable
- PR interval: 0.16 to 0.20 second
- QRS complex: 0.08 second
- T wave: Normal
- QT interval: 0.40 second
- Other: None
- Interpretation: NSR with wandering pacemaker and a run of VT

PRACTICE 6-64
- Rhythm: Chaotic
- Rate: Unmeasurable
- P wave: Indiscernible
- PR interval: Unmeasurable
- QRS complex: Abnormal
- T wave: Indiscernible
- QT interval: Unmeasurable
- Other: Complex size increases and decreases
- Interpretation: Torsades de pointes

PRACTICE 6-65
- Rhythm: Irregular
- Rate: 90 beats/minute
- P wave: Normal with sinus beats
- PR interval: 0.12 second
- QRS complex: 0.06 second
- T wave: Normal
- QT interval: 0.34 second
- Other: None
- Interpretation: NSR with PVC

PRACTICE 6-66
- Rhythm: Chaotic
- Rate: Greater than 300 beats/minute
- P wave: Indiscernible
- PR interval: Unmeasurable
- QRS complex: Abnormal
- T wave: Indiscernible
- QT interval: Unmeasurable
- Other: None
- Interpretation: VT

PRACTICE 6-67
- Rhythm: Irregular
- Rate: 60 beats/minute
- P wave: Normal with sinus beats
- PR interval: 0.24 second
- QRS complex: 0.12 second
- T wave: Normal
- QT interval: 0.56 second
- Other: None
- Interpretation: Sinus bradycardia with first-degree AV block and PVC

PRACTICE 6-68
- Rhythm: Irregular
- Rate: 90 beats/minute
- P wave: Normal with sinus beats
- PR interval: 0.16 second
- QRS complex: 0.06 second
- T wave: Normal
- QT interval: 0.28 second
- Other: None
- Interpretation: NSR with PVCs (trigemipy)

PRACTICE 6-69
- Rhythm: Regular
- Rate: 125 beats/minute
- P wave: Indiscernible
- PR interval: Unmeasurable
- QRS complex: 0.08 second
- T wave: Indiscernible
- QT interval: Unmeasurable
- Other: None
- Interpretation: AIVR

PRACTICE 6-70
- Rhythm: Irregular
- Rate: 170 beats/minute
- P wave: Normal with sinus beats
- PR interval: 0.12 second
- QRS complex: 0.04 second
- T wave: Normal
- QT interval: 0.20 second
- Other: None
- Interpretation: Sinus tachycardia with multifocal PVCs

PRACTICE 6-71
- Rhythm: Chaotic
- Rate: Unmeasurable
- P wave: Indiscernible
- PR interval: Unmeasurable
- QRS complex: Indiscernible
- T wave: Indiscernible
- QT interval: Unmeasurable
- Other: None
- Interpretation: VF

PRACTICE 6-72
- Rhythm: Irregular
- Rate: 90 beats/minute
- P wave: Normal with sinus beats
- PR interval: 0.16 second
- QRS complex: 0.06 second
- T wave: Normal
- QT interval: 0.28 second
- Other: None
- Interpretation: NSR with PVCs (trigeminy)

PRACTICE 6-73
- Rhythm: Chaotic
- Rate: Unmeasurable
- P wave: Indiscernible
- PR interval: Unmeasurable
- QRS complex: Abnormal
- T wave: Indiscernible
- QT interval: Unmeasurable
- Other: None
- Interpretation: VT leading into VF

PRACTICE 6-74
- Rhythm: Irregular
- Rate: 160 beats/minute
- P wave: Normal with sinus beats
- PR interval: 0.10 second
- QRS complex: 0.04 second
- T wave: Normal
- QT interval: 0.20 second
- Other: None
- Interpretation: Sinus tachycardia with PVCs

PRACTICE 6-75
- Rhythm: Chaotic
- Rate: Unmeasurable
- P wave: Indiscernible
- PR interval: Unmeasurable
- QRS complex: Indiscernible
- T wave: Indiscernible
- QT interval: Unmeasurable
- Other: None
- Interpretation: VF

PRACTICE 6-76
- Rhythm: Irregular
- Rate: 160 beats/minute
- P wave: Normal with sinus beats
- PR interval: 0.12 second
- QRS complex: 0.04 second
- T wave: Normal
- QT interval: 0.16 second
- Other: None
- Interpretation: Sinus tachycardia with PVCs (couplet)

PRACTICE 6-77
- Rhythm: Irregular
- Rate: 120 beats/minute
- P wave: Normal
- PR interval: 0.12 second
- QRS complex: 0.08 second
- T wave: Normal
- QT interval: 0.24 second
- Other: None
- Interpretation: NSR with PVCs (bigeminy)

PRACTICE 6-78
- Rhythm: Chaotic
- Rate: Unmeasurable
- P wave: Indiscernible
- PR interval: Unmeasurable
- QRS complex: Abnormal
- T wave: Indiscernible
- QT interval: Unmeasurable
- Other: Complex size increases and decreases
- Interpretation: Torsades de pointes

PRACTICE 6-79
- Rhythm: Chaotic
- Rate: Unmeasurable
- P wave: Indiscernible
- PR interval: Unmeasurable
- QRS complex: Indiscernible
- T wave: Indiscernible
- QT interval: Unmeasurable
- Other: None
- Interpretation: VF

PRACTICE 6-80
- Rhythm: Regular
- Rate: 60 beats/minute
- P wave: Indiscernible
- PR interval: Unmeasurable
- QRS complex: 0.20 second
- T wave: Inverted
- QT interval: 0.40 second
- Other: None
- Interpretation: AIVR

PRACTICE 6-81
- Rhythm: Irregular
- Rate: 140 beats/minute
- P wave: Normal with sinus beats
- PR interval: 0.16 second
- QRS complex: 0.06 second
- T wave: Normal
- QT interval: 0.24 second
- Other: None
- Interpretation: Sinus tachycardia with PVCs (pair)

PRACTICE 6-82
- Rhythm: Regular
- Rate: 250 beats/minute
- P wave: Indiscernible
- PR interval: Unmeasurable
- QRS complex: 0.14 second
- T wave: Indiscernible
- QT interval: Unmeasurable
- Other: None
- Interpretation: VT

PRACTICE 6-83
- Rhythm: Chaotic
- Rate: Unmeasurable
- P wave: Indiscernible
- PR interval: Unmeasurable
- QRS complex: Indiscernible
- T wave: Indiscernible
- QT interval: Unmeasurable
- Other: None
- Interpretation: VF

PRACTICE 6-84
- Rhythm: Irregular
- Rate: 100 beats/minute
- P wave: Normal with sinus beats
- PR interval: 0.16 second
- QRS complex: 0.08 second
- T wave: Normal
- QT interval: 0.28 second
- Other: None
- Interpretation: Sinus tachycardia with PVCs

PRACTICE 6-85
- Rhythm: Chaotic
- Rate: Unmeasurable
- P wave: Indiscernible
- PR interval: Unmeasurable
- QRS complex: Abnormal
- T wave: Indiscernible
- QT interval: Unmeasurable
- Other: None
- Interpretation: Torsades de pointes

PRACTICE 6-86
- Rhythm: Irregular
- Rate: 270 beats/minute with ventricular rhythm
- P wave: Normal with sinus beats
- PR interval: 0.12 second
- QRS complex: 0.06 second
- T wave: Normal
- QT interval: 0.24 second
- Other: None
- Interpretation: Sinus tachycardia leading to VT

PRACTICE 6-87
- Rhythm: Chaotic
- Rate: Unmeasurable
- P wave: Indiscernible
- PR interval: Unmeasurable
- QRS complex: Indiscernible
- T wave: Indiscernible
- QT interval: Unmeasurable
- Other: None
- Interpretation: VF

PRACTICE 6-88
- Rhythm: Regular
- Rate: 215 beats/minute
- P wave: Indiscernible
- PR interval: Unmeasurable
- QRS complex: 0.16 second
- T wave: Indiscernible
- QT interval: Unmeasurable
- Other: None
- Interpretation: VT

PRACTICE 6-89
- Rhythm: Irregular
- Rate: 140 beats/minute
- P wave: Flattened
- PR interval: 0.12 second
- QRS complex: 0.04 second
- T wave: Indiscernible
- QT interval: Unmeasurable
- Other: None
- Interpretation: NSR with PVCs (bigeminy)

PRACTICE 6-90
- Rhythm: Chaotic
- Rate: Unmeasurable
- P wave: Indiscernible
- PR interval: Unmeasurable
- QRS complex: Indiscernible
- T wave: Indiscernible
- QT interval: Unmeasurable
- Other: None
- Interpretation: VF

PRACTICE 6-91
- Rhythm: Irregular
- Rate: 260 beats/minute
- P wave: Normal with sinus beats
- PR interval: 0.08 second
- QRS complex: 0.08 second
- T wave: Flattened with sinus beats
- QT interval: Unmeasurable
- Other: None
- Interpretation: Sinus tachycardia leading to VT

PRACTICE 6-92
- Rhythm: Chaotic
- Rate: Unmeasurable
- P wave: Indiscernible
- PR interval: Unmeasurable
- QRS complex: Indiscernible
- T wave: Indiscernible
- QT interval: Unmeasurable
- Other: None
- Interpretation: VF

PRACTICE 6-93
- Rhythm: Irregular
- Rate: 150 beats/minute
- P wave: Normal with sinus beats
- PR interval: 0.12 second
- QRS complex: 0.04 second
- T wave: Normal
- QT interval: 0.20 second
- Other: None
- Interpretation: Sinus tachycardia with multifocal PVCs

PRACTICE 6-94
- Rhythm: Regular
- Rate: 250 beats/minute
- P wave: Indiscernible
- PR interval: Unmeasurable
- QRS complex: 0.12 second
- T wave: Indiscernible
- QT interval: Unmeasurable
- Other: None
- Interpretation: VT

PRACTICE 6-95
- Rhythm: Regular
- Rate: 50 beats/minute
- P wave: Indiscernible
- PR interval: Unmeasurable
- QRS complex: 0.12 second
- T wave: Distorted
- QT interval: Unmeasurable
- Other: None
- Interpretation: AIVR

PRACTICE 6-96
- Rhythm: Irregular
- Rate: 170 beats/minute
- P wave: Normal with sinus beats
- PR interval: 0.12 second
- QRS complex: 0.06 second
- T wave: Flattened
- QT interval: 0.20 second
- Other: None
- Interpretation: NSR with PVCs (couplet)

PRACTICE 6-97
- Rhythm: Regular
- Rate: Greater than 300 beats/minute
- P wave: Indiscernible
- PR interval: Unmeasurable
- QRS complex: 0.08 second
- T wave: Indiscernible
- QT interval: Unmeasurable
- Other: None
- Interpretation: VT

PRACTICE 6-98
- Rhythm: Irregular
- Rate: 130 beats/minute
- P wave: Normal with sinus beats
- PR interval: 0.12 second
- QRS complex: 0.06 second
- T wave: Flattened
- QT interval: 0.22 second
- Other: None
- Interpretation: Sinus tachycardia with multifocal PVCs

PRACTICE 6-99
- Rhythm: Irregular
- Rate: 167 beats/minute
- P wave: Normal with sinus beats
- PR interval: 0.12 second
- QRS complex: 0.06 second
- T wave: Inverted
- QT interval: 0.16 second
- Other: None
- Interpretation: Sinus tachycardia with PVCs

PRACTICE 6-100
- Rhythm: Chaotic
- Rate: Unmeasurable
- P wave: Indiscernible
- PR interval: Unmeasurable
- QRS complex: Indiscernible
- T wave: Indiscernible
- QT interval: Unmeasurable
- Other: None
- Interpretation: VF

PRACTICE 6-101
- Rhythm: Regular
- Rate: 300 beats/minute
- P wave: Indiscernible
- PR interval: Unmeasurable
- QRS complex: 0.08 second
- T wave: Indiscernible
- QT interval: Unmeasurable
- Other: None
- Interpretation: VT

PRACTICE 6-102
- Rhythm: Irregular
- Rate: 190 beats/minute
- P wave: Normal with sinus beats
- PR interval: 0.08 second
- QRS complex: 0.04 second
- T wave: Flattened
- QT interval: Unmeasurable
- Other: None
- Interpretation: Sinus tachycardia with PVCs (triplets)

PRACTICE 6-103
- Rhythm: Irregular
- Rate: 140 beats/minute
- P wave: Normal with sinus beats
- PR interval: 0.12 second
- QRS complex: 0.08 second
- T wave: Normal
- QT interval: 0.20 second
- Other: None
- Interpretation: Sinus tachycardia with PVCs (couplets)

PRACTICE 6-104
- Rhythm: Chaotic
- Rate: Unmeasurable
- P wave: Indiscernible
- PR interval: Unmeasurable
- QRS complex: Indiscernible
- T wave: Indiscernible
- QT interval: Unmeasurable
- Other: None
- Interpretation: VF

PRACTICE 6-105
- Rhythm: Irregular
- Rate: 200 beats/minute
- P wave: Normal with sinus beats
- PR interval: 0.12 second
- QRS complex: 0.06 second
- T wave: Inverted
- QT interval: 0.16 second
- Other: Artifact present
- Interpretation: Sinus tachycardia with PVCs

PRACTICE 6-106
- Rhythm: Regular
- Rate: 150 beats/minute
- P wave: Indiscernible
- PR interval: Unmeasurable
- QRS complex: Abnormal
- T wave: Indiscernible
- QT interval: Unmeasurable
- Other: None
- Interpretation: VT

PRACTICE 6-107
- Rhythm: Chaotic
- Rate: Greater than 300 beats/minute
- P wave: Indiscernible
- PR interval: Unmeasurable
- QRS complex: Abnormal
- T wave: Indiscernible
- QT interval: Unmeasurable
- Other: None
- Interpretation: Torsades de pointes

PRACTICE 6-108
- Rhythm: Irregular
- Rate: 40 beats/minute
- P wave: Indiscernible
- PR interval: Unmeasurable
- QRS complex: 0.06 second
- T wave: Normal
- QT interval: 0.24 second
- Other: None
- Interpretation: Atrial fibrillation with periods of asystole

PRACTICE 6-109
- Rhythm: Regular
- Rate: Greater than 300 beats/minute
- P wave: Indiscernible
- PR interval: Unmeasurable
- QRS complex: Abnormal
- T wave: Indiscernible
- QT interval: Unmeasurable
- Other: None
- Interpretation: VT

PRACTICE 6-110
- Rhythm: Irregular
- Rate: 220 beats/minute
- P wave: Normal with sinus beats
- PR interval: 0.08 second
- QRS complex: 0.06 second
- T wave: Normal
- QT interval: 0.06 second
- Other: None
- Interpretation: Junctional tachycardia with PVCs (or runs of VT)

PRACTICE 6-111
- Rhythm: Irregular
- Rate: 110 beats/minute
- P wave: Normal with sinus beats
- PR interval: 0.12 second
- QRS complex: 0.08 second
- T wave: Peaked
- QT interval: 0.28 second
- Other: None
- Interpretation: Sinus tachycardia leading to AIVR

PRACTICE 6-112
- Rhythm: Chaotic
- Rate: Unmeasurable
- P wave: Indiscernible
- PR interval: Unmeasurable
- QRS complex: Indiscernible
- T wave: Indiscernible
- QT interval: Unmeasurable
- Other: None
- Interpretation: VF

PRACTICE 6-113
- Rhythm: Absent
- Rate: None
- P wave: None
- PR interval: Unmeasurable
- QRS complex: Unmeasurable
- T wave: None
- QT interval: Unmeasurable
- Other: None
- Interpretation: Asystole

PRACTICE 6-114
- Rhythm: Irregular
- Rate: 100 beats/minute
- P wave: Normal with sinus beats
- PR interval: 0.12 second
- QRS complex: 0.08 second
- T wave: Normal
- QT interval: 0.36 second
- Other: None
- Interpretation: Sinus tachycardia with PVCs (bigeminy)

PRACTICE 6-115
- Rhythm: Regular
- Rate: 214 beats/minute
- P wave: Indiscernible
- PR interval: Unmeasurable
- QRS complex: Abnormal
- T wave: Indiscernible
- QT interval: Unmeasurable
- Other: None
- Interpretation: VT

PRACTICE 6-116
- Rhythm: Irregular
- Rate: 230 beats/minute
- P wave: Distorted
- PR interval: Unmeasurable
- QRS complex: 0.04 second
- T wave: Inverted
- QT interval: 0.12 second
- Other: None
- Interpretation: Atrial tachycardia with PVCs

PRACTICE 6-117
- Rhythm: Irregular
- Rate: 120 beats/minute
- P wave: Normal with sinus beats
- PR interval: 0.12 second
- QRS complex: 0.08 second
- T wave: Normal
- QT interval: 0.28 second
- Other: None
- Interpretation: NSR with PVCs (bigeminy)

PRACTICE 6-118
- Rhythm: Absent
- Rate: None
- P wave: None
- PR interval: Unmeasurable
- QRS complex: Unmeasurable
- T wave: None
- QT interval: Unmeasurable
- Other: None
- Interpretation: Asystole

PRACTICE 6-119
- Rhythm: Regular
- Rate: 214 beats/minute
- P wave: Indiscernible
- PR interval: Unmeasurable
- QRS complex: Abnormal
- T wave: Indiscernible
- QT interval: Unmeasurable
- Other: None
- Interpretation: VT

PRACTICE 6-120
- Rhythm: Chaotic
- Rate: Unmeasurable
- P wave: Indiscernible
- PR interval: Unmeasurable
- QRS complex: Unmeasurable
- T wave: Indiscernible
- QT interval: Unmeasurable
- Other: None
- Interpretation: VF

7

Atrioventricular blocks

Atrioventricular (AV) heart block refers to an interruption or delay in the conduction of electrical impulses between the atria and the ventricles. The block can occur at the AV node, the bundle of His, or the bundle branches. When the site of the block is the bundle of His or the bundle branches, the block is referred to as *infranodal AV block*. AV block can be partial (first or second degree) or complete (third degree).

The heart's electrical impulses normally originate in the sinoatrial (SA) node, so when those impulses are blocked at the AV node, atrial rates are usually normal (60 to 100 beats/minute). The clinical significance of the block depends on the number of impulses completely blocked and the resulting ventricular rate. A slow ventricular rate can decrease cardiac output and cause such symptoms as light-headedness, hypotension, and confusion.

AV blocks are classified according to the site of block and the severity of the conduction abnormality. The sites of AV block include the AV node, bundle of His, and bundle branches.

Severity of AV block is classified in degrees: first-degree AV block; second-degree AV block, type I (Wenckebach or Mobitz I); second-degree AV block, type II (Mobitz II); and third-degree (complete) AV block. The classification system for AV blocks aids in determining the patient's treatment and prognosis.

Atrioventricular blocks

There is an interruption or delay in conduction of electrical impulses between the atria and ventricles. The block can occur at the atrioventricular (AV) node, the bundle of His, or the bundle branches.

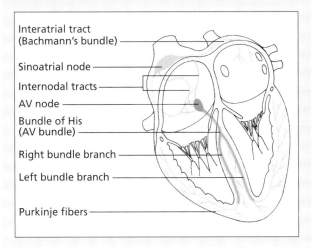

Interatrial tract (Bachmann's bundle)
Sinoatrial node
Internodal tracts
AV node
Bundle of His (AV bundle)
Right bundle branch
Left bundle branch
Purkinje fibers

First-degree atrioventricular block

First-degree AV block occurs when conduction of electrical impulses from the atria to the ventricles is delayed. This delay usually occurs at the level of the AV node, or bundle of His. First-degree AV block is characterized by a PR interval greater than 0.20 second. This interval remains constant beat to beat. Electrical impulses are conducted through the normal conduction pathway. However, conduction of these impulses takes longer than normal. In general, a rhythm strip with this block looks like normal sinus rhythm except that the PR interval is longer than normal. (See *Identifying first-degree AV block*.)

DEFINING CHARACTERISTICS

Identifying first-degree AV block

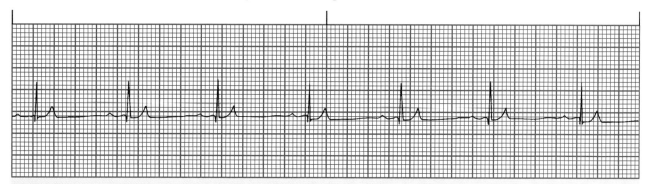

Rhythm
- Regular

Rate
- Within normal limits
- Atrial the same as ventricular

P wave
- Normal size
- Normal configuration
- Each followed by a QRS complex

PR interval
- Prolonged
- More than 0.20 second
- Constant

QRS complex
- Within normal limits (0.08 second) if conduction delay occurs in AV node
- If more than 0.12 second, conduction delay may be in His-Purkinje system

T wave
- Normal size
- Normal configuration
- May be abnormal if QRS complex is prolonged

QT interval
- Within normal limits

Other
- None

PRACTICE # First-degree atrioventricular block

Use the 8-step method to interpret the following rhythm strip. Place your answers on the blank lines. See the answer key below.

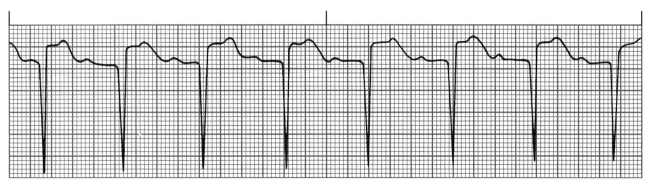

Rhythm:

Rate:

P wave:

PR interval:

QRS complex:

T wave:

QT interval:

Other:

■ **ANSWER KEY**

Rhythm: **Regular**

Rate: **75 beats/minute**

P wave: **Normal**

PR interval: **0.32 second**

QRS complex: **0.08 second**

T wave: **Normal**

QT interval: **0.40 second**

Other: **PR interval prolonged but constant**

Second-degree atrioventricular block

Second-degree AV block occurs when some of the electrical impulses from the AV node are blocked and some are conducted through normal conduction pathways. Second-degree AV block is subdivided into type I second-degree AV block and type II second-degree AV block.

Type I second-degree AV block

Also called *Wenckebach* or *Mobitz I block*, type I second-degree AV block occurs when each successive impulse from the SA node is delayed slightly longer than the pre-vious impulse. This pattern of progressive prolongation of the PR interval continues until an impulse fails to be conducted to the ventricles.

Usually only a single impulse is blocked from reaching the ventricles, and following this nonconducted P wave or dropped beat, the pattern is repeated. This repetitive sequence of two or more consecutive beats followed by a dropped beat results in "group beating." Type I second-degree AV block generally occurs at the level of the AV node. (See *Identifying second-degree AV block, type I.*)

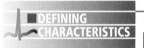
DEFINING CHARACTERISTICS

Identifying second-degree AV block, type I

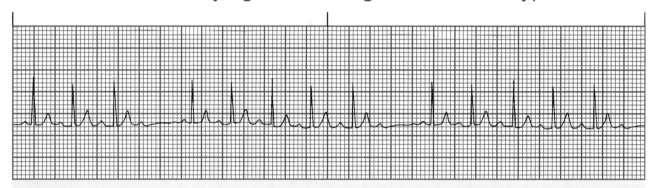

Rhythm
- Atrial: Regular
- Ventricular: Irregular

Rate
- Atrial rate exceeds ventricular rate because of nonconducted beats
- Both rates usually within normal limits

P wave
- Normal size
- Normal configuration
- Each followed by a QRS complex, except blocked P wave

PR interval
- Progressively longer with each cycle until a P wave appears without a QRS complex
- Commonly described as "long, longer, dropped"
- Slight variation in delay from cycle to cycle
- After the nonconducted beat, shorter than the interval preceding it

QRS complex
- Usually within normal limits
- Periodically absent

T wave
- Normal size
- Normal configuration
- Deflection may be opposite that of the QRS complex

QT interval
- Usually within normal limits

Other
- Wenckebach pattern of grouped beats (footprints of Wenckebach)
- R-R interval shortens until a P wave appears without a QRS complex; cycle then repeats

Second-degree atrioventricular block, type I

Use the 8-step method to interpret the following rhythm strip. Place your answers on the blank lines. See the answer key below.

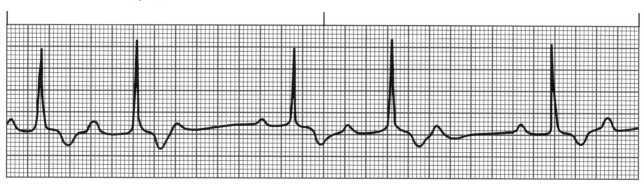

Rhythm:

Rate:

P wave:

PR interval:

QRS complex:

T wave:

QT interval:

Other:

■ **ANSWER KEY**

Rhythm: Atrial—regular; ventricular—irregular

Rate: Atrial—80 beats/minute; ventricular—50 beats/minute

P wave: Normal

PR interval: Progressively prolonged

QRS complex: 0.08 second

T wave: Inverted

QT interval: 0.46 second

Other: Wenckebach pattern of grouped beats; PR interval gets progressively longer until a QRS complex is dropped

Type II second-degree AV block

Type II second-degree AV block (also known as *Mobitz II block*) is less common than type I, but more serious. It occurs when impulses from the SA node occasionally fail to conduct to the ventricles. This form of second-degree AV block occurs below the level of the AV node, either at the bundle of His or, more commonly, at the bundle branches.

One hallmark of this type of block is that, unlike type I second- degree AV block, the PR interval doesn't lengthen before a dropped beat. In addition, more than one non-conducted beat can occur in succession. (See *Identifying second-degree AV block, type II.*)

It may be difficult to distinguish nonconducted premature atrial contractions from type II second-degree AV block. (See *Distinguishing nonconducted PACs from type II second-degree AV block.*)

Identifying second-degree AV block, type II

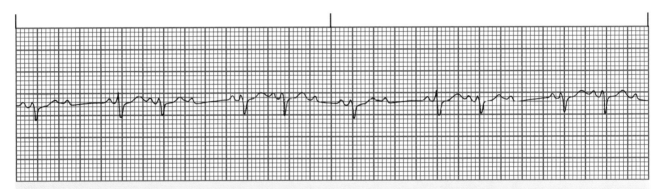

Rhythm

- Atrial: Regular
- Ventricular: Irregular
- Pauses correspond to dropped beat
- Irregular when block is intermittent or conduction ratio is variable
- Regular when conduction ratio is constant, such as 2:1 or 3:1

Rate

- Atrial exceeds ventricular
- Both may be within normal limits

P wave

- Normal size
- Normal configuration
- Some not followed by a QRS complex

PR interval

- Usually within normal limits but may be prolonged
- Constant for conducted beats

QRS complex

- Within normal limits or narrow if block occurs at bundle of His
- Widened and similar to bundle-branch block if block occurs at bundle branches
- Periodically absent

T wave

- Normal size
- Normal configuration

QT interval

- Within normal limits

Other

- PR and R-R intervals don't vary before a dropped beat, so no warning occurs
- R-R interval that contains nonconducted P wave equals two normal R-R intervals
- Must be a complete block in one bundle branch and intermittent interruption in conduction in the other bundle for a dropped beat to occur

Distinguishing nonconducted PACs from type II second-degree AV block

An isolated P wave that doesn't conduct through to the ventricle (P wave without a QRS complex following it; see shaded areas below) may occur with a nonconducted premature atrial contraction (PAC) or may indicate type II second-degree atrioventricular (AV) block. Mistakenly identifying AV block as nonconducted PACs may have serious consequences. The latter is generally benign; the former can be life-threatening.

Nonconducted PAC

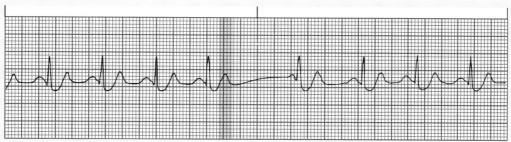

If the P-P interval, including the extra P wave, isn't constant, it's a nonconducted PAC.

Type II second-degree AV block

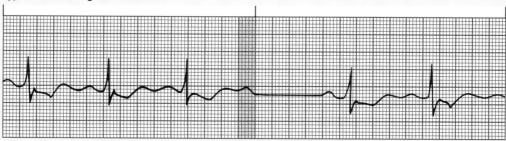

If the P-P interval is constant, including the extra P wave, it's type II second-degree AV block.

PRACTICE

Second-degree atrioventricular block, type II

Use the 8-step method to interpret the following rhythm strip. Place your answers on the blank lines. See the answer key below.

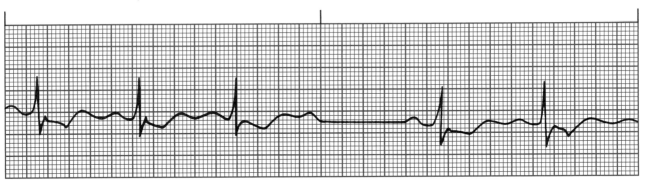

Rhythm:

Rate:

P wave:

PR interval:

QRS complex:

T wave:

QT interval:

Other:

■ **ANSWER KEY**

Rhythm: Atrial—regular; ventricular—irregular

Rate: Atrial—60 beats/minute; ventricular—50 beats/minute

P wave: Normal

PR interval: 0.28 second; constant for the conducted beats

QRS complex: 0.10 second

T wave: Normal

QT interval: 0.60 second

Other: PR and R-R intervals don't vary before a dropped beat, so no warning occurs

Third-degree atrioventricular block

Also called *complete heart block,* third-degree AV block indicates the complete absence of impulse conduction between the atria and ventricles. In complete heart block, the atrial rate is generally faster than the ventricular rate.

Third-degree AV block may occur at the level of the AV node, the bundle of His, or the bundle branches. The patient's treatment and prognosis vary depending on the anatomic level of the block.

When third-degree AV block occurs at the level of the AV node, ventricular depolarization is typically initiated by a junctional escape pacemaker. This pacemaker is typically stable, with a rate of 40 to 60 beats/minute. The sequence of ventricular depolarization is usually normal because the block is located above the bifurcation of the bundle of His, which results in a normal-appearing QRS complex.

On the other hand, when third-degree AV block occurs at the infranodal level, a block involving the right and left bundle branches is most commonly the cause. In this case, extensive disease exists in the infranodal conduction system, and the only available escape mechanism is located distal to the site of block in the ventricle. This unstable, ventricular escape pacemaker has a slow intrinsic rate of less than 40 beats/minute. Because these depolarizations originate in the ventricle, the QRS complex will have a wide and bizarre appearance. (See *Identifying third-degree AV block.*)

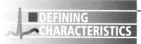

DEFINING CHARACTERISTICS

Identifying third-degree AV block

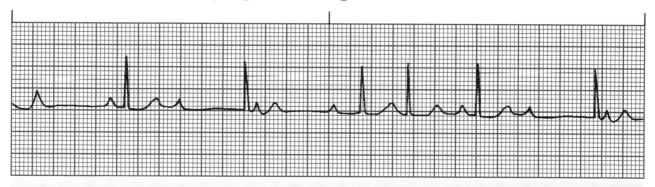

Rhythm

- Atrial: Regular
- Ventricular: Regular

Rate

- Atrial: 60 to 100 beats/minute (atria act independently under control of SA node)
- Ventricular: Usually 40 to 60 beats/minute in an intranodal block (a junctional escape rhythm)
- Ventricular: Usually less than 40 beats/minute in intranodal block (a ventricular escape rhythm)

P wave

- Normal size
- Normal configuration
- May be buried in QRS complex or T wave

PR interval

- Unmeasurable

QRS complex

- Configuration depends on location of escape mechanism and origin of ventricular depolarization
- Appears normal if the block is at the level of the AV node or bundle of His
- Widened if the block is at the level of the bundle branches

T wave

- Normal size
- Normal configuration
- May be abnormal if QRS complex originates in ventricle

QT interval

- Within normal limits

Other

- Atria and ventricles are depolarized from different pacemaker sites and beat independently of each other
- P waves occur without QRS complexes

Third-degree atrioventricular block

Use the 8-step method to interpret the following rhythm strip. Place your answers on the blank lines. See the answer key below.

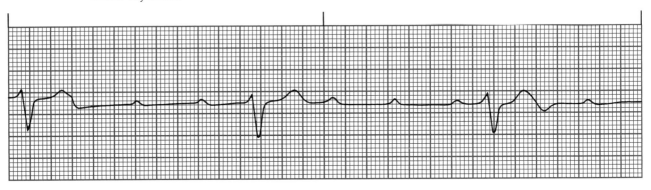

Rhythm: _____

Rate: _____

P wave: _____

PR interval: _____

QRS complex: _____

T wave: _____

QT interval: _____

Other: _____

■ **ANSWER KEY**

Rhythm: Regular

Rate: Atrial—90 beats/minute; ventricular—30 beats/minute

P wave: Normal

PR interval: Variable

QRS complex: 0.16 second

T wave: Normal

QT interval: 0.56 second

Other: P wave occurs without a QRS complex

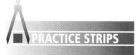

■ PRACTICE 7-1

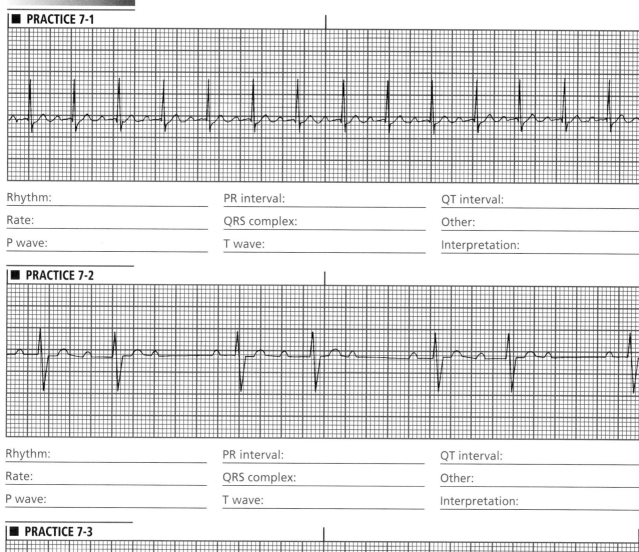

Rhythm: _____   PR interval: _____   QT interval: _____

Rate: _____   QRS complex: _____   Other: _____

P wave: _____   T wave: _____   Interpretation: _____

■ PRACTICE 7-2

Rhythm: _____   PR interval: _____   QT interval: _____

Rate: _____   QRS complex: _____   Other: _____

P wave: _____   T wave: _____   Interpretation: _____

■ PRACTICE 7-3

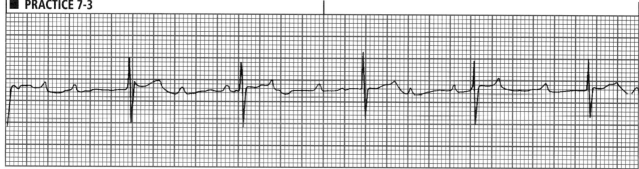

Rhythm: _____   PR interval: _____   QT interval: _____

Rate: _____   QRS complex: _____   Other: _____

P wave: _____   T wave: _____   Interpretation: _____

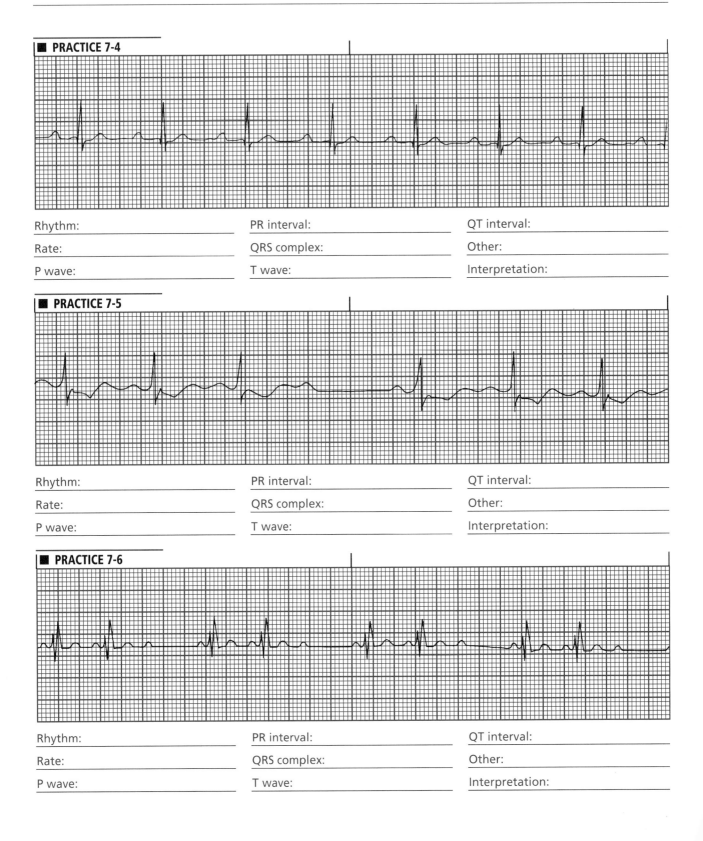

■ **PRACTICE 7-4**

Rhythm: _____   PR interval: _____   QT interval: _____

Rate: _____   QRS complex: _____   Other: _____

P wave: _____   T wave: _____   Interpretation: _____

■ **PRACTICE 7-5**

Rhythm: _____   PR interval: _____   QT interval: _____

Rate: _____   QRS complex: _____   Other: _____

P wave: _____   T wave: _____   Interpretation: _____

■ **PRACTICE 7-6**

Rhythm: _____   PR interval: _____   QT interval: _____

Rate: _____   QRS complex: _____   Other: _____

P wave: _____   T wave: _____   Interpretation: _____

■ PRACTICE 7-7

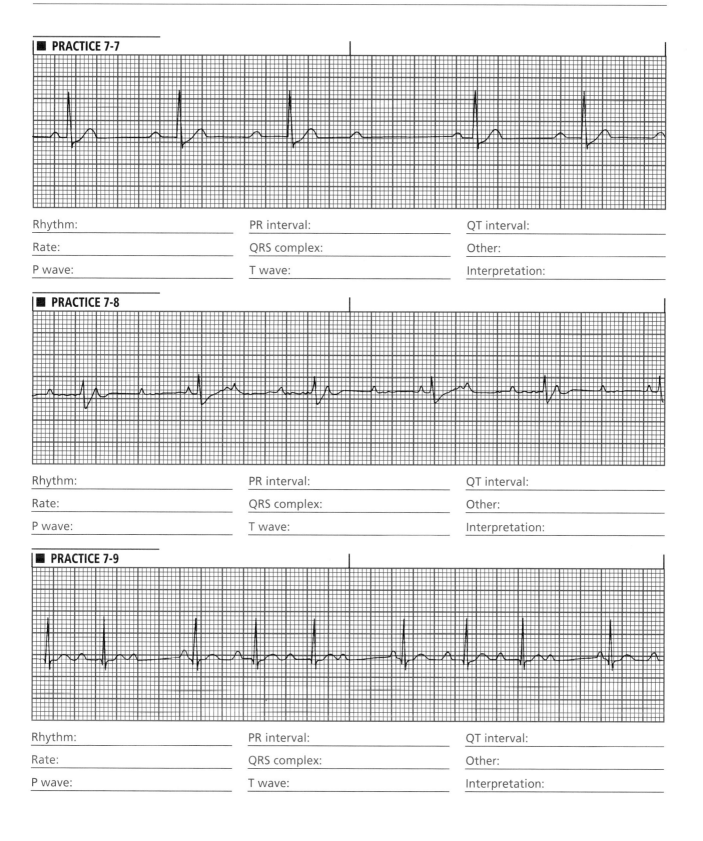

Rhythm: _____   PR interval: _____   QT interval: _____

Rate: _____   QRS complex: _____   Other: _____

P wave: _____   T wave: _____   Interpretation: _____

■ PRACTICE 7-8

Rhythm: _____   PR interval: _____   QT interval: _____

Rate: _____   QRS complex: _____   Other: _____

P wave: _____   T wave: _____   Interpretation: _____

■ PRACTICE 7-9

Rhythm: _____   PR interval: _____   QT interval: _____

Rate: _____   QRS complex: _____   Other: _____

P wave: _____   T wave: _____   Interpretation: _____

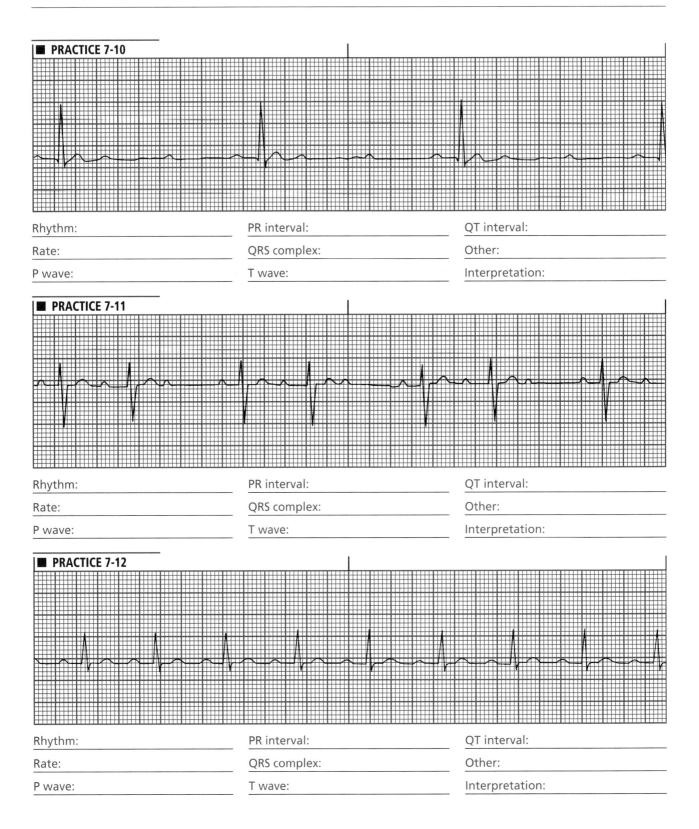

■ **PRACTICE 7-10**

Rhythm: _____   PR interval: _____   QT interval: _____

Rate: _____   QRS complex: _____   Other: _____

P wave: _____   T wave: _____   Interpretation: _____

■ **PRACTICE 7-11**

Rhythm: _____   PR interval: _____   QT interval: _____

Rate: _____   QRS complex: _____   Other: _____

P wave: _____   T wave: _____   Interpretation: _____

■ **PRACTICE 7-12**

Rhythm: _____   PR interval: _____   QT interval: _____

Rate: _____   QRS complex: _____   Other: _____

P wave: _____   T wave: _____   Interpretation: _____

■ **PRACTICE 7-13**

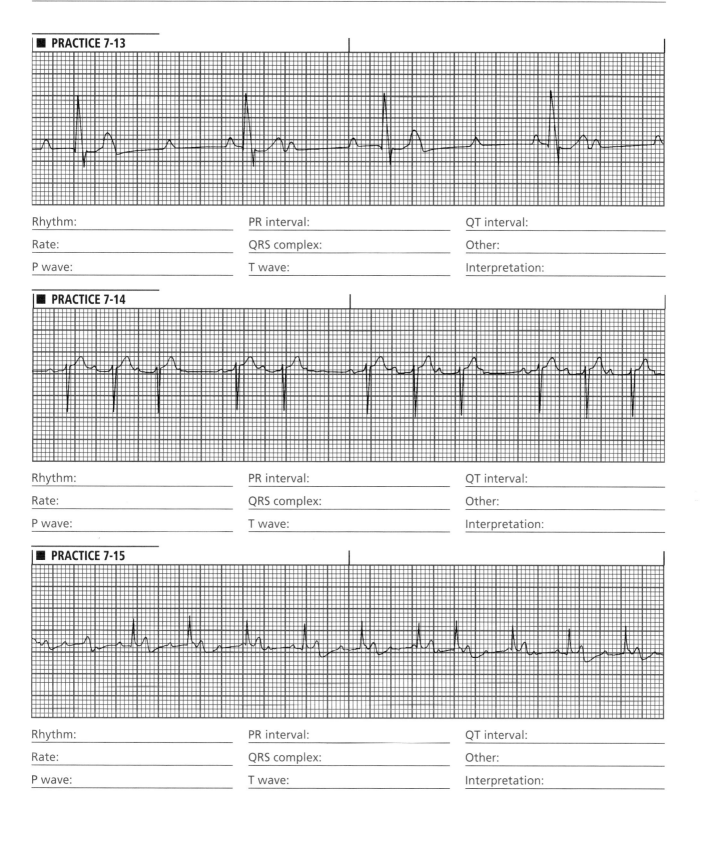

Rhythm: _____   PR interval: _____   QT interval: _____

Rate: _____   QRS complex: _____   Other: _____

P wave: _____   T wave: _____   Interpretation: _____

■ **PRACTICE 7-14**

Rhythm: _____   PR interval: _____   QT interval: _____

Rate: _____   QRS complex: _____   Other: _____

P wave: _____   T wave: _____   Interpretation: _____

■ **PRACTICE 7-15**

Rhythm: _____   PR interval: _____   QT interval: _____

Rate: _____   QRS complex: _____   Other: _____

P wave: _____   T wave: _____   Interpretation: _____

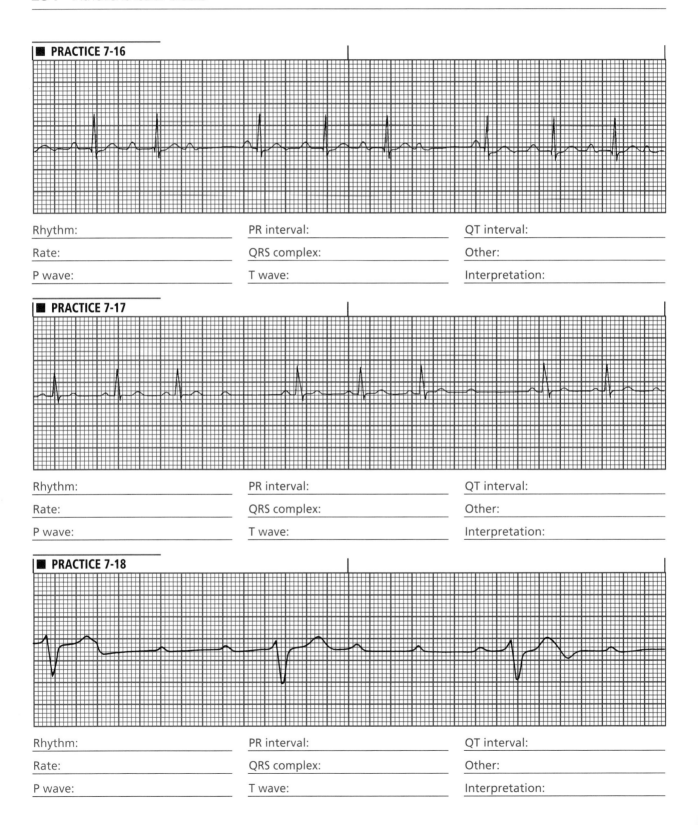

■ **PRACTICE 7-16**

Rhythm: _____ PR interval: _____ QT interval: _____

Rate: _____ QRS complex: _____ Other: _____

P wave: _____ T wave: _____ Interpretation: _____

■ **PRACTICE 7-17**

Rhythm: _____ PR interval: _____ QT interval: _____

Rate: _____ QRS complex: _____ Other: _____

P wave: _____ T wave: _____ Interpretation: _____

■ **PRACTICE 7-18**

Rhythm: _____ PR interval: _____ QT interval: _____

Rate: _____ QRS complex: _____ Other: _____

P wave: _____ T wave: _____ Interpretation: _____

■ **PRACTICE 7-19**

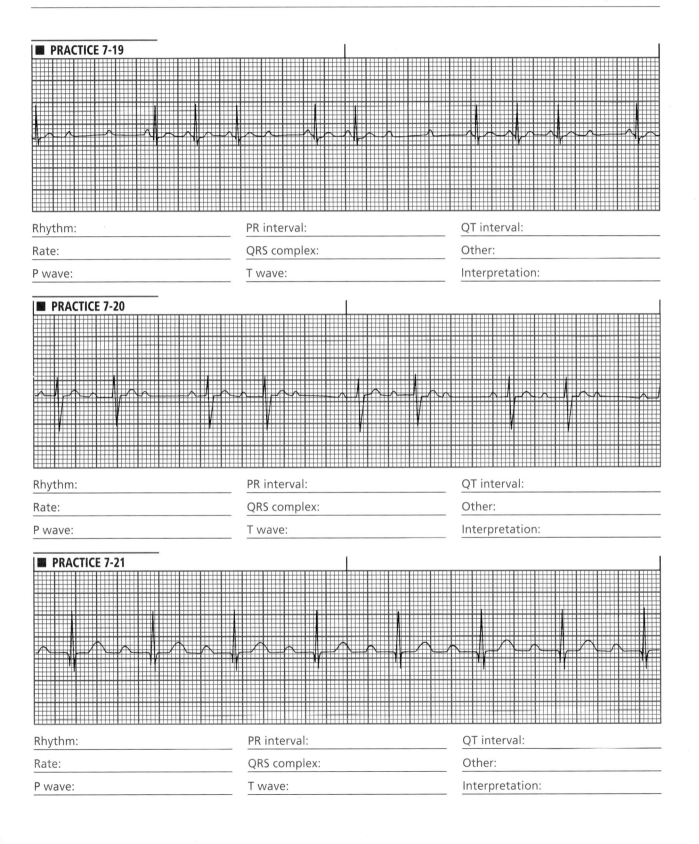

Rhythm: _____   PR interval: _____   QT interval: _____

Rate: _____   QRS complex: _____   Other: _____

P wave: _____   T wave: _____   Interpretation: _____

■ **PRACTICE 7-20**

Rhythm: _____   PR interval: _____   QT interval: _____

Rate: _____   QRS complex: _____   Other: _____

P wave: _____   T wave: _____   Interpretation: _____

■ **PRACTICE 7-21**

Rhythm: _____   PR interval: _____   QT interval: _____

Rate: _____   QRS complex: _____   Other: _____

P wave: _____   T wave: _____   Interpretation: _____

■ **PRACTICE 7-22**

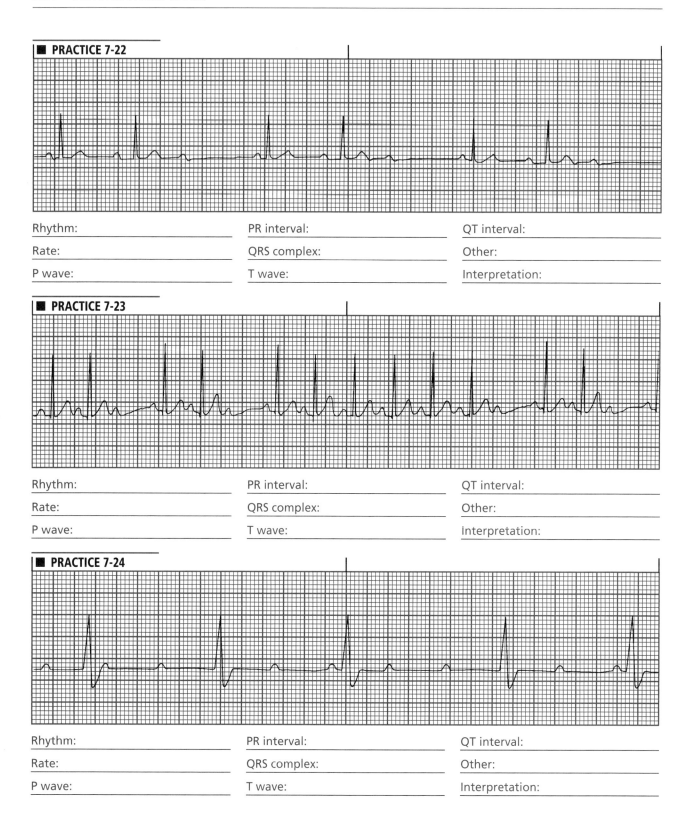

Rhythm: _____   PR interval: _____   QT interval: _____

Rate: _____   QRS complex: _____   Other: _____

P wave: _____   T wave: _____   Interpretation: _____

■ **PRACTICE 7-23**

Rhythm: _____   PR interval: _____   QT interval: _____

Rate: _____   QRS complex: _____   Other: _____

P wave: _____   T wave: _____   Interpretation: _____

■ **PRACTICE 7-24**

Rhythm: _____   PR interval: _____   QT interval: _____

Rate: _____   QRS complex: _____   Other: _____

P wave: _____   T wave: _____   Interpretation: _____

■ PRACTICE 7-25

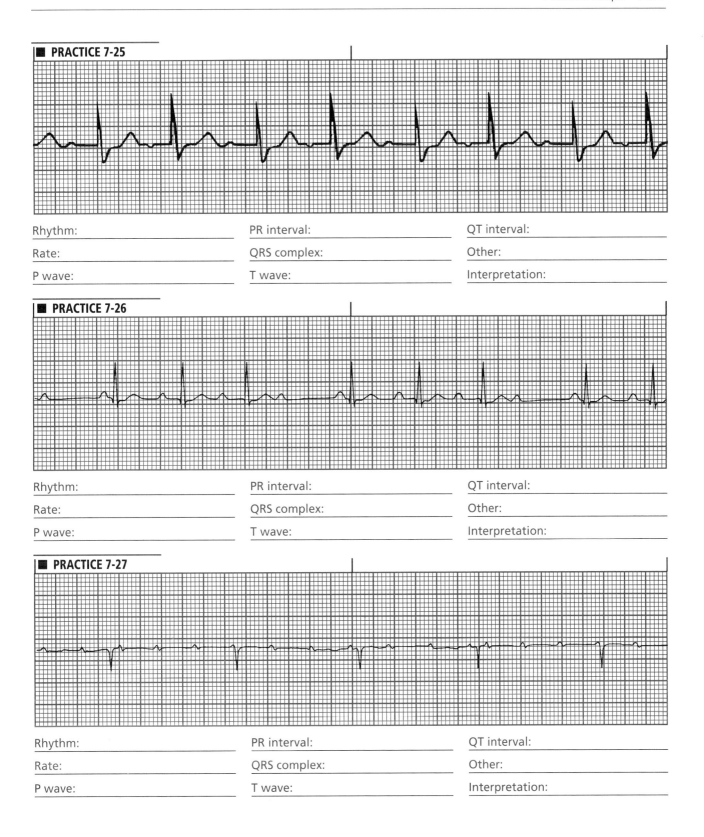

Rhythm: _____

Rate: _____

P wave: _____

PR interval: _____

QRS complex: _____

T wave: _____

QT interval: _____

Other: _____

Interpretation: _____

■ PRACTICE 7-26

Rhythm: _____

Rate: _____

P wave: _____

PR interval: _____

QRS complex: _____

T wave: _____

QT interval: _____

Other: _____

Interpretation: _____

■ PRACTICE 7-27

Rhythm: _____

Rate: _____

P wave: _____

PR interval: _____

QRS complex: _____

T wave: _____

QT interval: _____

Other: _____

Interpretation: _____

■ **PRACTICE 7-28**

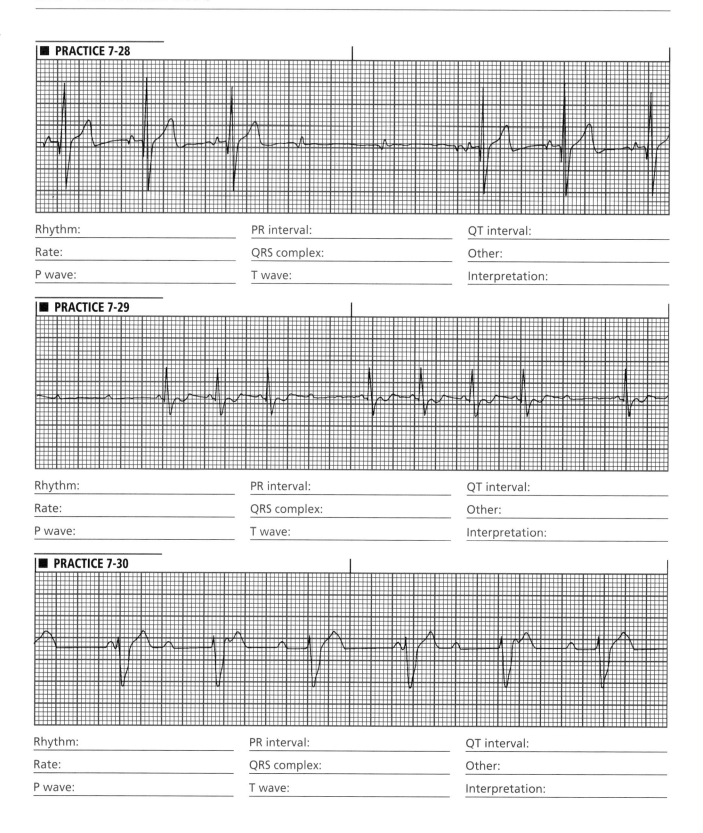

Rhythm: _____ PR interval: _____ QT interval: _____

Rate: _____ QRS complex: _____ Other: _____

P wave: _____ T wave: _____ Interpretation: _____

■ **PRACTICE 7-29**

Rhythm: _____ PR interval: _____ QT interval: _____

Rate: _____ QRS complex: _____ Other: _____

P wave: _____ T wave: _____ Interpretation: _____

■ **PRACTICE 7-30**

Rhythm: _____ PR interval: _____ QT interval: _____

Rate: _____ QRS complex: _____ Other: _____

P wave: _____ T wave: _____ Interpretation: _____

■ **PRACTICE 7-31**

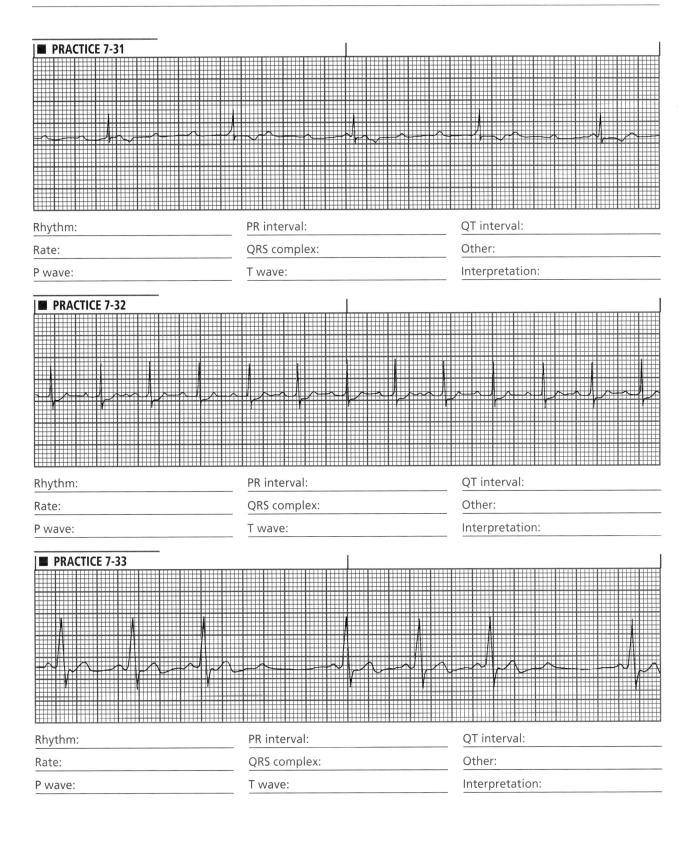

Rhythm: _____

Rate: _____

P wave: _____

PR interval: _____

QRS complex: _____

T wave: _____

QT interval: _____

Other: _____

Interpretation: _____

■ **PRACTICE 7-32**

Rhythm: _____

Rate: _____

P wave: _____

PR interval: _____

QRS complex: _____

T wave: _____

QT interval: _____

Other: _____

Interpretation: _____

■ **PRACTICE 7-33**

Rhythm: _____

Rate: _____

P wave: _____

PR interval: _____

QRS complex: _____

T wave: _____

QT interval: _____

Other: _____

Interpretation: _____

■ PRACTICE 7-34

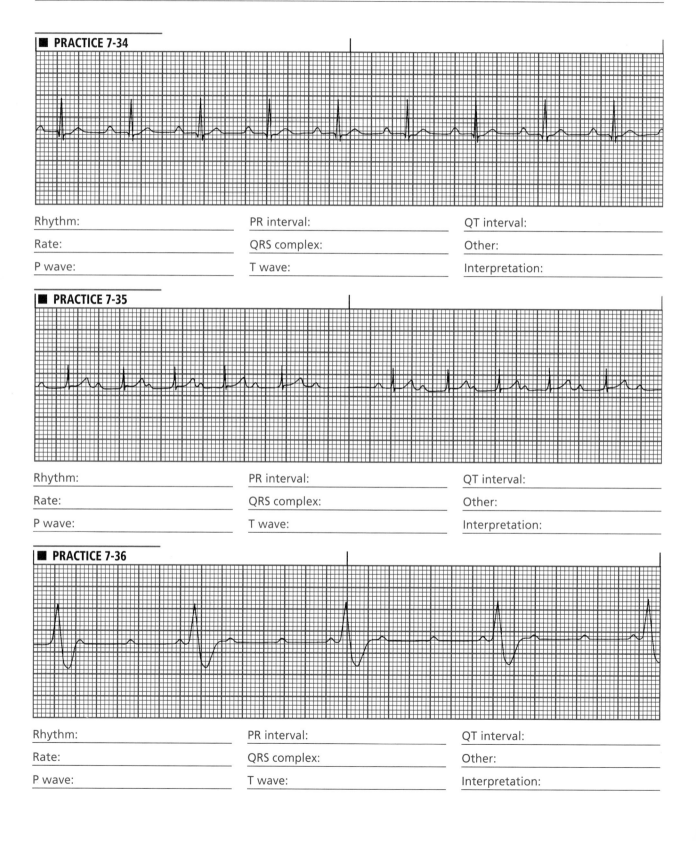

Rhythm: _____

Rate: _____

P wave: _____

PR interval: _____

QRS complex: _____

T wave: _____

QT interval: _____

Other: _____

Interpretation: _____

■ PRACTICE 7-35

Rhythm: _____

Rate: _____

P wave: _____

PR interval: _____

QRS complex: _____

T wave: _____

QT interval: _____

Other: _____

Interpretation: _____

■ PRACTICE 7-36

Rhythm: _____

Rate: _____

P wave: _____

PR interval: _____

QRS complex: _____

T wave: _____

QT interval: _____

Other: _____

Interpretation: _____

■ PRACTICE 7-37

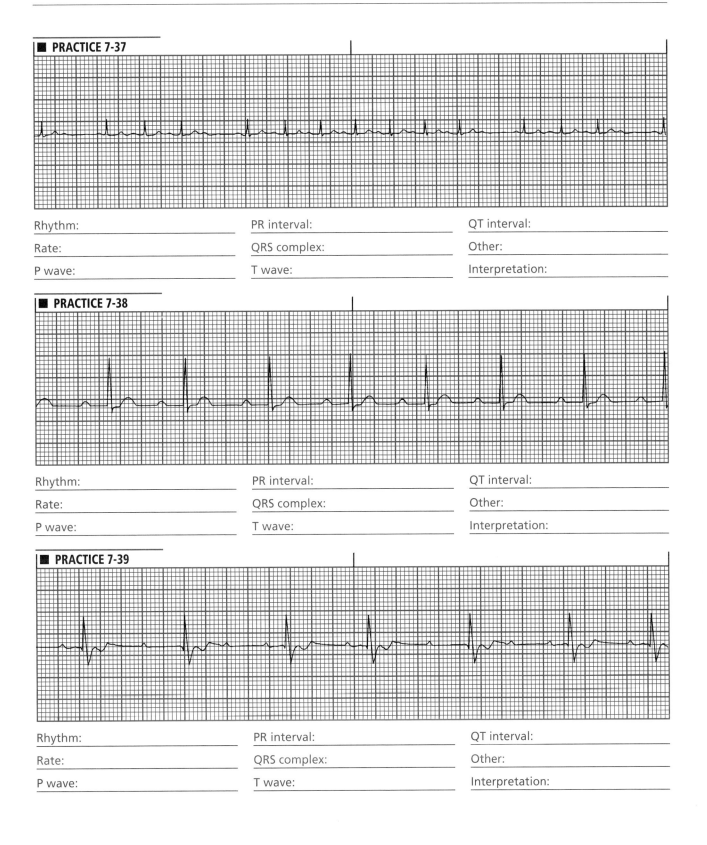

Rhythm: _____   PR interval: _____   QT interval: _____

Rate: _____   QRS complex: _____   Other: _____

P wave: _____   T wave: _____   Interpretation: _____

■ PRACTICE 7-38

Rhythm: _____   PR interval: _____   QT interval: _____

Rate: _____   QRS complex: _____   Other: _____

P wave: _____   T wave: _____   Interpretation: _____

■ PRACTICE 7-39

Rhythm: _____   PR interval: _____   QT interval: _____

Rate: _____   QRS complex: _____   Other: _____

P wave: _____   T wave: _____   Interpretation: _____

■ PRACTICE 7-40

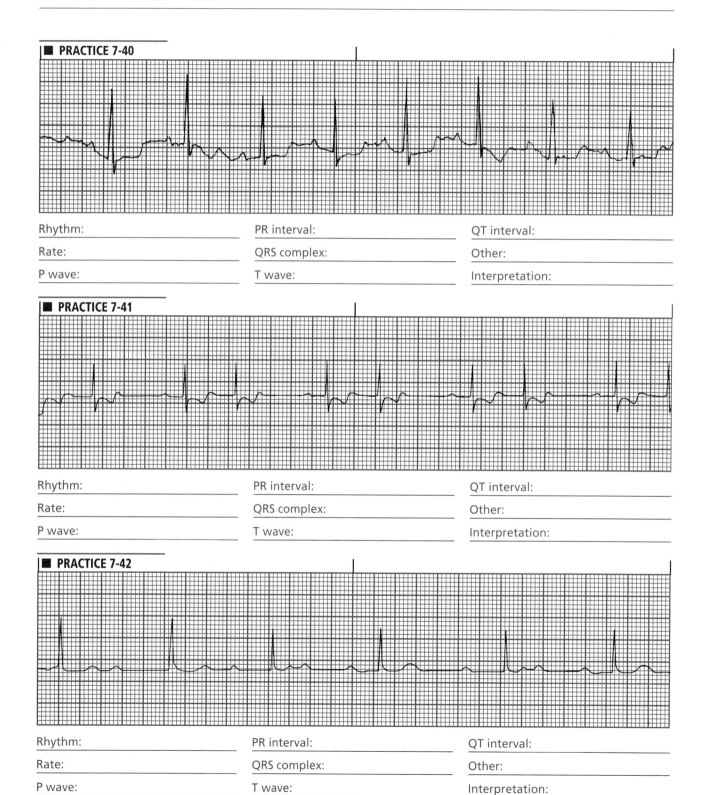

Rhythm: _____

Rate: _____

P wave: _____

PR interval: _____

QRS complex: _____

T wave: _____

QT interval: _____

Other: _____

Interpretation: _____

■ PRACTICE 7-41

Rhythm: _____

Rate: _____

P wave: _____

PR interval: _____

QRS complex: _____

T wave: _____

QT interval: _____

Other: _____

Interpretation: _____

■ PRACTICE 7-42

Rhythm: _____

Rate: _____

P wave: _____

PR interval: _____

QRS complex: _____

T wave: _____

QT interval: _____

Other: _____

Interpretation: _____

■ PRACTICE 7-43

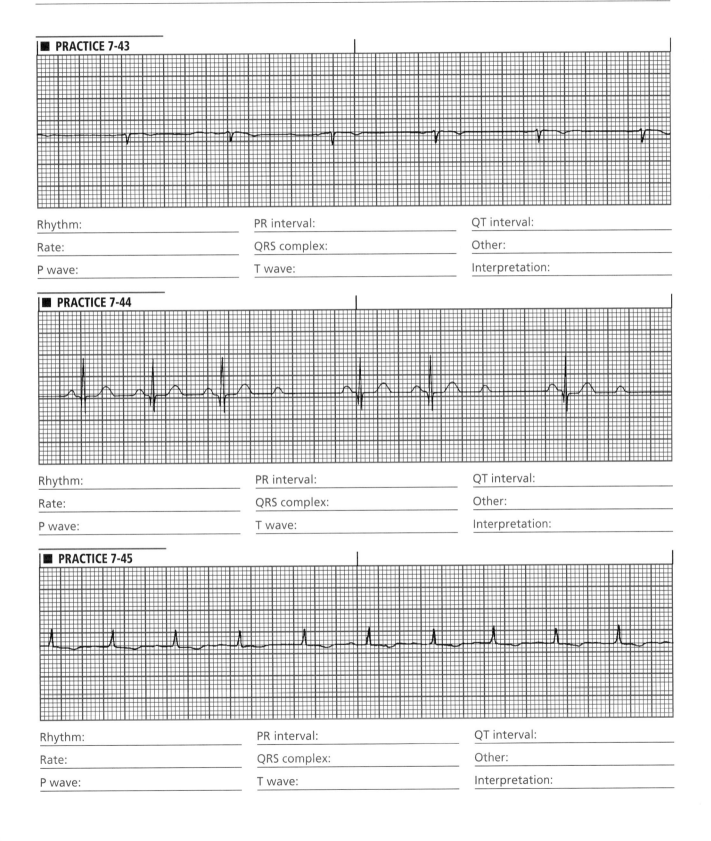

Rhythm: _____   PR interval: _____   QT interval: _____

Rate: _____   QRS complex: _____   Other: _____

P wave: _____   T wave: _____   Interpretation: _____

■ PRACTICE 7-44

Rhythm: _____   PR interval: _____   QT interval: _____

Rate: _____   QRS complex: _____   Other: _____

P wave: _____   T wave: _____   Interpretation: _____

■ PRACTICE 7-45

Rhythm: _____   PR interval: _____   QT interval: _____

Rate: _____   QRS complex: _____   Other: _____

P wave: _____   T wave: _____   Interpretation: _____

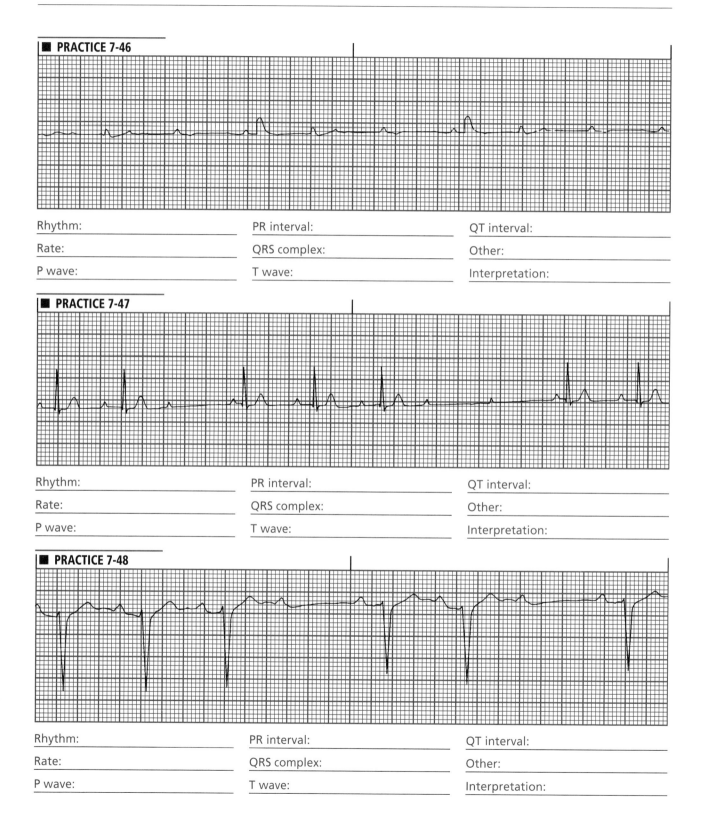

■ **PRACTICE 7-46**

Rhythm: _____   PR interval: _____   QT interval: _____

Rate: _____   QRS complex: _____   Other: _____

P wave: _____   T wave: _____   Interpretation: _____

■ **PRACTICE 7-47**

Rhythm: _____   PR interval: _____   QT interval: _____

Rate: _____   QRS complex: _____   Other: _____

P wave: _____   T wave: _____   Interpretation: _____

■ **PRACTICE 7-48**

Rhythm: _____   PR interval: _____   QT interval: _____

Rate: _____   QRS complex: _____   Other: _____

P wave: _____   T wave: _____   Interpretation: _____

■ **PRACTICE 7-49**

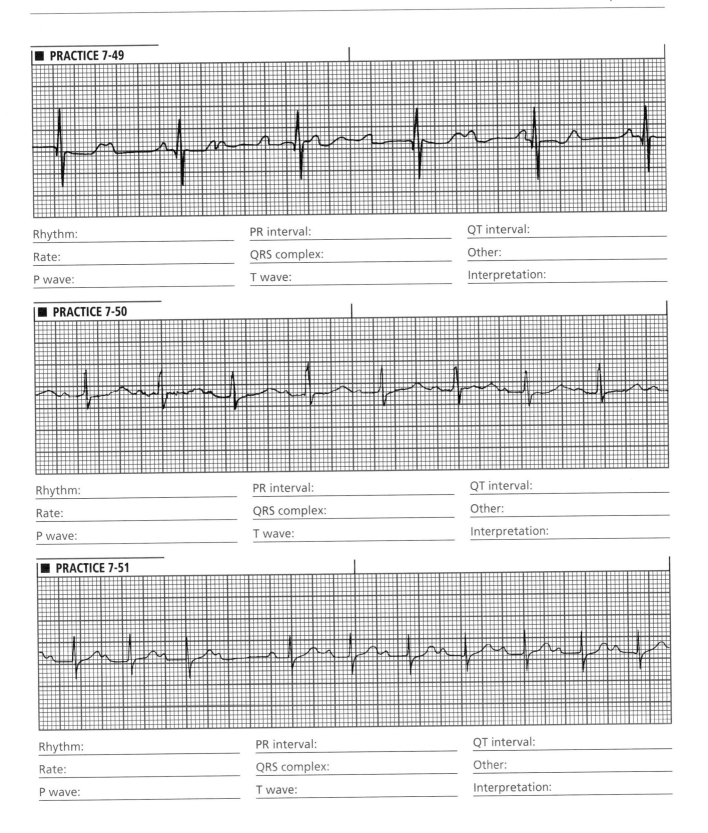

Rhythm: _____

Rate: _____

P wave: _____

PR interval: _____

QRS complex: _____

T wave: _____

QT interval: _____

Other: _____

Interpretation: _____

■ **PRACTICE 7-50**

Rhythm: _____

Rate: _____

P wave: _____

PR interval: _____

QRS complex: _____

T wave: _____

QT interval: _____

Other: _____

Interpretation: _____

■ **PRACTICE 7-51**

Rhythm: _____

Rate: _____

P wave: _____

PR interval: _____

QRS complex: _____

T wave: _____

QT interval: _____

Other: _____

Interpretation: _____

■ PRACTICE 7-52

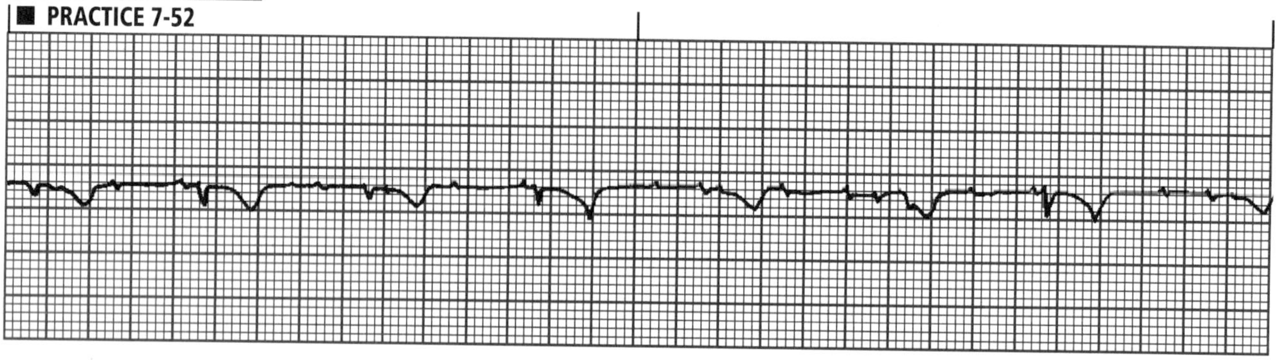

Rhythm: _____

Rate: _____

P wave: _____

PR interval: _____

QRS complex: _____

T wave: _____

QT interval: _____

Other: _____

Interpretation: _____

■ PRACTICE 7-53

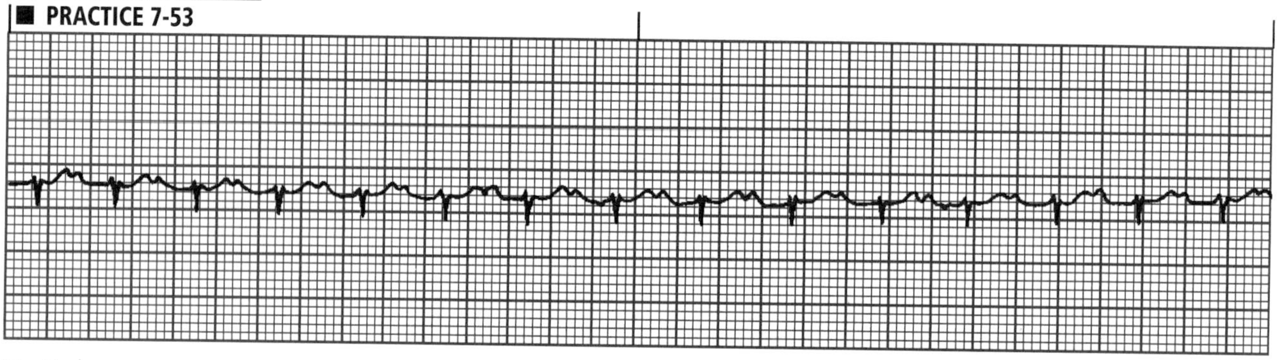

Rhythm: _____

Rate: _____

P wave: _____

PR interval: _____

QRS complex: _____

T wave: _____

QT interval: _____

Other: _____

Interpretation: _____

■ PRACTICE 7-54

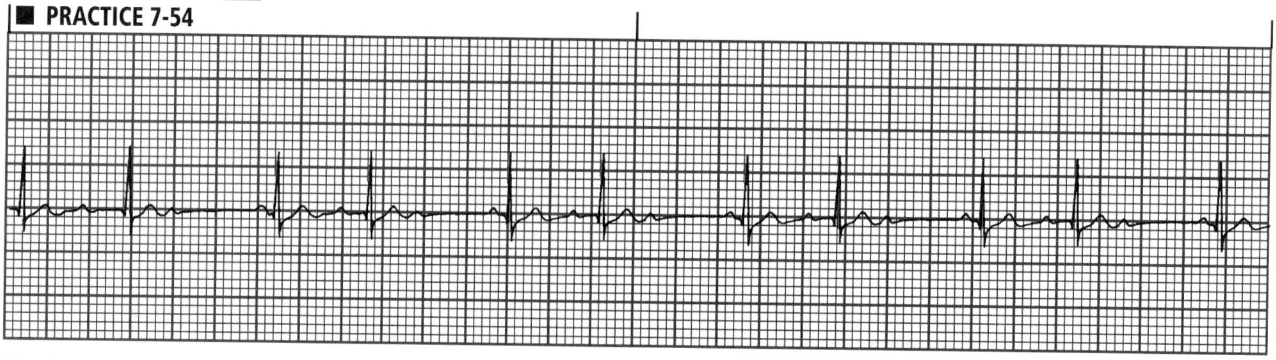

Rhythm: _____

Rate: _____

P wave: _____

PR interval: _____

QRS complex: _____

T wave: _____

QT interval: _____

Other: _____

Interpretation: _____

■ **PRACTICE 7-55**

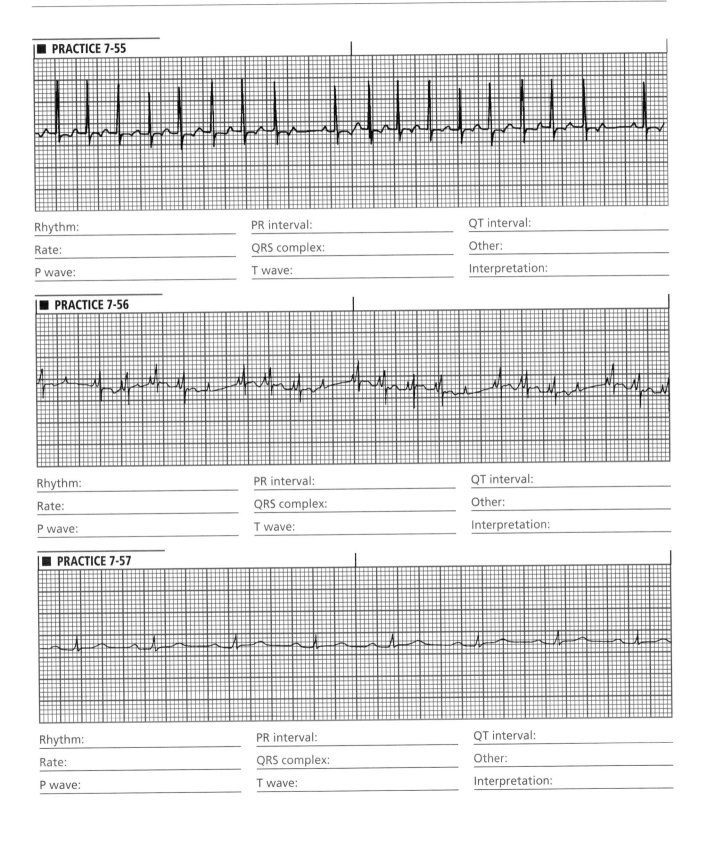

Rhythm: _____

Rate: _____

P wave: _____

PR interval: _____

QRS complex: _____

T wave: _____

QT interval: _____

Other: _____

Interpretation: _____

■ **PRACTICE 7-56**

Rhythm: _____

Rate: _____

P wave: _____

PR interval: _____

QRS complex: _____

T wave: _____

QT interval: _____

Other: _____

Interpretation: _____

■ **PRACTICE 7-57**

Rhythm: _____

Rate: _____

P wave: _____

PR interval: _____

QRS complex: _____

T wave: _____

QT interval: _____

Other: _____

Interpretation: _____

■ **PRACTICE 7-58**

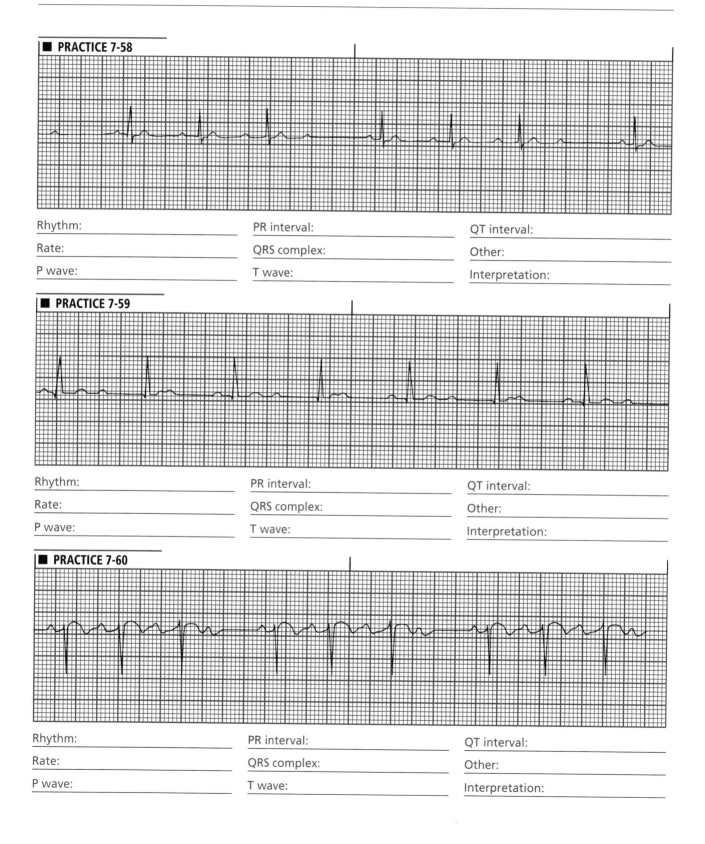

Rhythm: _____   PR interval: _____   QT interval: _____

Rate: _____   QRS complex: _____   Other: _____

P wave: _____   T wave: _____   Interpretation: _____

■ **PRACTICE 7-59**

Rhythm: _____   PR interval: _____   QT interval: _____

Rate: _____   QRS complex: _____   Other: _____

P wave: _____   T wave: _____   Interpretation: _____

■ **PRACTICE 7-60**

Rhythm: _____   PR interval: _____   QT interval: _____

Rate: _____   QRS complex: _____   Other: _____

P wave: _____   T wave: _____   Interpretation: _____

■ PRACTICE STRIP ANSWERS

PRACTICE 7-1
- Rhythm: Regular
- Rate: 136 beats/minute
- P wave: Normal
- PR interval: 0.20 second
- QRS complex: 0.08 second
- T wave: Normal
- QT interval: 0.20 second
- Other: None
- Interpretation: Sinus tachycardia with first-degree AV block

PRACTICE 7-2
- Rhythm: Irregular
- Rate: 70 beats/minute
- P wave: Normal
- PR interval: Variable
- QRS complex: 0.12 second
- T wave: Normal
- QT interval: 0.30 second
- Other: PR interval increases until dropped beat
- Interpretation: Second-degree AV block, type I

PRACTICE 7-3
- Rhythm: Slightly irregular
- Rate: 75 beats/minute
- P wave: Normal
- PR interval: Unmeasurable
- QRS complex: 0.08 second
- T wave: Distorted by P waves
- QT interval: 0.32 second
- Other: P wave not related to QRS complex
- Interpretation: Third-degree AV block

PRACTICE 7-4
- Rhythm: Regular
- Rate: 75 beats/minute
- P wave: Normal
- PR interval: 0.28 second
- QRS complex: 0.08 second
- T wave: Normal
- QT interval: 0.28 second
- Other: None
- Interpretation: Normal sinus rhythm (NSR) with first-degree AV block

PRACTICE 7-5
- Rhythm: Irregular
- Rate: 60 beats/minute
- P wave: Flattened
- PR interval: 0.24 second
- QRS complex: 0.12 second
- T wave: Inverted
- QT interval: 0.52 second
- Other: None
- Interpretation: Second-degree AV block, type II

PRACTICE 7-6
- Rhythm: Irregular
- Rate: 88 beats/minute
- P wave: Normal
- PR interval: 0.12 second
- QRS complex: 0.12 second
- T wave: Normal
- QT interval: 0.32 second
- Other: None
- Interpretation: Second-degree AV block, type II

PRACTICE 7-7
- Rhythm: Irregular
- Rate: 50 beats/minute
- P wave: Normal
- PR interval: Variable
- QRS complex: 0.06 second
- T wave: Normal
- QT interval: 0.28 second
- Other: PR interval increases until dropped beat
- Interpretation: Second-degree AV block, type I

PRACTICE 7-8
- Rhythm: Regular
- Rate: 56 beats/minute
- P wave: Normal
- PR interval: Unmeasurable
- QRS complex: 0.12 second
- T wave: Distorted by P waves
- QT interval: Unmeasurable
- Other: P wave not related to QRS complex
- Interpretation: Third-degree AV block

PRACTICE 7-9
- Rhythm: Irregular
- Rate: 90 beats/minute
- P wave: Normal
- PR interval: Variable
- QRS complex: 0.06 second
- T wave: Normal
- QT interval: 0.26 second
- Other: PR interval increases until dropped beat
- Interpretation: Second-degree AV block, type I

PRACTICE 7-10
- Rhythm: Regular
- Rate: 32 beats/minute
- P wave: Normal
- PR interval: 0.28 second
- QRS complex: 0.08 second
- T wave: Normal
- QT interval: 0.28 second
- Other: None
- Interpretation: Second-degree AV block, type II

PRACTICE 7-11
- Rhythm: Irregular
- Rate: 70 beats/minute
- P wave: Normal
- PR interval: Variable
- QRS complex: 0.08 second
- T wave: Normal
- QT interval: 0.28 second
- Other: PR interval increases until dropped beat
- Interpretation: Second-degree AV block, type I

PRACTICE 7-12
- Rhythm: Regular
- Rate: 88 beats/minute
- P wave: Normal
- PR interval: 0.24 second
- QRS complex: 0.08 second
- T wave: Normal
- QT interval: 0.32 second
- Other: None
- Interpretation: NSR with first-degree AV block

PRACTICE 7-13
- Rhythm: Slightly irregular
- Rate: 40 beats/minute
- P wave: Normal
- PR interval: Unmeasurable
- QRS complex: 0.12 second
- T wave: Distorted by P waves
- QT interval: 0.40 second
- Other: P wave not related to QRS complex
- Interpretation: Third-degree AV block

PRACTICE 7-14
- Rhythm: Irregular
- Rate: 110 beats/minute
- P wave: Normal
- PR interval: Variable
- QRS complex: 0.06 second
- T wave: Normal
- QT interval: 0.22 second
- Other: PR interval increases until dropped beat
- Interpretation: Second-degree AV block, type I

PRACTICE 7-15
- Rhythm: Slightly irregular
- Rate: 110 beats/minute
- P wave: Normal
- PR interval: Unmeasurable
- QRS complex: 0.06 second
- T wave: Occasionally distorted by P waves
- QT interval: 0.16 second
- Other: P wave not related to QRS complex
- Interpretation: Third-degree AV block

PRACTICE 7-16
- Rhythm: Irregular
- Rate: 80 beats/minute
- P wave: Normal
- PR interval: Variable
- QRS complex: 0.06 second
- T wave: Normal
- QT interval: 0.28 second
- Other: PR interval increases until dropped beat
- Interpretation: Second-degree AV block, type I

PRACTICE 7-17
- Rhythm: Irregular
- Rate: 80 beats/minute
- P wave: Normal
- PR interval: 0.16 second
- QRS complex: 0.08 second
- T wave: Normal
- QT interval: 0.32 second
- Other: None
- Interpretation: Second-degree AV block, type II

PRACTICE 7-18
- Rhythm: Regular
- Rate: 30 beats/minute
- P wave: Normal
- PR interval: Unmeasurable
- QRS complex: 0.20 second
- T wave: Distorted by P waves
- QT interval: 0.50 second
- Other: None
- Interpretation: Third-degree AV block

PRACTICE 7-19
- Rhythm: Irregular
- Rate: 100 beats/minute
- P wave: Normal
- PR interval: 0.12 second
- QRS complex: 0.06 second
- T wave: Normal
- QT interval: 0.20 second
- Other: None
- Interpretation: Second-degree AV block, type II

PRACTICE 7-20
- Rhythm: Irregular
- Rate: 80 beats/minute
- P wave: Normal
- PR interval: Variable
- QRS complex: 0.08 second
- T wave: Normal
- QT interval: 0.28 second
- Other: PR interval increases until dropped beat
- Interpretation: Second-degree AV block, type I

PRACTICE 7-21
- Rhythm: Regular
- Rate: 75 beats/minute
- P wave: Normal
- PR interval: 0.32 second
- QRS complex: 0.08 second
- T wave: Normal
- QT interval: 0.36 second
- Other: None
- Interpretation: NSR with first-degree AV block

PRACTICE 7-22
- Rhythm: Irregular
- Rate: 60 beats/minute
- P wave: Normal
- PR interval: Variable
- QRS complex: 0.08 second
- T wave: Normal
- QT interval: 0.28 second
- Other: PR interval increases until dropped beat
- Interpretation: Second-degree AV block, type I

PRACTICE 7-23
- Rhythm: Irregular
- Rate: 120 beats/minute
- P wave: Normal
- PR interval: 0.12 second
- QRS complex: 0.06 second
- T wave: Normal
- QT interval: 0.20 second
- Other: None
- Interpretation: Second-degree AV block, type II

PRACTICE 7-24
- Rhythm: Irregular
- Rate: 50 beats/minute
- P wave: Normal
- PR interval: Unmeasurable
- QRS complex: 0.18 second
- T wave: Flattened
- QT interval: Unmeasurable
- Other: P wave not related to QRS complex
- Interpretation: Third-degree AV block

PRACTICE 7-25
- Rhythm: Irregular
- Rate: 80 beats/minute
- P wave: Normal in sinus beats; inverted in PACs
- PR interval: 0.28 second in sinus beats
- QRS complex: 0.10 second
- T wave: Normal
- QT interval: 0.40 second
- Other: None
- Interpretation: First-degree AV block with PACs

PRACTICE 7-26
- Rhythm: Irregular
- Rate: 80 beats/minute
- P wave: Normal
- PR interval: Variable
- QRS complex: 0.08 second
- T wave: Normal
- QT interval: 0.28 second
- Other: PR interval increases until dropped beat
- Interpretation: Second-degree AV block, type I

PRACTICE 7-27
- Rhythm: Regular
- Rate: 50 beats/minute
- P wave: Normal
- PR interval: Unmeasurable
- QRS complex: 0.06 second
- T wave: Flattened or distorted by P wave
- QT interval: Unmeasurable
- Other: P wave not related to QRS complex
- Interpretation: Third-degree AV block

PRACTICE 7-28
- Rhythm: Irregular
- Rate: 60 beats/minute
- P wave: Biphasic
- PR interval: 0.12 second
- QRS complex: 0.12 second
- T wave: Normal
- QT interval: 0.34 second
- Other: None
- Interpretation: Second-degree AV block, type II

PRACTICE 7-29
- Rhythm: Irregular
- Rate: 80 beats/minute
- P wave: Normal
- PR interval: 0.08 second
- QRS complex: 0.10 second
- T wave: Inverted
- QT interval: 0.24 second
- Other: None
- Interpretation: Second-degree AV block, type II

PRACTICE 7-30
- Rhythm: Regular
- Rate: 65 beats/minute
- P wave: Normal
- PR interval: Unmeasurable
- QRS complex: 0.12 second
- T wave: Normal
- QT interval: 0.32 second
- Other: P wave not related to QRS complex
- Interpretation: Third-degree AV block

PRACTICE 7-31
- Rhythm: Regular
- Rate: 50 beats/minute
- P wave: Normal
- PR interval: Unmeasurable
- QRS complex: 0.08 second
- T wave: Flattened or distorted by P wave
- QT interval: 0.28 second
- Other: P wave not related to QRS complex
- Interpretation: Third-degree AV block

PRACTICE 7-32
- Rhythm: Regular
- Rate: 125 beats/minute
- P wave: Normal
- PR interval: 0.20 second
- QRS complex: 0.08 second
- T wave: Normal
- QT interval: 0.20 second
- Other: ST-segment depression
- Interpretation: Sinus tachycardia with first-degree AV block

PRACTICE 7-33
- Rhythm: Irregular
- Rate: 70 beats/minute
- P wave: Normal
- PR interval: 0.16 second
- QRS complex: 0.12 second
- T wave: Normal
- QT interval: 0.36 second
- Other: None
- Interpretation: Second-degree AV block, type II

PRACTICE 7-34
- Rhythm: Regular
- Rate: 94 beats/minute
- P wave: Normal
- PR interval: 0.20 second
- QRS complex: 0.08 second
- T wave: Normal
- QT interval: 0.28 second
- Other: None
- Interpretation: NSR with first-degree AV block

PRACTICE 7-35
- Rhythm: Irregular
- Rate: 100 beats/minute
- P wave: Normal
- PR interval: Variable
- QRS complex: 0.04 second
- T wave: Normal
- QT interval: 0.24 second
- Other: None
- Interpretation: Second-degree AV block, type I

PRACTICE 7-36
- Rhythm: Regular
- Rate: 42 beats/minute
- P wave: Normal
- PR interval: Unmeasurable
- QRS complex: 0.26 second
- T wave: Indiscernible
- QT interval: Unmeasurable
- Other: P wave not related to QRS complex
- Interpretation: Third-degree AV block

PRACTICE 7-37
- Rhythm: Irregular
- Rate: 150 beats/minute
- P wave: Normal
- PR interval: Variable
- QRS complex: 0.06 second
- T wave: Normal
- QT interval: 0.20 second
- Other: None
- Interpretation: Second-degree AV block, type II

PRACTICE 7-38
- Rhythm: Regular
- Rate: 84 beats/minute
- P wave: Normal
- PR interval: 0.24 second
- QRS complex: 0.06 second
- T wave: Normal
- QT interval: 0.26 second
- Other: None
- Interpretation: NSR with first-degree AV block

PRACTICE 7-39
- Rhythm: Slightly irregular
- Rate: 70 beats/minute
- P wave: Normal
- PR interval: Unmeasurable
- QRS complex: 0.12 second
- T wave: Inverted
- QT interval: 0.24 second
- Other: P wave not related to QRS complex
- Interpretation: Third-degree AV block

PRACTICE 7-40
- Rhythm: Regular
- Rate: 80 beats/minute
- P wave: Normal
- PR interval: 0.22 second
- QRS complex: 0.80 second
- T wave: Inverted
- QT interval: 0.36 second
- Other: None
- Interpretation: NSR with first-degree AV block

PRACTICE 7-41
- Rhythm: Irregular
- Rate: 90 beats/minute
- P wave: Normal
- PR interval: 0.24 second
- QRS complex: 0.08 second
- T wave: Inverted
- QT interval: 0.28 second
- Other: None
- Interpretation: NSR with first-degree AV block and premature junctional contractions (bigeminy)

PRACTICE 7-42
- Rhythm: Slightly irregular
- Rate: 60 beats/minute
- P wave: Normal
- PR interval: Unmeasurable
- QRS complex: 0.08 second
- T wave: Normal
- QT interval: 0.40 second
- Other: P wave not related to QRS complex
- Interpretation: Third-degree AV block

PRACTICE 7-43
- Rhythm: Regular
- Rate: 63 beats/minute
- P wave: Flattened
- PR interval: 0.20 second
- QRS complex: 0.06 second
- T wave: Inverted
- QT interval: 0.32 second
- Other: None
- Interpretation: NSR

PRACTICE 7-44
- Rhythm: Irregular
- Rate: 60 beats/minute
- P wave: Normal
- PR interval: 0.12 second
- QRS complex: 0.08 second
- T wave: Normal
- QT interval: 0.32 second
- Other: None
- Interpretation: Second-degree AV block, type II

PRACTICE 7-45
- Rhythm: Regular
- Rate: 100 beats/minute
- P wave: Flattened
- PR interval: 0.22 second
- QRS complex: 0.06 second
- T wave: Inverted
- QT interval: 0.30 second
- Other: None
- Interpretation: Sinus tachycardia with first-degree AV block

PRACTICE 7-46
- Rhythm: Unknown from strip
- Rate: 20 beats/minute
- P wave: Normal
- PR interval: Unmeasurable
- QRS complex: 0.12 second
- T wave: Indiscernible
- QT interval: Unmeasurable
- Other: P wave not related to QRS complex
- Interpretation: Third-degree AV block

PRACTICE 7-47
- Rhythm: Irregular
- Rate: 70 beats/minute
- P wave: Normal
- PR interval: Variable
- QRS complex: 0.08 second
- T wave: Normal
- QT interval: 0.26 second
- Other: PR interval increases until dropped beat
- Interpretation: Second-degree AV block, type I

PRACTICE 7-48
- Rhythm: Irregular
- Rate: 60 beats/minute
- P wave: Normal
- PR interval: 0.28 second
- QRS complex: 0.12 second
- T wave: Normal
- QT interval: 0.38 second
- Other: None
- Interpretation: Second-degree AV block, type II

PRACTICE 7-49
- Rhythm: Regular
- Rate: 60 beats/minute
- P wave: Normal
- PR interval: Unmeasurable
- QRS complex: 0.08 second
- T wave: Distorted by P waves
- QT interval: Unmeasurable
- Other: P wave not related to QRS complex
- Interpretation: Third-degree AV block

PRACTICE 7-50
- Rhythm: Regular
- Rate: 83 beats/minute
- P wave: Normal
- PR interval: 0.22 second
- QRS complex: 0.08 second
- T wave: Normal
- QT interval: 0.48 second
- Other: None
- Interpretation: NSR with first-degree AV block

PRACTICE 7-51
- Rhythm: Irregular
- Rate: 100 beats/minute
- P wave: Normal
- PR interval: 0.26 second
- QRS complex: 0.08 second
- T wave: Normal
- QT interval: 0.32 second
- Other: ST-segment depression
- Interpretation: Sinus tachycardia with first-degree AV block and blocked PAC

PRACTICE 7-52
- Rhythm: Regular
- Rate: 80 beats/minute
- P wave: Normal
- PR interval: Unmeasurable
- QRS complex: 0.04 second
- T wave: Inverted
- QT interval: 0.28 second
- Other: P wave not related to QRS complex
- Interpretation: Third-degree AV block

PRACTICE 7-53
- Rhythm: Regular
- Rate: 150 beats/minute
- P wave: Normal
- PR interval: 0.20 second
- QRS complex: 0.04 second
- T wave: Inverted
- QT interval: 0.20 second
- Other: None
- Interpretation: Sinus tachycardia with first-degree AV block

PRACTICE 7-54
- Rhythm: Irregular
- Rate: 110 beats/minute
- P wave: Normal
- PR interval: Variable
- QRS complex: 0.06 second
- T wave: Normal
- QT interval: 0.20 second
- Other: PR interval increases until dropped beat
- Interpretation: Second-degree AV block, type I

PRACTICE 7-55
- Rhythm: Irregular
- Rate: 180 beats/minute
- P wave: Normal
- PR interval: Variable
- QRS complex: 0.06 second
- T wave: Inverted
- QT interval: 0.12 second
- Other: None
- Interpretation: Second-degree AV block, type II

PRACTICE 7-56
- Rhythm: Irregular
- Rate: 170 beats/minute
- P wave: Peaked
- PR interval: 0.08 second
- QRS complex: 0.08 second
- T wave: Flattened
- QT interval: 0.20 second
- Other: None
- Interpretation: Second-degree AV block, type II

PRACTICE 7-57
- Rhythm: Regular
- Rate: 84 beats/minute
- P wave: Normal
- PR interval: 0.24 second
- QRS complex: 0.06 second
- T wave: Normal
- QT interval: 0.36 second
- Other: None
- Interpretation: NSR with first-degree AV block

PRACTICE 7-58
- Rhythm: Irregular
- Rate: 70 beats/minute
- P wave: Normal
- PR interval: Variable
- QRS complex: 0.06 second
- T wave: Normal
- QT interval: 0.20 second
- Other: PR interval increases until dropped beat
- Interpretation: Second-degree AV block, type I

PRACTICE 7-59
- Rhythm: Regular
- Rate: 72 beats/minute
- P wave: Normal
- PR interval: Unmeasurable
- QRS complex: 0.08 second
- T wave: Occasionally distorted by P waves
- QT interval: 0.28 second
- Other: P wave not related to QRS complex
- Interpretation: Third-degree AV block

PRACTICE 7-60
- Rhythm: Irregular
- Rate: 90 beats/minute
- P wave: Peaked
- PR interval: Variable
- QRS complex: 0.08 second
- T wave: Elevated
- QT interval: 0.20 second
- Other: PR interval increases until dropped beat
- Interpretation: Second-degree AV block, type I

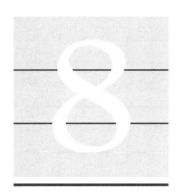

Pacemakers

A pacemaker is an artificial device that electrically stimulates the myocardium to depolarize, initiating mechanical contractions. It works by generating an impulse from a power source and transmitting that impulse to the heart muscle. The impulse flows throughout the heart and causes the heart muscle to depolarize.

A pacemaker may be used when a patient has an arrhythmia, such as certain bradyarrhythmias and tachyarrhythmias, sick sinus syndrome, or second- and third-degree atrioventricular (AV) block. The device may be used as a temporary measure or a permanent one, depending on the patient's condition. Pacemakers are typically necessary following myocardial infarction or cardiac surgery.

This chapter examines electrocardiogram (ECG) characteristics, pacemaker function assessment, and troubleshooting pacemaker problems.

ECG characteristics

The most prominent characteristic of a pacemaker on an ECG is the *pacemaker spike*. (See *Identifying pacemaker spikes*.) It occurs when the pacemaker sends an electrical impulse to the heart muscle. The impulse appears as a vertical line, or spike. The collective group of spikes on an ECG is called *pacemaker artifact*.

Depending on the electrode's position, the spike appears in different locations on the waveform:
■ When the pacemaker stimulates the atria, the spike is followed by a P wave and the patient's baseline QRS complex and T wave. This series of waveforms represents successful pacing, or *capture,* of the myocardium. The P wave appears different from the patient's normal P wave.

Identifying pacemaker spikes

Pacemaker impulses—the stimuli that travel from the pacemaker to the heart—are visible on an electrocardiogram tracing as spikes. Large or small, pacemaker spikes appear above or below the isoelectric line. This rhythm strip shows an atrial and a ventricular pacemaker spike.

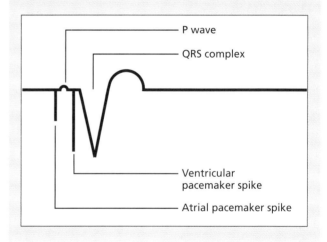

■ When the ventricles are stimulated by a pacemaker, the spike is followed by a QRS complex and T wave. The QRS complex appears wider than the patient's QRS complex because of how the pacemaker depolarizes the ventricles.
■ When the pacemaker stimulates both the atria and ventricles, the spike is followed by a P wave, then a spike, and then a QRS complex. Be aware that the type of pacemaker used and the patient's condition may affect whether every beat is paced.

Pacemaker programming

Pacemakers are commonly known by their programmed function and by the number of heart chambers that have a pacing lead. Common programmable functions include rate, mode, output, sensitivity, AV interval, and upper and lower rate limits.

Synchronous and asynchronous pacing

Pacemakers can be classified according to sensitivity. In synchronous, or *demand*, pacing, the pacemaker initiates electrical impulses only when the heart's intrinsic heart rate falls below the preset rate of the pacemaker. In asynchronous, or *fixed*, pacing, the pacemaker constantly initiates electrical impulses at a preset rate without regard to the patient's intrinsic electrical activity or heart rate. This type of pacemaker is rarely used.

Pacemaker description codes

The capabilities of permanent pacemakers are described by a five-letter coding system that details the device's function by the site of pacing and the pacing mode. The first three letters describe basic functions, and the last two describe more complicated functions. (See *Pacemaker coding system.*)

Pacing modes

A pacemaker's mode indicates its functions. Several different modes may be used during pacing, and they may not mimic the normal cardiac cycle. A three-letter code, rather than a five-letter code, is typically used to describe pacemaker function. Modes include AAI, VVI, DVI, and DDD. (See *AAI and VVI pacemakers*, page 276; *DVI pacemakers*, page 277; and *DDD pacemakers*, page 278.)

Pacemaker coding system

The capabilities of permanent pacemakers can be described by a five-letter coding system. Typically, only the first three letters are used.

First letter

The first letter identifies which heart chambers are paced:
- V = Ventricle
- A = Atrium
- D = Dual—ventricle and atrium
- 0 = None

Second letter

The second letter signifies the heart chamber where the pacemaker senses intrinsic activity:
- V = Ventricle
- A = Atrium
- D = Dual
- 0 = None

Third letter

The third letter indicates the pacemaker's mode of response to the intrinsic electrical activity it senses in the atrium or ventricle:
- T = Triggers pacing
- I = Inhibits pacing
- D = Dual—can trigger or inhibit depending on the mode and where intrinsic activity occurs
- 0 = None—doesn't change mode in response to sensed activity

Fourth letter

The fourth letter describes the degree of programmability and the presence or absence of an adaptive rate response:
- P = Basic functions programmable
- M = Multiprogrammable parameters
- C = Communicating functions such as telemetry
- R = Rate responsiveness—rate adjusts to fit the patient's metabolic needs and to achieve normal hemodynamic status
- 0 = None

Fifth letter

The fifth letter denotes the pacemaker's response to a tachyarrhythmia:
- P = Pacing ability—pacemaker's rapid burst paces the heart at a rate above its intrinsic rate to override the tachycardia source
- S = Shock—implantable cardioverter-defibrillator identifies ventricular tachycardia and delivers a shock to stop the arrhythmia
- D = Dual ability to shock and pace
- 0 = None

AAI and VVI pacemakers

AAI and VVI pacemakers are single-chamber pacemakers. The electrode is placed in the atrium for an AAI pacemaker and in the ventricle for a VVI pacemaker. The rhythm strips here show how each pacemaker works.

AAI pacemaker

An AAI pacemaker senses and paces only the atria. As shown in the shaded area below, a P wave follows each atrial spike (atrial depolarization).The QRS complexes reflect the heart's own conduction.

This pacemaker requires a functioning atrioventricular node and an intact conduction system. It may be used in patients who have symptom-producing sinus bradycardia or sick sinus syndrome.

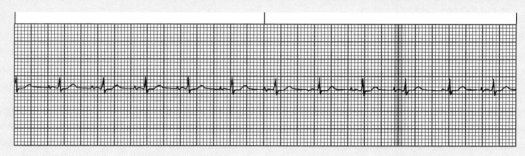

VVI pacemaker

A VVI pacemaker senses and paces the ventricles. When each spike is followed by a QRS complex (depolarization), as shown below, the rhythm is said to reflect 100% capture.

This pacemaker may be used in patients who have chronic atrial fibrillation with slow ventricular response and in those who need infrequent pacing.

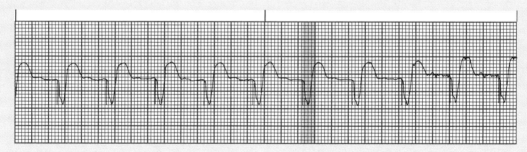

Types of pacemakers

A pacemaker can be permanent or temporary.

▨ Permanent pacemakers

A permanent pacemaker is used to treat chronic heart conditions such as second- and third-degree AV block. It's surgically implanted, usually under local anesthesia. The leads are placed transvenously, positioned in the appropriate chambers, and anchored to the endocardium.

Biventricular pacing, also referred to as *cardiac resynchronization therapy,* is a permanent pacemaker used to treat patients with moderate or severe heart failure who have left ventricular dyssynchrony. These patients have intraventricular conduction defects, which result in uncoordinated contraction of the right and left ventricles and a wide QRS complex on an ECG. To coordinate ventricular contractions and improve hemodynamic status, biventricular pacemakers use three leads—one in the

DVI pacemakers

A committed DVI pacemaker (also known as an *atrioventricular [AV] sequential pacemaker*) senses ventricular activity and paces the atria and ventricles, firing despite the intrinsic QRS complex.

    The rhythm strip here shows the effects of a committed DVI pacemaker. Notice that in two of the complexes (shaded areas), the pacemaker didn't sense the intrinsic QRS complex because the complex occurred during the AV interval, when the pacemaker was already committed to fire.

    With a noncommitted DVI pacemaker, spikes wouldn't appear after the QRS complex because the stimulus to pace the ventricles would be inhibited.

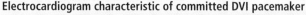

Electrocardiogram characteristic of committed DVI pacemaker

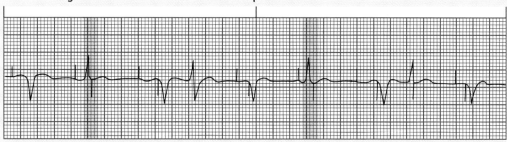

■ Ventricular pacemaker: fires despite the intrinsic QRS complex

right atrium and one in each ventricle. Both ventricles are paced at the same time, causing them to contract simultaneously, thereby increasing cardiac output.

    Unlike traditional lead placement, the electrode tip for the left ventricle is placed in the coronary sinus to a branch of the inferior cardiac vein. Because this electrode tip isn't anchored in place, lead displacement may occur. (See *Biventricular lead placement,* page 279.)

■ Temporary pacemakers

A temporary pacemaker is commonly inserted in an emergency. It can also serve as a bridge until a permanent pacemaker is inserted or the cause of an arrhythmia is resolved. These pacemakers are used for patients with high-grade heart block, bradycardia, or low cardiac output. Several types of temporary pacemakers are available, including transvenous, epicardial, transcutaneous, and transthoracic.

Transvenous pacemakers

Physicians usually use the transvenous approach—inserting the pacemaker through a vein, such as the subclavian or internal jugular vein—when inserting a temporary

pacemaker. The transvenous pacemaker is probably the most common and reliable type of temporary pacemaker. It's usually inserted at the bedside or in a fluoroscopy suite. The leadwires are advanced through a catheter into the right ventricle or atrium and then connected to the pulse generator.

Epicardial pacemakers

Epicardial pacemakers are commonly used for patients undergoing cardiac surgery. The tips of the leadwires are attached to the heart's surface, and then the wires are brought through the chest wall, below the incision. They're then attached to the pulse generator. The leadwires are usually removed several days after surgery or when the patient no longer requires them.

Transcutaneous pacemakers

Transcutaneous pacing is a quick, noninvasive, and effective method of pacing heart rhythm that's commonly used in emergencies until a transvenous pacemaker can be inserted or the cause of an arrhythmia is resolved. With transcutaneous pacing, electrode pads are placed

DDD pacemakers

When evaluating the rhythm strip of a patient with a DDD pacemaker, keep several points in mind:
■ If the patient has an adequate intrinsic rhythm, the pacemaker won't fire; it doesn't need to.

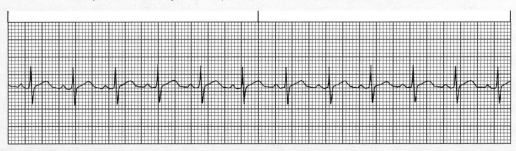

■ If you see an intrinsic P wave followed by a ventricular pacemaker spike, the pacemaker is tracking the atrial rate and ensuring a ventricular response.

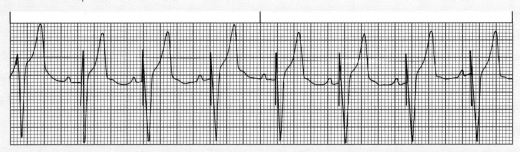

■ If you see a pacemaker spike before a P wave, followed by an intrinsic ventricular QRS complex, the atrial rate is falling below the lower rate limit, causing the atrial channel to fire. Normal conduction to the ventricles follows.

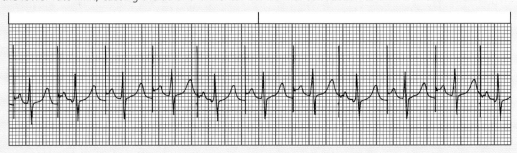

■ If you see a pacemaker spike before a P wave and before the QRS complex, no intrinsic activity is taking place in either the atria or ventricles.

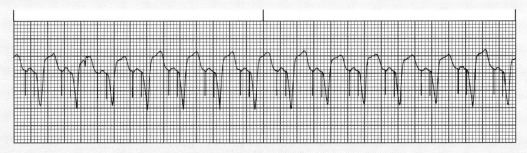

Biventricular lead placement

The biventricular pacemaker uses three leads: one to pace the right atrium, one to pace the right ventricle, and one to pace the left ventricle. The left ventricular lead is placed in the coronary sinus. Both ventricles are paced at the same time, causing them to contract simultaneously, improving cardiac output.

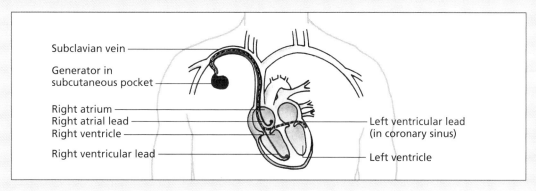

Subclavian vein

Generator in subcutaneous pocket

Right atrium
Right atrial lead
Right ventricle

Right ventricular lead

Left ventricular lead
(in coronary sinus)

Left ventricle

on the chest wall and back to deliver pacing impulses through the patient's skin to the heart muscle.

Transthoracic pacemakers

A transthoracic pacemaker is a type of temporary ventricular pacemaker used only during cardiac emergencies as a last resort. Transthoracic pacing requires insertion of a long needle into the right ventricle, using a subxiphoid approach. A pacing wire is then guided directly into the endocardium.

Troubleshooting pacemaker problems

A malfunctioning pacemaker can lead to arrhythmias, hypotension, syncope, and other signs and symptoms of decreased cardiac output. After placement of a pacemaker, its function should be evaluated. (See *Assessing pacemaker function.*)

Sometimes it's difficult to distinguish intermittent ventricular pacing from premature ventricular contractions. (See *Distinguishing intermittent ventricular pacing from PVCs,* page 280.)

There are many situations in which a patient may be exposed to electromagnetic interference (EMI). Prolonged exposure or close exposure to potential sources of electromagnetic sources can interfere with pacemaker function.

Assessing pacemaker function

When you apply a magnet to a patient's pacemaker, the device reverts to a predefined (asynchronous) response mode that allows you to assess various aspects of pacemaker function. Specifically, you can:
- determine which chambers are being paced
- assess capture
- provide emergency pacing if the device malfunctions
- ensure pacing despite electromagnetic interference
- assess battery life by checking the magnet rate—a predetermined rate that indicates the need for battery replacement.

Keep in mind, however, that you must know which implanted device the patient has before you consider using a magnet on it. The patient might have an implantable cardioverter-defibrillator (ICD), which is only rarely an appropriate target for magnet application.

What's more, because pacemakers and ICDs are similar in generator size and implant location, it isn't as easy to differentiate between the two. In addition, a single device may perform multiple functions.

In general, you shouldn't apply a magnet to an ICD or a pacemaker-ICD combination. Applying a magnet to an ICD can cause an unexpected response because various responses can be programmed or determined by the manufacturer. When directed, applying a magnet to an ICD usually suspends therapies for ventricular tachycardia and fibrillation while leaving bradycardia pacing active, which may be helpful in patients who receive multiple, inappropriate shocks. Some models may beep when exposed to a magnetic field.

Distinguishing intermittent ventricular pacing from PVCs

Knowing whether your patient has an artificial pacemaker will help you avoid mistaking a ventricular paced beat for a premature ventricular contraction (PVC). If your facility uses a monitoring system that eliminates artifact, make sure that the monitor is set up correctly for a patient with a pacemaker. Otherwise, the pacemaker spikes may be eliminated as well.

If your patient has intermittent ventricular pacing, the paced ventricular complex will have a pacemaker spike preceding it as shown in the shaded area of the top electrocardiogram (ECG) strip. You may need to look in different leads for a bipolar pacemaker spike because it's small and may be difficult to see. What's more, the paced ventricular complex of a properly functioning pacemaker won't occur early or prematurely; it will occur only when the patient's own ventricular rate falls below the rate set for the pacemaker.

If your patient is having PVCs, they'll occur prematurely and won't have pacemaker spikes preceding them. Examples are shown in the shaded areas of the bottom ECG strip.

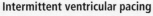

Intermittent ventricular pacing

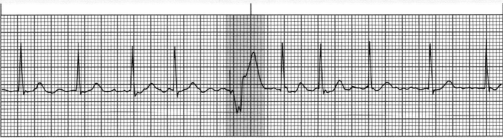

PVCs

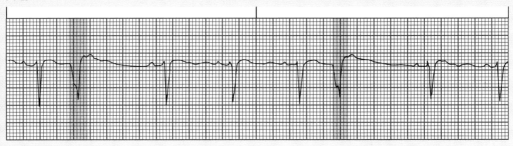

Common problems with pacemakers include:
- failure to capture
- failure to pace
- undersensing
- oversensing. (*See Recognizing a malfunctioning pacemaker,* pages 281 and 282.)

Failure to capture

Failure to capture appears on an ECG as a pacemaker spike without the appropriate atrial or ventricular response—a spike without a complex. Think of failure to capture as the pacemaker's inability to stimulate the heart chamber.

Recognizing a malfunctioning pacemaker

Occasionally, pacemakers fail to function properly. When this happens, you'll need to take immediate action to correct the problem. The rhythm strips below show examples of problems that can occur with a temporary or permanent pacemaker.

Failure to capture

- Electrocardiogram (ECG) shows a pacemaker spike without the appropriate atrial or ventricular response (spike without a complex), as shown at right.
- Patient may be asymptomatic or have signs of decreased cardiac output.
- Pacemaker can't stimulate the chamber.
- Problem may be caused by increased pacing thresholds related to certain situations:
  - metabolic or electrolyte imbalance
  - antiarrhythmic use
  - fibrosis or edema at electrode tip.
- Problem may be caused by lead malfunction:
  - dislodged lead
  - broken or damaged lead
  - perforation of myocardium by lead
  - loose connection between lead and pulse generator.
- Related interventions may solve the problem:
  - Treat metabolic disturbance.
  - Replace damaged lead.
  - Change pulse generator battery.
  - Slowly increase output setting on the temporary pacemaker until capture occurs.
  - Determine electrode placement with a chest X-ray, if needed.

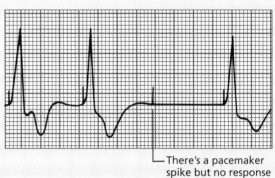

There's a pacemaker spike but no response from the heart.

Failure to pace

- ECG shows no pacemaker activity when pacemaker activity should be evident, as shown at right.
- Magnet application yields no response. (It should cause asynchronous pacing.)
- Problem has several common causes, including:
  - depleted battery
  - circuit failure
  - lead malfunction
  - inappropriate programming of sensing function
  - electromagnetic interference (EMI).
- Failure to pace can lead to asystole or a severe decrease in cardiac output in the patient who's pacemaker dependent.
- If you think a pacemaker is failing to pace, a temporary pacemaker (transcutaneous or transvenous) should be used to prevent asystole.
- Related interventions may solve the problem:
  - Replace the pulse generator battery.
  - Replace the pulse generator unit.
  - Adjust the sensitivity setting.
  - Remove the source of EMI.

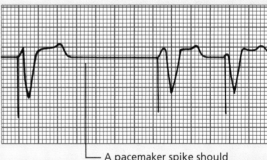

A pacemaker spike should appear here but doesn't.

(continued)

Recognizing a malfunctioning pacemaker *(continued)*

Failure to sense intrinsic beats (undersensing)

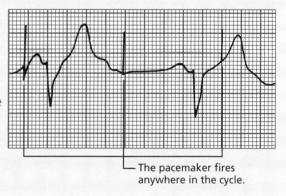

The pacemaker fires anywhere in the cycle.

- ECG may show pacing spikes anywhere in the cycle, as shown at right.
- A pacemaker spike may appear where intrinsic cardiac activity is present.
- Patient may report feeling palpitations or skipped beats.
- Spikes are especially dangerous if they fall on the T wave because ventricular tachycardia or ventricular fibrillation may result.
- Problem has several common causes, including:
  - battery failure
  - fracture of pacing leadwire
  - displacement of electrode tip
  - "cross-talk" between atrial and ventricular channels
  - EMI mistaken for intrinsic signals.
- Related interventions may solve the problem:
  - Replace the pulse generator battery.
  - Replace the leadwires.
  - Adjust the sensitivity setting.

Failure to pace

Failure to pace is indicated by the absence of pacemaker activity on an ECG when pacemaker activity is appropriately expected. This problem may be caused by battery or circuit failure, cracked or broken leads, or interference between atrial and ventricular sensing in a dual-chambered pacemaker. Failure to pace can lead to asystole.

Undersensing

Undersensing is indicated by a pacemaker spike when intrinsic cardiac activity is present. In asynchronous pacemakers that have codes, such as VOO or DOO, undersensing is a programming limitation.

When undersensing occurs in synchronous pacemakers, pacing spikes occur on the ECG where they shouldn't. Although they may appear in any part of the cardiac cycle, the spikes are especially dangerous if they fall on the T wave, where they can cause ventricular tachycardia or ventricular fibrillation.

In synchronous pacemakers, undersensing may be caused by electrolyte imbalances, disconnection or dislodgment of a lead, improper lead placement, increased sensing threshold from edema or fibrosis at the electrode tip, drug interactions, or a depleted pacemaker battery.

Oversensing

Oversensing occurs if the pacemaker is too sensitive and can misinterpret muscle movements or other events in the cardiac cycle as intrinsic cardiac electrical activity. Pacing won't occur when it's needed, and the heart rate and AV synchrony won't be maintained.

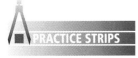

■ PRACTICE 8-1

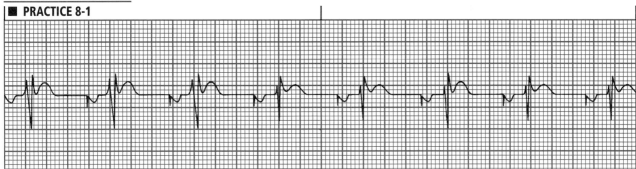

Rhythm: _____   PR interval: _____   QT interval: _____

Rate: _____   QRS complex: _____   Other: _____

P wave: _____   T wave: _____   Interpretation: _____

■ PRACTICE 8-2

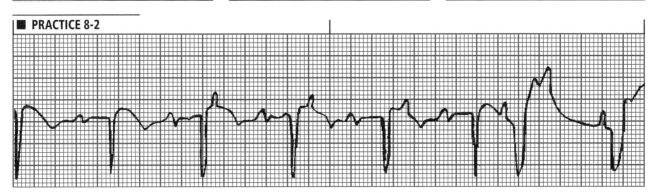

Rhythm: _____   PR interval: _____   QT interval: _____

Rate: _____   QRS complex: _____   Other: _____

P wave: _____   T wave: _____   Interpretation: _____

■ PRACTICE 8-3

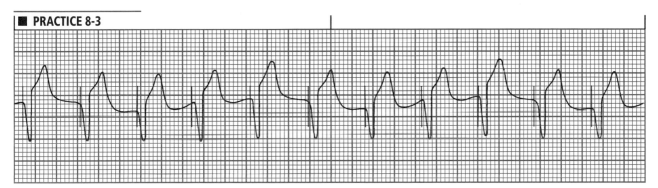

Rhythm: _____   PR interval: _____   QT interval: _____

Rate: _____   QRS complex: _____   Other: _____

P wave: _____   T wave: _____   Interpretation: _____

■ **PRACTICE 8-4**

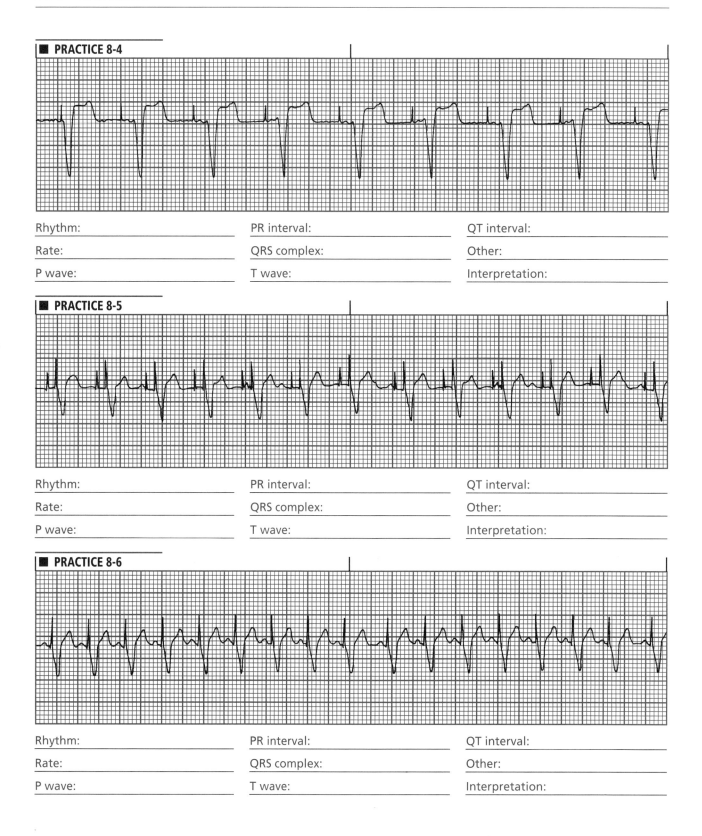

Rhythm: _____

Rate: _____

P wave: _____

PR interval: _____

QRS complex: _____

T wave: _____

QT interval: _____

Other: _____

Interpretation: _____

■ **PRACTICE 8-5**

Rhythm: _____

Rate: _____

P wave: _____

PR interval: _____

QRS complex: _____

T wave: _____

QT interval: _____

Other: _____

Interpretation: _____

■ **PRACTICE 8-6**

Rhythm: _____

Rate: _____

P wave: _____

PR interval: _____

QRS complex: _____

T wave: _____

QT interval: _____

Other: _____

Interpretation: _____

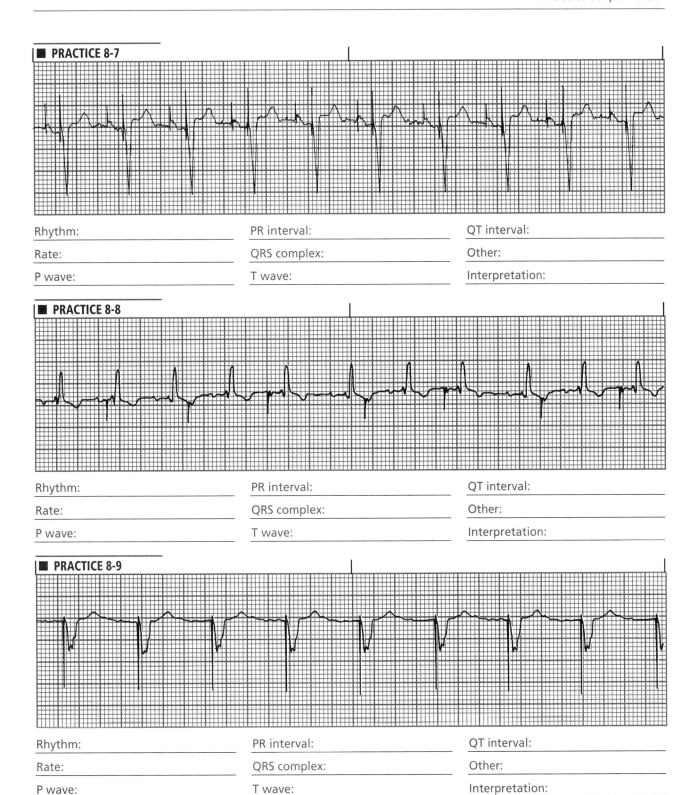

■ PRACTICE 8-7

Rhythm: _____

Rate: _____

P wave: _____

PR interval: _____

QRS complex: _____

T wave: _____

QT interval: _____

Other: _____

Interpretation: _____

■ PRACTICE 8-8

Rhythm: _____

Rate: _____

P wave: _____

PR interval: _____

QRS complex: _____

T wave: _____

QT interval: _____

Other: _____

Interpretation: _____

■ PRACTICE 8-9

Rhythm: _____

Rate: _____

P wave: _____

PR interval: _____

QRS complex: _____

T wave: _____

QT interval: _____

Other: _____

Interpretation: _____

■ **PRACTICE 8-10**

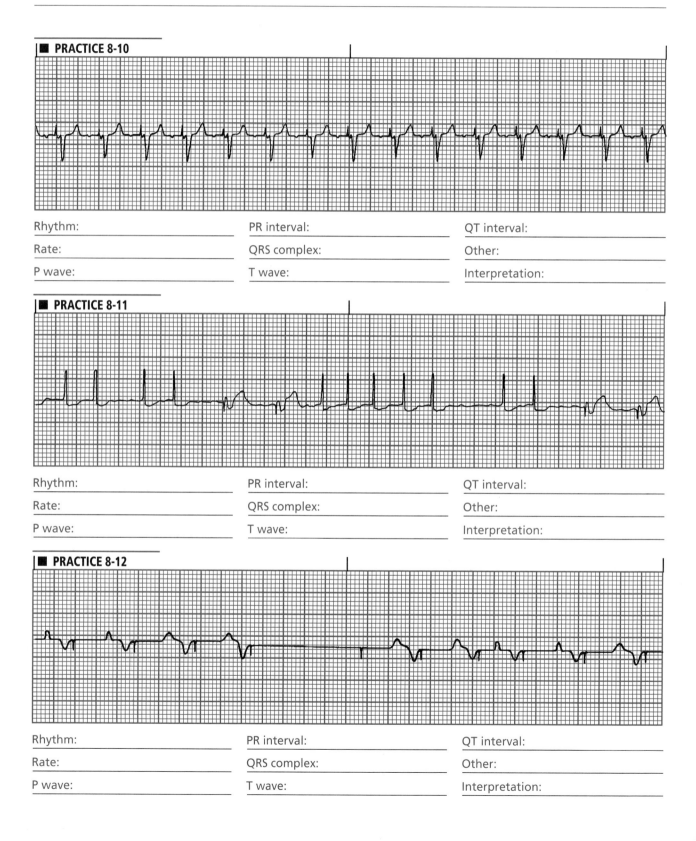

Rhythm: _____   PR interval: _____   QT interval: _____

Rate: _____   QRS complex: _____   Other: _____

P wave: _____   T wave: _____   Interpretation: _____

■ **PRACTICE 8-11**

Rhythm: _____   PR interval: _____   QT interval: _____

Rate: _____   QRS complex: _____   Other: _____

P wave: _____   T wave: _____   Interpretation: _____

■ **PRACTICE 8-12**

Rhythm: _____   PR interval: _____   QT interval: _____

Rate: _____   QRS complex: _____   Other: _____

P wave: _____   T wave: _____   Interpretation: _____

■ **PRACTICE 8-13**

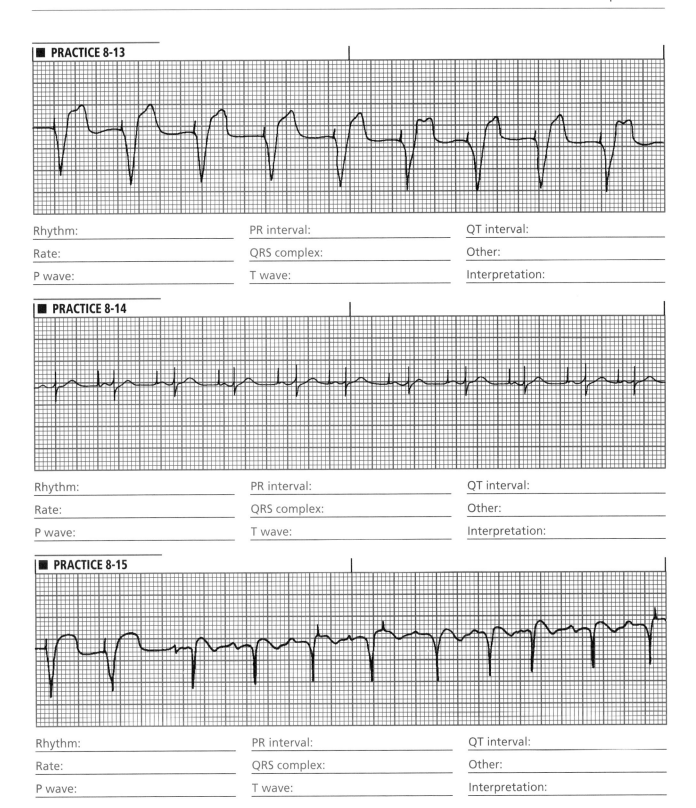

Rhythm: _____   PR interval: _____   QT interval: _____

Rate: _____   QRS complex: _____   Other: _____

P wave: _____   T wave: _____   Interpretation: _____

■ **PRACTICE 8-14**

Rhythm: _____   PR interval: _____   QT interval: _____

Rate: _____   QRS complex: _____   Other: _____

P wave: _____   T wave: _____   Interpretation: _____

■ **PRACTICE 8-15**

Rhythm: _____   PR interval: _____   QT interval: _____

Rate: _____   QRS complex: _____   Other: _____

P wave: _____   T wave: _____   Interpretation: _____

■ **PRACTICE 8-16**

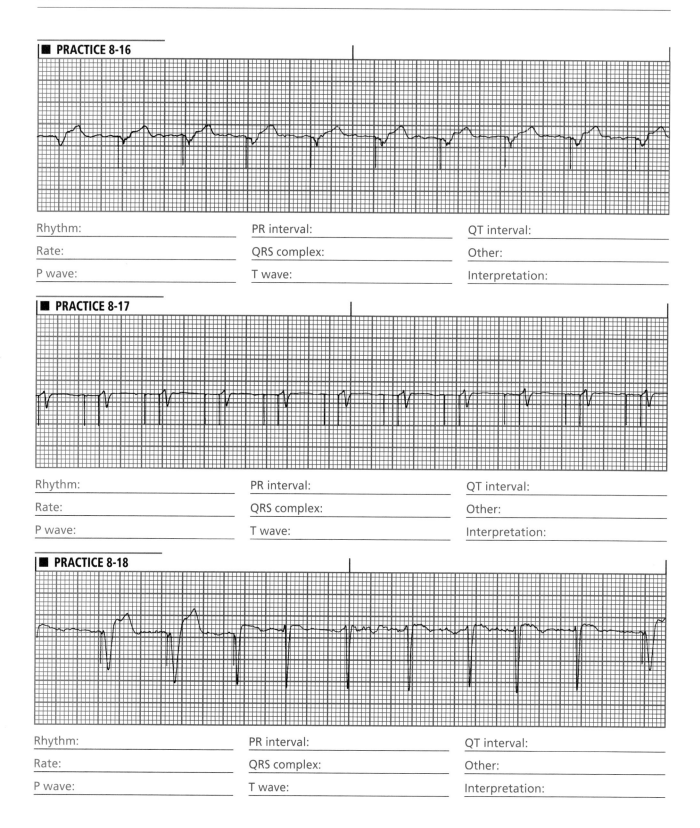

Rhythm: _____   PR interval: _____   QT interval: _____

Rate: _____   QRS complex: _____   Other: _____

P wave: _____   T wave: _____   Interpretation: _____

■ **PRACTICE 8-17**

Rhythm: _____   PR interval: _____   QT interval: _____

Rate: _____   QRS complex: _____   Other: _____

P wave: _____   T wave: _____   Interpretation: _____

■ **PRACTICE 8-18**

Rhythm: _____   PR interval: _____   QT interval: _____

Rate: _____   QRS complex: _____   Other: _____

P wave: _____   T wave: _____   Interpretation: _____

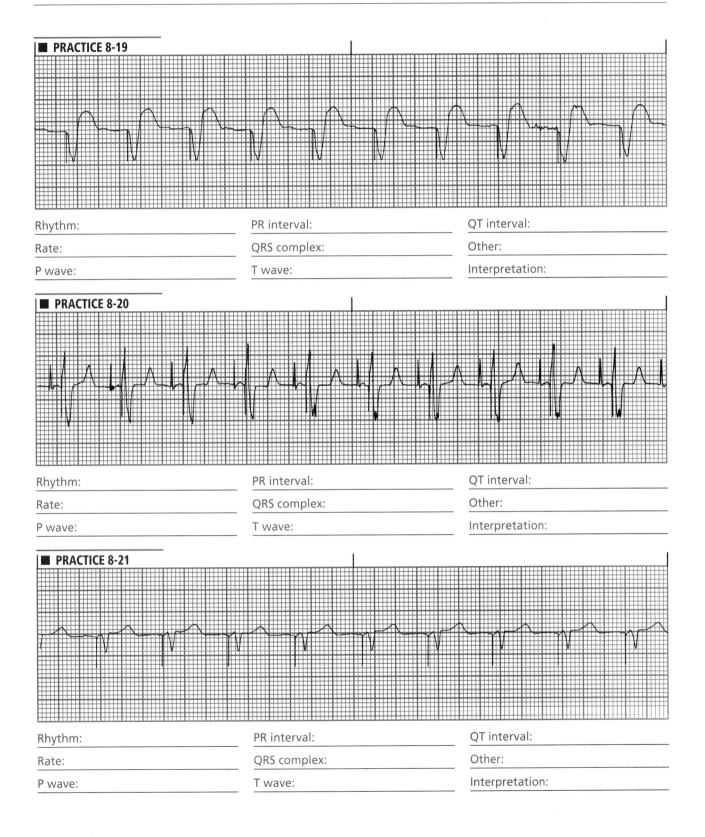

■ PRACTICE 8-19

Rhythm: _____

Rate: _____

P wave: _____

PR interval: _____

QRS complex: _____

T wave: _____

QT interval: _____

Other: _____

Interpretation: _____

■ PRACTICE 8-20

Rhythm: _____

Rate: _____

P wave: _____

PR interval: _____

QRS complex: _____

T wave: _____

QT interval: _____

Other: _____

Interpretation: _____

■ PRACTICE 8-21

Rhythm: _____

Rate: _____

P wave: _____

PR interval: _____

QRS complex: _____

T wave: _____

QT interval: _____

Other: _____

Interpretation: _____

■ **PRACTICE 8-22**

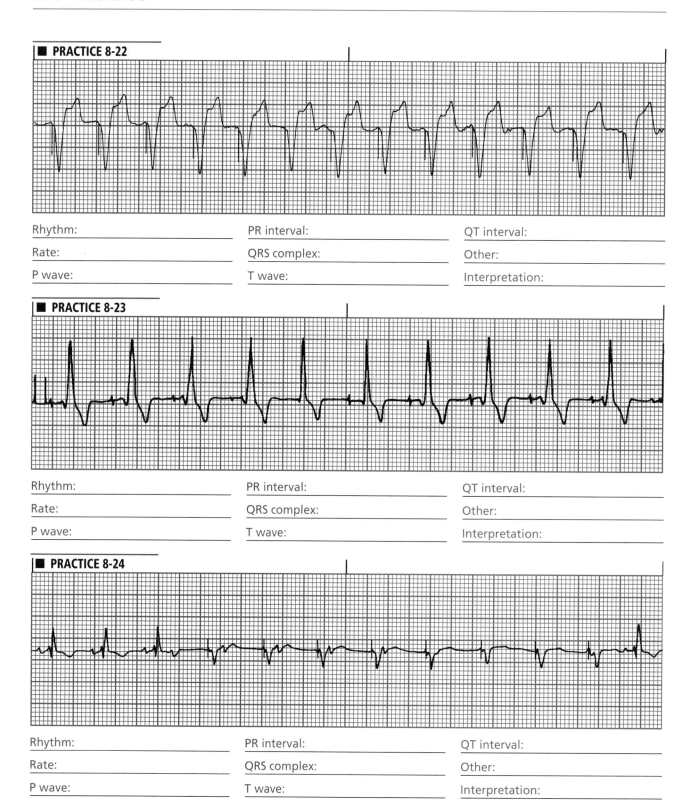

Rhythm: _____   PR interval: _____   QT interval: _____

Rate: _____   QRS complex: _____   Other: _____

P wave: _____   T wave: _____   Interpretation: _____

■ **PRACTICE 8-23**

Rhythm: _____   PR interval: _____   QT interval: _____

Rate: _____   QRS complex: _____   Other: _____

P wave: _____   T wave: _____   Interpretation: _____

■ **PRACTICE 8-24**

Rhythm: _____   PR interval: _____   QT interval: _____

Rate: _____   QRS complex: _____   Other: _____

P wave: _____   T wave: _____   Interpretation: _____

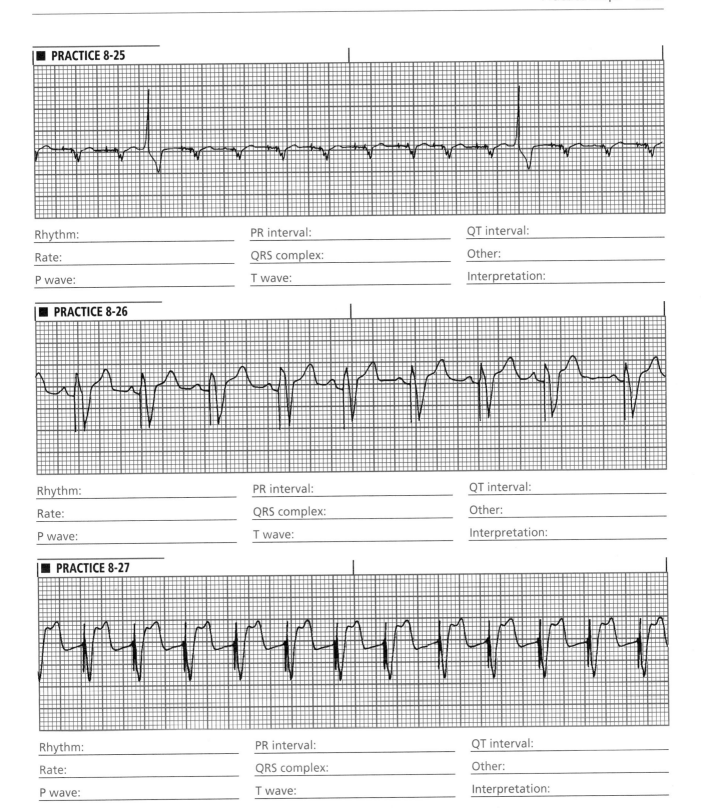

■ PRACTICE 8-25

Rhythm: _____

Rate: _____

P wave: _____

PR interval: _____

QRS complex: _____

T wave: _____

QT interval: _____

Other: _____

Interpretation: _____

■ PRACTICE 8-26

Rhythm: _____

Rate: _____

P wave: _____

PR interval: _____

QRS complex: _____

T wave: _____

QT interval: _____

Other: _____

Interpretation: _____

■ PRACTICE 8-27

Rhythm: _____

Rate: _____

P wave: _____

PR interval: _____

QRS complex: _____

T wave: _____

QT interval: _____

Other: _____

Interpretation: _____

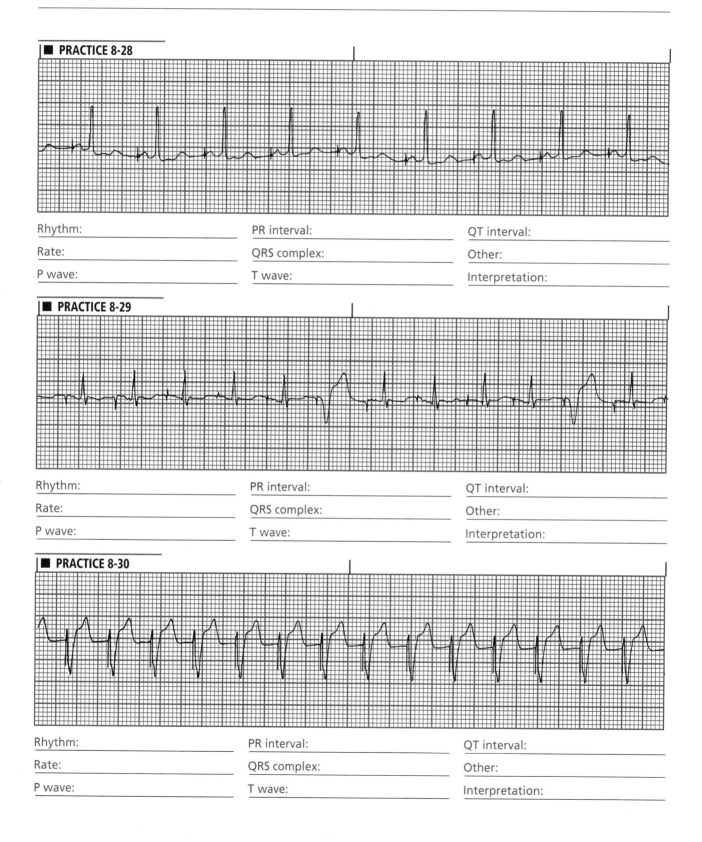

■ **PRACTICE 8-28**

Rhythm: _____ PR interval: _____ QT interval: _____

Rate: _____ QRS complex: _____ Other: _____

P wave: _____ T wave: _____ Interpretation: _____

■ **PRACTICE 8-29**

Rhythm: _____ PR interval: _____ QT interval: _____

Rate: _____ QRS complex: _____ Other: _____

P wave: _____ T wave: _____ Interpretation: _____

■ **PRACTICE 8-30**

Rhythm: _____ PR interval: _____ QT interval: _____

Rate: _____ QRS complex: _____ Other: _____

P wave: _____ T wave: _____ Interpretation: _____

■ PRACTICE STRIP ANSWERS

PRACTICE 8-1
- Rhythm: Regular
- Rate: 75 beats/minute
- P wave: Pacemaker generated
- PR interval: 0.24 second
- QRS complex: 0.08 second
- T wave: Normal
- QT interval: 0.28 second
- Other: None
- Interpretation: Atrial pacing

PRACTICE 8-2
- Rhythm: Irregular
- Rate: 80 beats/minute
- P wave: Normal when present
- PR interval: 0.32 second
- QRS complex: 0.08 second
- T wave: Normal; occasionally distorted by spike
- QT interval: 0.36 second
- Other: ST-segment elevation; erratic pacer spikes present
- Interpretation: Failure to sense

PRACTICE 8-3
- Rhythm: Regular
- Rate: 115 beats/minute
- P wave: None
- PR interval: Unmeasurable
- QRS complex: 0.08 second; pacemaker generated
- T wave: Normal
- QT interval: Unmeasurable
- Other: None
- Interpretation: Ventricular pacing

PRACTICE 8-4
- Rhythm: Regular
- Rate: 88 beats/minute
- P wave: None
- PR interval: Unmeasurable
- QRS complex: 0.10 second
- T wave: Normal
- QT interval: 0.32 second
- Other: None
- Interpretation: Atrial pacing

PRACTICE 8-5
- Rhythm: Regular
- Rate: 125 beats/minute
- P wave: None
- PR interval: Unmeasurable
- QRS complex: 0.10 second; pacemaker generated
- T wave: Normal
- QT interval: Unmeasurable
- Other: None
- Interpretation: AV pacing

PRACTICE 8-6
- Rhythm: Regular
- Rate:167 beats/minute
- P wave: Normal
- PR interval: 0.12 second
- QRS complex: 0.12 second
- T wave: Normal
- QT interval: 0.24 second
- Other: None
- Interpretation: Sinus tachycardia with tracking

PRACTICE 8-7
- Rhythm: Regular
- Rate: 100 beats/minute
- P wave: Pacemaker generated
- PR interval: 0.12 second
- QRS complex: 0.10 second; pacemaker generated
- T wave: Normal
- QT interval: Unmeasurable
- Other: None
- Interpretation: AV pacing

PRACTICE 8-8
- Rhythm: Irregular
- Rate: 110 beats/minute
- P wave: Inverted
- PR interval: 0.16 second
- QRS complex: 0.08 second
- T wave: Inverted; occasionally distorted by spike
- QT interval: 0.24 second
- Other: Erratic pacer spikes present
- Interpretation: Failure to sense

PRACTICE 8-9
- Rhythm: Regular
- Rate: 88 beats/minute
- P wave: None
- PR interval: Unmeasurable
- QRS complex: 0.12 second; pacemaker generated
- T wave: Normal
- QT interval: 0.32 second
- Other: None
- Interpretation: Ventricular pacing

PRACTICE 8-10
- Rhythm: Regular
- Rate: 150 beats/minute
- P wave: None
- PR interval: Unmeasurable
- QRS complex: 0.08 second; pacemaker generated
- T wave: Normal
- QT interval: Unmeasurable
- Other: None
- Interpretation: Ventricular pacing

PRACTICE 8-11
- Rhythm: Irregular
- Rate: 150 beats/minute
- P wave: None
- PR interval: Unmeasurable
- QRS complex: 0.04 second in non-paced beats
- T wave: Flattened
- QT interval: Unmeasurable
- Other: ST-segment depression
- Interpretation: Atrial fibrillation with ventricular pacing

PRACTICE 8-12
- Rhythm: Irregular
- Rate: 90 beats/minute
- P wave: Abnormal
- PR interval: 0.38 second
- QRS complex: Unmeasurable
- T wave: Indiscernible
- QT interval: Unmeasurable
- Other: None
- Interpretation: Failure to capture

PRACTICE 8-13
- Rhythm: Regular
- Rate: 90 beats/minute
- P wave: None
- PR interval: Unmeasurable
- QRS complex: 0.16 second; pacemaker generated
- T wave: Normal
- QT interval: 0.40 second
- Other: None
- Interpretation: Ventricular pacing

PRACTICE 8-14
- Rhythm: Regular
- Rate: 107 beats/minute
- P wave: Pacemaker generated
- PR interval: 0.12 second; pacemaker generated
- QRS complex: Unmeasurable
- T wave: Normal
- QT interval: 0.28 second
- Other: None
- Interpretation: AV pacing

PRACTICE 8-15
- Rhythm: Regular
- Rate: 110 beats/minute
- P wave: Indiscernible
- PR interval: Unmeasurable
- QRS complex: Variable
- T wave: Indiscernible
- QT interval: Unmeasurable
- Other: None
- Interpretation: Ventricular pacing leading to atrial fibrillation with failure to sense

PRACTICE 8-16
- Rhythm: Regular
- Rate: 100 beats/minute
- P wave: None
- PR interval: Unmeasurable
- QRS complex: 0.12 second
- T wave: Normal
- QT interval: 0.28 second
- Other: None
- Interpretation: Atrial pacing

PRACTICE 8-17
- Rhythm: Regular
- Rate: 107 beats/minute
- P wave: None
- PR interval: Unmeasurable
- QRS complex: 0.16 second; pacemaker generated
- T wave: Flattened
- QT interval: Unmeasurable
- Other: None
- Interpretation: AV pacing

PRACTICE 8-18
- Rhythm: Irregular
- Rate: 100 beats/minute
- P wave: None
- PR interval: Unmeasurable
- QRS complex: 0.12 second in paced beats; 0.08 second in underlying rhythm
- T wave: Normal with paced beats
- QT interval: 0.30 second
- Other: None
- Interpretation: Ventricular pacing with period of atrial fibrillation

PRACTICE 8-19
- Rhythm: Regular
- Rate: 100 beats/minute
- P wave: None
- PR interval: Unmeasurable
- QRS complex: 0.12 second; pacemaker generated
- T wave: Normal
- QT interval: 0.28 second
- Other: None
- Interpretation: Ventricular pacing

PRACTICE 8-20
- Rhythm: Regular
- Rate: 107 beats/minute
- P wave: None
- PR interval: Variable; pacemaker generated
- QRS complex: 0.12 second; pacemaker generated
- T wave: Normal
- QT interval: 0.32 second
- Other: None
- Interpretation: AV pacing

PRACTICE 8-21
- Rhythm: Regular
- Rate: 94 beats/minute
- P wave: None
- PR interval: Unmeasurable
- QRS complex: 0.08 second
- T wave: Normal
- QT interval: 0.32 second
- Other: None
- Interpretation: Atrial pacing

PRACTICE 8-22
- Rhythm: Regular
- Rate: 125 beats/minute
- P wave: None
- PR interval: Unmeasurable
- QRS complex: 0.12 second; pacemaker generated
- T wave: Normal
- QT interval: 0.28 second
- Other: None
- Interpretation: Ventricular pacing

PRACTICE 8-23
- Rhythm: Regular
- Rate: 100 beats/minute
- P wave: None
- PR interval: Unmeasurable
- QRS complex: 0.10 second; pacemaker generated
- T wave: Inverted
- QT interval: 0.28 second
- Other: None
- Interpretation: AV pacing

PRACTICE 8-24
- Rhythm: Regular
- Rate: 125 beats/minute
- P wave: Normal with sinus beats
- PR interval: 0.12 second
- QRS complex: 0.08 second with sinus beats
- T wave: Inverted with sinus beats
- QT interval: 0.24 second with sinus beats
- Other: None
- Interpretation: Normal sinus rhythm (NSR) leading to ventricular pacing, then back to NSR

PRACTICE 8-25
- Rhythm: Irregular
- Rate: 150 beats/minute
- P wave: None
- PR interval: Unmeasurable
- QRS complex: 0.12 second; pacemaker generated
- T wave: Normal
- QT interval: 0.22 second
- Other: None
- Interpretation: AV pacing with premature ventricular contractions (PVCs)

PRACTICE 8-26
- Rhythm: Regular
- Rate: 94 beats/minute
- P wave: Normal
- PR interval: 0.16 second
- QRS complex: 0.16 second; pacemaker generated
- T wave: Normal
- QT interval: 0.36 second
- Other: None
- Interpretation: Ventricular pacing

PRACTICE 8-27
- Rhythm: Regular
- Rate: 125 beats/minute
- P wave: None
- PR interval: Unmeasurable
- QRS complex: 0.16 second; pacemaker generated
- T wave: Normal
- QT interval: 0.32 second
- Other: None
- Interpretation: Ventricular pacing

PRACTICE 8-28
- Rhythm: Regular
- Rate: 90 beats/minute
- P wave: Normal
- PR interval: 0.16 second; pacemaker generated
- QRS complex: 0.12 second
- T wave: Normal
- QT interval: 0.32 second
- Other: None
- Interpretation: Atrial pacing

PRACTICE 8-29
- Rhythm: Irregular
- Rate: 120 beats/minute
- P wave: None
- PR interval: Unmeasurable
- QRS complex: 0.08 second
- T wave: Flattened
- QT interval: 0.32 second
- Other: None
- Interpretation: Atrial pacing with PVCs

PRACTICE 8-30
- Rhythm: Regular
- Rate: 150 beats/minute
- P wave: None
- PR interval: Unmeasurable
- QRS complex: 0.08 second; pacemaker generated
- T wave: Normal
- QT interval: 0.28 second
- Other: None
- Interpretation: Ventricular pacing

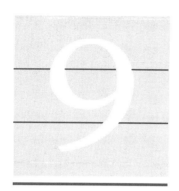

12-lead ECGs

The 12-lead electrocardiogram (ECG) is a diagnostic test that helps identify pathologic conditions, especially ischemia and acute myocardial infarction (MI). This chapter reviews the normal 12-lead ECG and abnormal 12-lead ECG findings with acute MI.

The 12-lead ECG provides a more complete view of the heart's electrical activity than a rhythm strip does and can be used to assess left ventricular function more effectively.

Patients with conditions that affect the heart's electrical system may also benefit from a 12-lead ECG, including those with:
- cardiac arrhythmias
- heart chamber enlargement or hypertrophy
- digoxin or other drug toxicity
- electrolyte imbalances
- pulmonary embolism
- pericarditis
- pacemakers
- hypothermia.

Like other diagnostic tests, a 12-lead ECG must be viewed in conjunction with other clinical data. Therefore, always correlate the patient's ECG results with the history, physical assessment findings, and results of laboratory and other diagnostic studies as well as the drug regimen.

The 12-lead ECG records the heart's electrical activity using a series of electrodes placed on the patient's extremities and chest wall. The 12 leads include three bipolar limb leads (I, II, and III), three unipolar augmented limb leads (aV$_R$, aV$_L$, and aV$_F$), and six unipolar precordial, or chest, leads (V$_1$, V$_2$, V$_3$, V$_4$, V$_5$, and V$_6$). These leads provide 12 different views of the heart's electrical activity. (See *Viewing ECG leads.*)

Scanning up, down, and across, each lead transmits information about a different area of the heart. The waveforms obtained from each lead vary depending on the lead's location in relation to the wave of depolarization passing through the myocardium.

Limb leads

The six limb leads record electrical activity in the heart's frontal plane, a view through the middle of the heart from top to bottom and from right to left.

Precordial leads

The six precordial leads provide information on electrical activity in the heart's horizontal plane, a transverse view through the middle of the heart, dividing it into upper and lower portions.

Electrical axes

As well as assessing 12 different leads, a 12-lead ECG records the heart's electrical axis. The term *axis* refers to the direction of depolarization as it spreads through the heart. As impulses travel through the heart, they generate small electrical forces called *instantaneous vectors*. The mean of these vectors represents the force and direction of the wave of depolarization through the heart—the electrical axis. The electrical axis is also called the *mean instantaneous vector* and the *mean QRS vector*.

In a healthy heart, impulses originate in the sinoatrial node, travel through the atria to the atrioventricular (AV) node, and then travel to the ventricles. Most of the movement of the impulses is downward and to the left, the direction of a normal axis.

In an unhealthy heart, axis direction varies. That's because the direction of electrical activity travels away from areas of damage or necrosis and toward areas of

Viewing ECG leads

Each of the leads on a 12-lead electrocardiogram (ECG) views the heart from a different angle. These illustrations show the direction of electrical activity (depolarization) monitored by each lead and the corresponding 12 views of the heart.

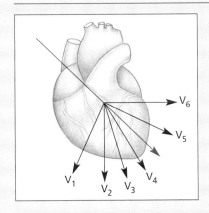

Views reflected on 12-lead ECG	Lead	View of the heart
	STANDARD LIMB LEADS (BIPOLAR)	
	I	Lateral wall
	II	Inferior wall
	III	Inferior wall
	AUGMENTED LIMB LEADS (UNIPOLAR)	
	aV_R	No specific view
	aV_L	Lateral wall
	aV_F	Inferior wall
	PRECORDIAL, OR CHEST, LEADS (UNIPOLAR)	
	V_1	Septal wall
	V_2	Septal wall
	V_3	Anterior wall
	V_4	Anterior wall
	V_5	Lateral wall
	V_6	Lateral wall

hypertrophy. Knowing the normal deflection of each lead will help you evaluate whether the electrical axis is normal or abnormal.

Obtaining a 12-lead ECG

To obtain an accurate 12-lead ECG recording, you'll need to properly prepare the patient, select appropriate electrode sites, and correctly apply the electrodes and leads.

◼ Preparation

Gather all necessary supplies, including the ECG machine, recording paper, electrodes, and gauze pads. Tell the patient that the physician has ordered an ECG, and explain the procedure. Emphasize that the test takes about 10 minutes and that it's a safe and painless way to evaluate the heart's electrical activity. Answer the patient's questions, and offer reassurance. Preparing the patient properly will help alleviate anxiety and promote cooperation.

Ask the patient to lie in a supine position in the center of the bed with arms at his sides. If he can't tolerate lying flat, raise the head of the bed to semi-Fowler's position. Document the patient's position during the procedure.

Precordial lead placement

The precordial leads complement the limb leads to provide a complete view of the heart. To record the precordial leads, place the electrodes as shown here.

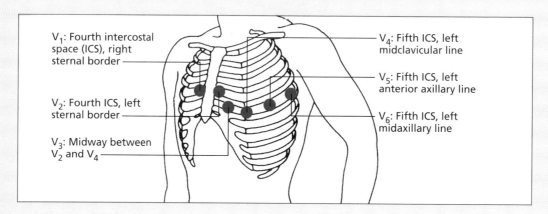

V_1: Fourth intercostal space (ICS), right sternal border

V_2: Fourth ICS, left sternal border

V_3: Midway between V_2 and V_4

V_4: Fifth ICS, left midclavicular line

V_5: Fifth ICS, left anterior axillary line

V_6: Fifth ICS, left midaxillary line

Ensure privacy, and expose the patient's arms, legs, and chest, draping for comfort.

When selecting the areas to which you'll apply the electrodes, choose areas that are flat and fleshy, not muscular or bony. Clip any excessive hair from the area. Remove excess oil and other substances, such as body lotion, from the skin to enhance electrode contact. Remember, the better the electrode contact is, the better the recording will be.

Electrode and lead placement

The 12-lead ECG provides 12 different views of the heart, just as 12 photographers snapping the same picture would produce 12 different photographs. Taking all of those snapshots requires placing four electrodes on the limbs and six across the front of the chest wall.

To help ensure an accurate recording, the electrodes must be applied correctly. Inaccurate placement of an electrode by greater than ⅝″ (1.5 cm) from its standard position may lead to inaccurate waveforms and an incorrect ECG interpretation.

You'll need patience when obtaining a pediatric ECG. With the help of the parents, if possible, try distracting the attention of the child. If artifact from arm and leg movement is a problem, try placing the electrodes in a more proximal position on the extremity.

Limb lead placement

To record the bipolar limb leads I, II, and III and the unipolar limb leads aV_R, aV_L, and aV_F, place electrodes

on both of the patient's arms and on his left leg. The right leg also receives an electrode, but that electrode acts as a ground and doesn't contribute to the waveform.

Attaching the leads is typically easy because each lead-wire is labeled or color-coded. For example, a wire (usually white) might be labeled "RA" for right arm. Another (usually red) might be labeled "LL" for left leg.

Precordial lead placement

Precordial leads are also labeled or color-coded according to which wire corresponds to which lead. To record the six precordial leads (V_1 through V_6), position the electrodes on specific areas of the anterior chest wall:

■ Place lead V_1 over the fourth intercostal space at the right sternal border. To find the space, locate the sternal notch at the second rib and feel your way down the sternal border until you reach the fourth intercostal space.

■ Place lead V_2 just opposite V_1, over the fourth intercostal space at the left sternal border.

■ Place lead V_4 over the fifth intercostal space at the left midclavicular line. Placing lead V_4 before V_3 makes it easier to see where to place lead V_3.

■ Place lead V_3 midway between V_2 and V_4.

■ Place lead V_5 over the fifth intercostal space at the left anterior axillary line.

■ Place lead V_6 over the fifth intercostal space at the left midaxillary line. If you've placed leads V_4 through V_6 correctly, they should line up horizontally.

(See *Precordial lead placement*.) If they're placed too low, the ECG tracing will be inaccurate.

Reading the multichannel ECG recording

The top of a 12-lead electrocardiogram (ECG) recording usually shows patient identification information along with an interpretation by the machine. A rhythm strip is commonly included at the bottom of the recording.

Standardization

Look for standardization marks on the recording, normally 10 small squares high. If the patient has high voltage complexes, the marks will be half as high. You'll also notice that lead markers separate the lead recordings on the paper and that each lead is labeled.

Familiarize yourself with the order in which the leads are arranged on an ECG tracing. Getting accustomed to the layout of the tracing will help you interpret the ECG more quickly and accurately.

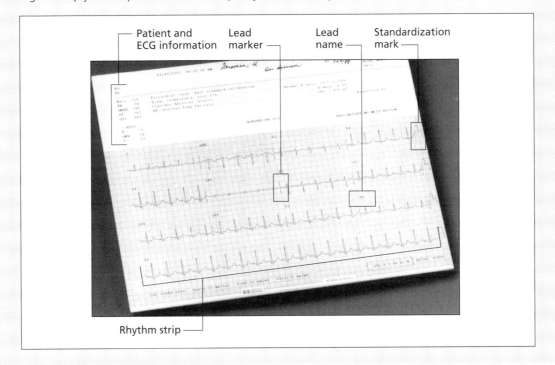

Patient and ECG information — Lead marker — Lead name — Standardization mark

Rhythm strip

▉ Recording the ECG

After properly placing the electrodes and leads, record the ECG. With a multichannel recorder, all leads are attached to the patient at the same time and the machine prints a simultaneous view of all leads.

To record a multichannel ECG, follow these steps:

- Plug the cord of the ECG machine into a grounded outlet. If the machine operates on a charged battery, it may not need to be plugged in.
- Place all of the electrodes on the patient.
- Attach all leads securely, and then turn on the machine.
- Instruct the patient to relax, lie still, and breathe normally. Ask him not to talk during the recording, to prevent distortion of the ECG tracing.

- Set the ECG paper speed selector to 25 mm per second. Enter the patient's identification data as prompted.
- Press the appropriate button on the ECG machine, and record the ECG.
- Observe the quality of the tracing. When the machine finishes the recording, turn it off.
- Remove the leads and electrodes, and clean the patient's skin.

ECG printout

Depending on the information entered, ECG printouts from a multichannel ECG machine will show the patient's name, room number and, possibly, medical record number. At the top of the printout, you'll see the patient's heart rate and wave durations, measured in seconds. (See *Reading the multichannel ECG recording*.)

Using the quadrant method

This chart will help you quickly determine the direction of a patient's electrical axis. Observe the deflections of the QRS complexes in leads I and aV$_F$. Then check the chart to determine whether the patient's axis is normal or has a left, right, or extreme right axis deviation.

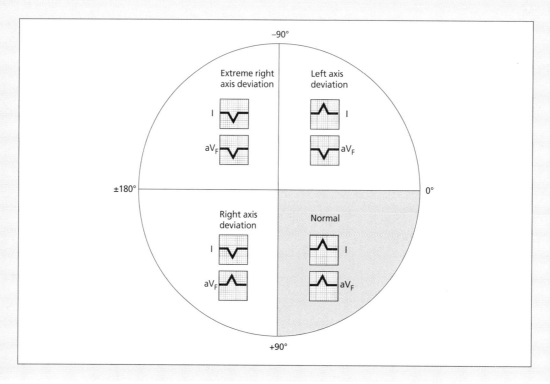

Some machines can record ST-segment elevation and depression. The name of the lead will appear next to each 6-second strip.

If it isn't already included on the printout, be sure to write the following information: date, time, physician's name, and special circumstances. For example, you might record an ECG with an episode of chest pain, abnormal electrolyte levels, related drug treatment, abnormal placement of the electrodes, or the presence of an artificial pacemaker. Also note whether a magnet was used while the ECG was obtained.

Remember, ECGs are legal documents. They belong in the patient's medical record and must be saved for future reference and comparison with baseline strips.

Interpreting 12-lead ECGs

To interpret a 12-lead ECG, follow these steps:

1. Check the ECG tracing to see if it's technically correct. Make sure the baseline is free from electrical interference and drift.

2. Scan leads I, II, and III. The R-wave voltage in lead II should equal the sum of the R-wave voltage in leads I and III. Lead aV$_R$ is typically negative. If these rules aren't met, the tracing may be recorded incorrectly.

3. Locate the lead markers on the waveform. Lead markers are the points where one lead changes to another.

4. Check the standardization markings (1 millivolt or 10 mm), usually located at the beginning of the strip, to make sure all leads were recorded with the ECG machine's amplitude at the same setting.

5. Assess the heart's rate and rhythm.

Using the degree method

The degree method of determining axis deviation allows you to identify a patient's electrical axis by degrees on the hexaxial system, not just by quadrant. To use this method, take the following steps.

Step 1

Identify the limb lead with the smallest QRS complex or the equiphasic QRS complex. In this example, it's lead III.

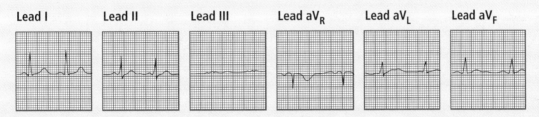

| Lead I | Lead II | Lead III | Lead aV$_R$ | Lead aV$_L$ | Lead aV$_F$ |

Step 2

Locate the axis for lead III on the hexaxial diagram. Then find the axis perpendicular to it, which is the axis for lead aV$_R$.

Step 3

Now, examine the QRS complex in lead aV$_R$, noting whether the deflection is positive or negative. As you can see, the QRS complex for this lead is negative, indicating that the current is moving toward the negative pole of aV$_R$, which is in the right lower quadrant at +30 degrees on the hexaxial diagram. So the electrical axis here is normal at +30 degrees.

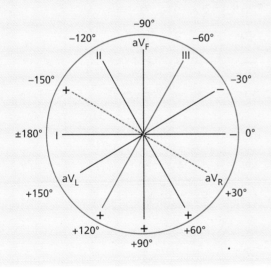

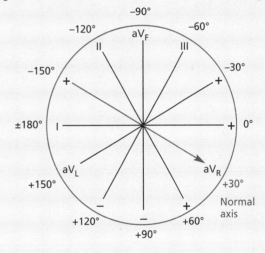

6. Determine the heart's electrical axis. Use either the quadrant method or the degree method. (See *Using the quadrant method* and *Using the degree method*.)

7. Examine leads I, II, and III. The R wave in lead II should be taller than the one in lead I. The R wave in lead III should be a smaller version of the R wave in lead I. The P wave or QRS complex may be inverted. Each lead should have flat ST segments and upright T waves. Pathologic Q waves should be absent.

8. Examine leads aV$_L$, aV$_F$, and aV$_R$. The tracings from leads aV$_L$ and aV$_F$ should be similar, but lead aV$_F$ should have taller P waves and R waves. Lead aV$_R$ has little di-

agnostic value. Its P wave, QRS complex, and T wave should be deflected downward.

9. Examine the R wave in the precordial leads. Normally, the R wave (the first positive deflection of the QRS complex) gets progressively taller from leads V$_1$ to V$_5$. It gets slightly smaller in lead V$_6$.

10. Examine the S wave (the negative deflection after an R wave) in the precordial leads. It should appear extremely deep in lead V$_1$ and become progressively more shallow, usually disappearing by lead V$_5$. (See *Normal findings in a 12-lead ECG*, pages 302 to 304.)

(Text continues on page 305.)

Normal findings in a 12-lead ECG

Each electrocardiogram (ECG) waveform (P wave, QRS complex, T wave) represents the electrical events occurring in one cardiac cycle. The 12-lead ECG provides 12 views of the electrical activity of the heart, which includes three bipolar leads (I, II, and III), three unipolar augmented leads (aV$_R$, aV$_L$, and aV$_F$), and six precordial, or chest, leads (V$_1$, V$_2$, V$_3$, V$_4$, V$_5$, and V$_6$). Each lead on a 12-lead ECG views the heart from a different angle. The tracings shown here represent normal findings of the heart's electrical activity in each of the 12 leads.

Lead I

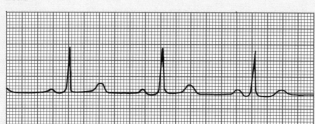

P wave: Upright
Q wave: Small or none
R wave: Largest wave
S wave: None present, or smaller than R wave
T wave: Upright
U wave: None present
ST segment: Usually isoelectric but may vary from +1 to –0.5 mm

Lead II

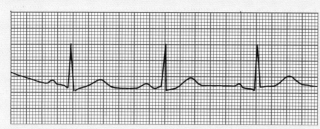

P wave: Upright
Q wave: Small or none
R wave: Large (vertical heart)
S wave: None present, or smaller than R wave
T wave: Upright
U wave: None present
ST segment: Usually isoelectric but may vary from +1 to –0.5 mm

Lead III

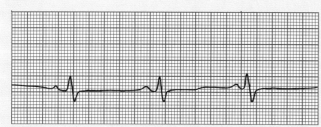

P wave: Upright, diphasic, or inverted
Q wave: Usually small or none (a Q wave must also be present in lead aV$_F$ to be considered diagnostic)
R wave: None present to large wave
S wave: None present to large wave, indicating horizontal heart
T wave: Upright, diphasic, or inverted
U wave: None present
ST segment: Usually isoelectric but may vary from +1 to –0.5 mm

Lead aV$_R$

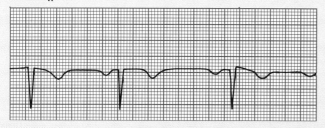

P wave: Inverted
Q wave: None, small wave, or large wave present
R wave: None, or small wave present
S wave: Large wave (may be QS)
T wave: Inverted
U wave: None present
ST segment: Usually isoelectric but may vary from +1 to –0.5 mm

Normal findings in a 12-lead ECG *(continued)*

Lead aV_L

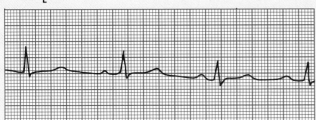

P wave: Upright, diphasic, or inverted
Q wave: None, small wave, or large wave present (a Q wave must also be present in lead I or precordial leads to be considered diagnostic)
R wave: None, small wave, or large wave present (large wave indicates horizontal heart)
S wave: None present to large wave (large wave indicates vertical heart)
T wave: Upright, diphasic, or inverted
U wave: None present
ST segment: Usually isoelectric but may vary from +1 to –0.5 mm

Lead aV_F

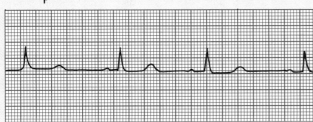

P wave: Upright
Q wave: None, or small wave present
R wave: None, small wave, or large wave present (large wave suggests vertical heart)
S wave: None present to large wave (large wave suggests horizontal heart)
T wave: Upright, diphasic, or inverted
U wave: None present
ST segment: Usually isoelectric but may vary from +1 to –0.5 mm

Lead V₁

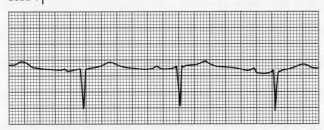

P wave: Upright, diphasic, or inverted
Q wave: Deep QS pattern possibly present
R wave: None present, or less than S wave
S wave: Large (part of QS pattern)
T wave: Usually inverted but may be upright and diphasic
U wave: None present
ST segment: May vary from 0 to +1 mm

Lead V₂

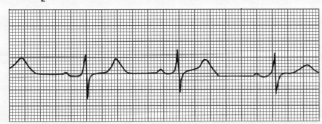

P wave: Upright
Q wave: Deep QS pattern possibly present
R wave: None present, or less than S wave (wave may become progressively larger)
S wave: Large (part of QS pattern)
T wave: Upright
U wave: Upright; lower amplitude than T wave
ST segment: May vary from 0 to +1 mm

(continued)

Normal findings in a 12-lead ECG *(continued)*

Lead V₃

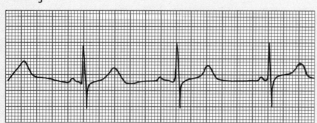

P wave: Upright
Q wave: None, or small wave present
R wave: Less than, greater than, or equal to S wave (wave may become progressively larger)
S wave: Large (greater than R wave, less than R wave, or equal to R wave)
T wave: Upright
U wave: Upright; lower amplitude than T wave
ST segment: May vary from 0 to +1 mm

Lead V₄

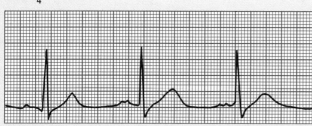

P wave: Upright
Q wave: None, or small wave present
R wave: Progressively larger wave; R wave greater than S wave
S wave: Progressively smaller (less than R wave)
T wave: Upright
U wave: Upright; lower amplitude than T wave
ST segment: Usually isoelectric but may vary from +1 to –0.5 mm

Lead V₅

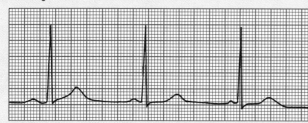

P wave: Upright
Q wave: Small
R wave: Progressively larger but less than 26 mm
S wave: Progressively smaller; less than the S wave in lead V₄
T wave: Upright
U wave: None present
ST segment: Usually isoelectric but may vary from +1 to –0.5 mm

Lead V₆

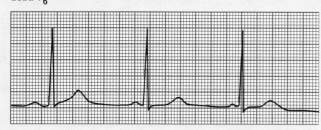

P wave: Upright
Q wave: Small
R wave: Largest wave but less than 26 mm
S wave: Smallest wave; less than the S wave in lead V₅
T wave: Upright
U wave: None present
ST segment: Usually isoelectric but may vary from +1 to –0.5 mm

ECG findings in acute MI

A 12-lead ECG is used to assist in the diagnosis of MI. If a patient complains of chest pain, obtain an ECG as quickly as possible. It's a crucial component in determining whether myocardial ischemia is present. Interpretation of the ECG will direct the patient's treatment plan. (See *Stages of myocardial ischemia, injury, and infarct.*)

The location of the MI is a critical factor in determining the most appropriate treatment and predicting possible complications. Characteristic ECG changes that oc-

---

Stages of myocardial ischemia, injury, and infarct

Three stages occur when occlusion of a vessel exists: ischemia, injury, and infarct.

Ischemia

Ischemia, the first stage, indicates that blood flow and oxygen demand are out of balance. It can be resolved by improving flow or reducing oxygen needs. Electrocardiogram (ECG) changes indicate ST-segment depression or T-wave changes.

Injury

The second stage, injury, occurs when the ischemia is prolonged enough to damage the area of the heart. ECG changes typically reveal ST-segment elevation (usually in two or more leads).

Infarct

Infarct, the third stage, occurs with the actual death of myocardial cells. Scar tissue eventually replaces the dead tissue, and the damage caused is irreversible.

In the earliest stage of a myocardial infarction (MI), hyperacute or very tall and narrow T waves may be seen on the ECG. Within hours, the T waves become inverted and ST-segment elevation occurs in the leads facing the area of damage. The last change to occur in the evolution of an MI is the development of a pathologic Q wave, which is the only permanent ECG evidence of myocardial necrosis. Q waves are considered pathologic when they appear greater than or equal to 0.04 second wide and their height is greater than 25% of the R-wave height in that lead. Pathologic Q waves develop in over 90% of patients with ST-segment elevation MI. Approximately 25% of patients with non-ST-segment elevation MI will develop pathologic Q waves, and the remaining patients will have a non-Q-wave MI.

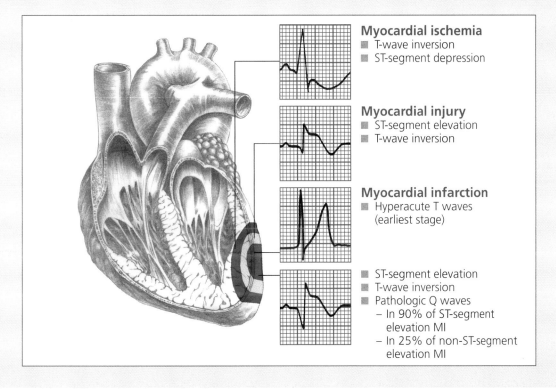

Myocardial ischemia
- T-wave inversion
- ST-segment depression

Myocardial injury
- ST-segment elevation
- T-wave inversion

Myocardial infarction
- Hyperacute T waves (earliest stage)

- ST-segment elevation
- T-wave inversion
- Pathologic Q waves
  - In 90% of ST-segment elevation MI
  - In 25% of non-ST-segment elevation MI

Locating myocardial damage

After you've noted characteristic electrocardiogram lead changes in an acute myocardial infarction, use this table to identify the areas of damage. Match the lead changes (ST elevation, abnormal Q waves) in the second column with the affected wall in the first column and the artery involved in the third column. The fourth column shows reciprocal lead changes.

Wall affected	Leads	Artery involved	Reciprocal changes
Anterior	V_2, V_3, V_4	Left coronary artery, left anterior descending (LAD) artery	II, III, aV_F
Anterolateral	I, aV_L, V_2, V_3, V_4, V_5, V_6	LAD artery and diagonal branches, circumflex and marginal branches	II, III, aV_F
Anteroseptal	V_1, V_2, V_3, V_4	LAD artery	None
Inferior	II, III, aV_F	Right coronary artery (RCA)	I, aV_L
Lateral	I, aV_L, V_5, V_6	Circumflex branch of left coronary artery	II, III, aV_F
Posterior	V_1, V_2	RCA or circumflex artery	V_1, V_2, V_3, V_4 (R greater than S in V_1 and V_2, ST-segment depression, elevated T wave)

cur with each type of MI are localized to the leads overlying the infarction site. (See *Locating myocardial damage.*)

This section reviews characteristic ECG changes that occur with different types of MI. By reviewing the sample ECGs, you'll know the classic signs to look for.

Anterior wall MI

The left anterior descending artery supplies blood to the anterior portion of the left ventricle, ventricular septum, and portions of the right and left bundle-branch systems. When the left anterior descending artery becomes occluded, an anterior wall MI occurs.

Complications include second-degree AV block, bundle-branch block, ventricular irritability, and left-sided heart failure.

ECG changes

In anterior wall MI, the R waves don't progress through the precordial leads. ST-segment elevation occurs in leads V_2 and V_3, and the reciprocal leads II, III, and aV_F show slight ST-segment depression.

Recognizing anterior wall MI

This 12-lead electrocardiogram shows typical characteristics of an anterior wall myocardial infarction (MI). Note that the R waves don't progress through the precordial leads. Also note the ST-segment elevation in leads V_2 and V_3. As expected, the reciprocal leads II, III, and aV_F show slight ST-segment depression. The axis is normal at +60 degrees.

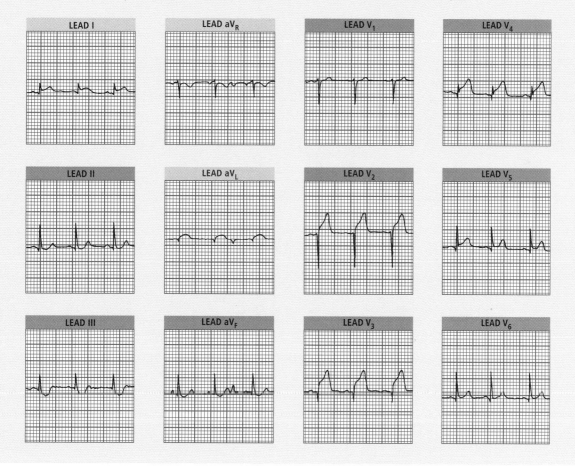

Septal wall MI

The patient with a septal wall MI is at increased risk for developing a ventricular septal defect. ECG changes are present in leads V_1 and V_2. In those leads, the R wave disappears, the ST segment rises, and the T wave inverts. Because the left anterior descending artery also supplies blood to the ventricular septum, a septal wall MI typically accompanies an anterior wall MI.

Lateral wall MI

A lateral wall MI is usually caused by a blockage in the left circumflex artery. This type of MI typically causes premature ventricular contractions (PVCs) and varying degrees of heart block. It usually accompanies an anterior or inferior wall MI.

ECG changes

With lateral wall MI, the ECG shows characteristic ST-segment elevation in leads I, aV_L, V_5, and V_6. The reciprocal leads for a lateral wall infarction are leads II, III, and aV_F.

Recognizing lateral wall MI

This 12-lead electrocardiogram shows typical characteristics of a lateral wall myocardial infarction (MI). Note the ST-segment elevation in leads I, aV_L, V_5, and V_6.

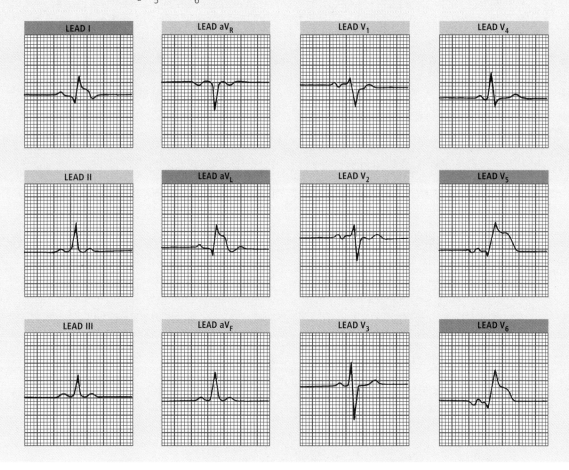

Inferior wall MI

An inferior wall MI is usually caused by occlusion of the right coronary artery. It's also called a *diaphragmatic MI* because the inferior wall of the heart lies over the diaphragm.

Patients with inferior wall MI are at risk for developing sinus bradycardia, sinus arrest, heart block, and PVCs. This type of MI occurs alone or with a lateral wall, posterior wall, or right ventricular MI.

ECG changes

ECG changes characteristic of inferior wall MI include T-wave inversion, ST-segment elevation, and pathologic Q waves in leads II, III, and aV$_F$.

Recognizing inferior wall MI

This 12-lead electrocardiogram (ECG) shows the characteristic changes of an inferior wall myocardial infarction (MI). In leads II, III, and aV$_F$, note the T-wave inversion, ST-segment elevation, and pathologic Q waves. In leads I and aV$_L$, note the slight ST-segment depression—a reciprocal change. This ECG shows left axis deviation at –60 degrees.

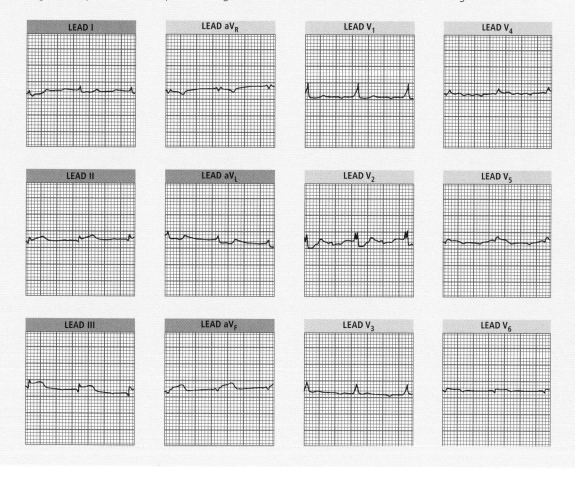

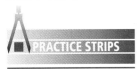

■ PRACTICE 9-1

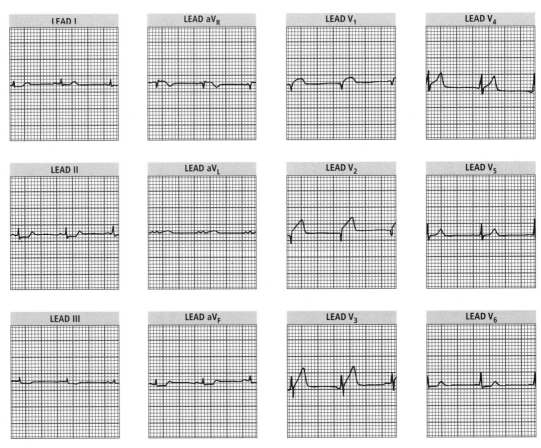

Rhythm: _____

Rate: _____

Axis: _____

Interpretation: _____

T wave: _____

ST segment: _____

Q wave: _____

Leads I, II, III: _____

Leads aV_R, aV_L, aV_F: _____

Leads V_1 to V_6: _____

■ **PRACTICE 9-2**

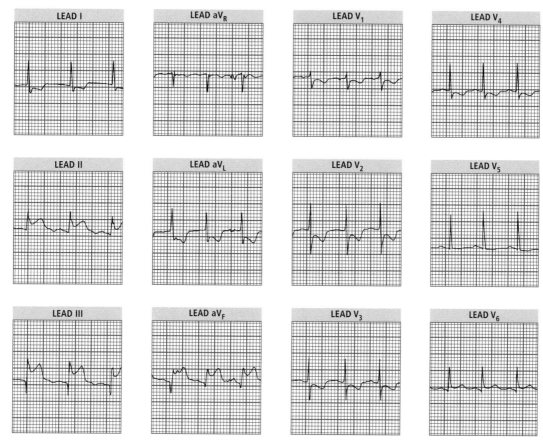

Rhythm: _____

Rate: _____

Axis: _____

Interpretation: _____

T wave: _____

ST segment: _____

Q wave: _____

Leads I, II, III: _____

Leads aV$_R$, aV$_L$, aV$_F$: _____

Leads V$_1$ to V$_6$: _____

■ **PRACTICE 9-3**

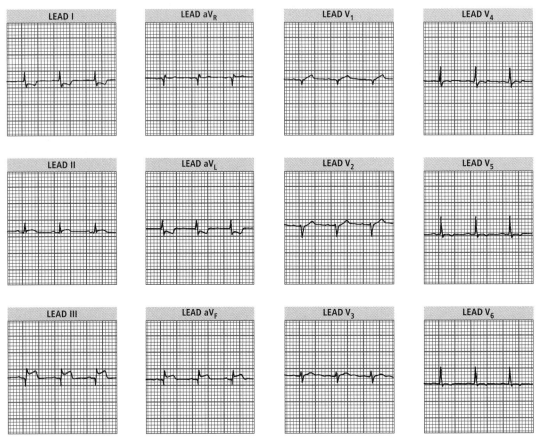

Rhythm: _____

Rate: _____

Axis: _____

Interpretation: _____

T wave: _____

ST segment: _____

Q wave: _____

Leads I, II, III: _____

Leads aV$_R$, aV$_L$, aV$_F$: _____

Leads V$_1$ to V$_6$: _____

■ **PRACTICE 9-4**

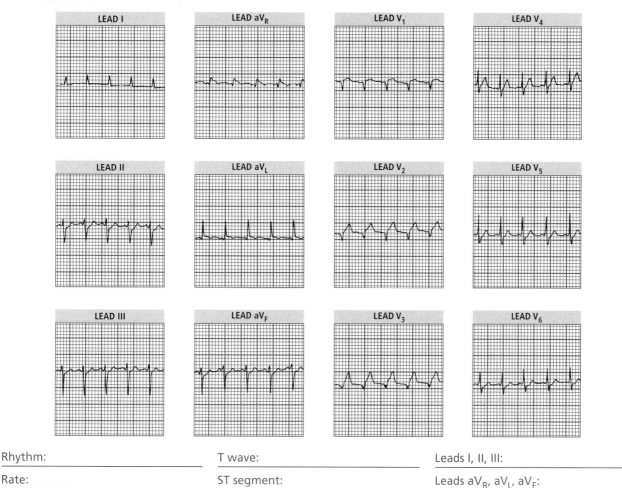

Rhythm: _____

Rate: _____

Axis: _____

Interpretation: _____

T wave: _____

ST segment: _____

Q wave: _____

Leads I, II, III: _____

Leads aV$_R$, aV$_L$, aV$_F$: _____

Leads V$_1$ to V$_6$: _____

■ PRACTICE 9-5

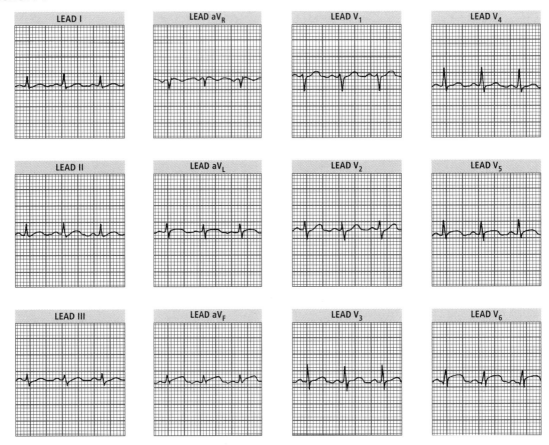

Rhythm: _____

Rate: _____

Axis: _____

Interpretation: _____

T wave: _____

ST segment: _____

Q wave: _____

Leads I, II, III: _____

Leads aV$_R$, aV$_L$, aV$_F$: _____

Leads V$_1$ to V$_6$: _____

■ **PRACTICE 9-6**

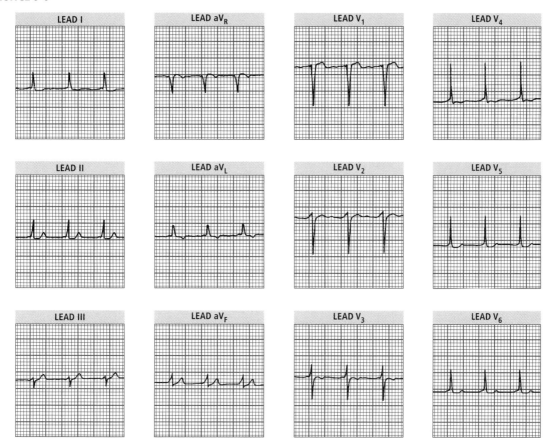

Rhythm: _____

Rate: _____

Axis: _____

Interpretation: _____

T wave: _____

ST segment: _____

Q wave: _____

Leads I, II, III: _____

Leads aV$_R$, aV$_L$, aV$_F$: _____

Leads V$_1$ to V$_6$: _____

■ PRACTICE STRIP ANSWERS

PRACTICE 9-1
- Rhythm. Regular
- Rate: 94 beats/minute
- Axis: Normal
- T wave: Inverted in leads II, III, and aV_F
- ST segment: Elevation in leads V_1, V_2, V_3, and V_4; depressed in leads II, III, and aV_F
- Q wave: Present in lead V_2
- Leads I, II, III: ST-segment depression in leads II and III
- Leads aV_R, aV_L, aV_F: ST-segment depression in lead aV_F
- Leads V_1 to V_6: ST-segment elevation in leads V_1, V_2, V_3, and V_4
- Interpretation: Normal sinus rhythm with acute anteroseptal MI

PRACTICE 9-2
- Rhythm: Regular
- Rate: 115 beats/minute
- Axis: Normal
- T wave: Inverted in leads V_2, V_3, V_4, I, and aV_L
- ST segment: Elevation in leads II, III, and aV_F; depressed in leads V_2, V_3, and V_4
- Q wave: Present in leads II, III and aV_F
- Leads I, II, III: Inverted T waves in lead I; ST-segment elevation and Q wave in leads II and III
- Leads aV_R, aV_L, aV_F: Inverted T waves, ST-segment elevation, and Q wave in lead aV_F
- Leads V_1 to V_6: ST-segment depression and inverted T waves in leads V_2, V_3, and aV_R
- Interpretation: Sinus tachycardia with acute inferior MI

PRACTICE 9-3
- Rhythm: Regular
- Rate: 136 beats/minute
- Axis: Normal
- T wave: Inverted T waves in leads I, aV_L, V_5, and V_6
- ST segment: Elevation in leads II, III, and aV_F
- Q wave: Present in leads III and aV_F
- Leads I, II, III: Inverted T waves in lead I; ST-segment elevation in leads II and III; Q wave in lead III
- Leads aV_R, aV_L, aV_F: Inverted T waves in lead aV_L; ST-segment elevation and Q wave in lead aV_F
- Leads V_1 to V_6: Inverted T waves in leads V_5 and V_6
- Interpretation: Sinus tachycardia with acute inferior MI

PRACTICE 9-4
- Rhythm: Regular
- Rate: 214 beats/minute
- Axis: Normal
- T wave: Within normal limits
- ST segment: Elevation in leads V_2 and V_3
- Q wave: Present in leads V_2 and V_3
- Leads I, II, III: Within normal limits
- Leads aV_R, aV_L, aV_F: Within normal limits
- Leads V_1 to V_6: ST-segment elevation and Q wave in leads V_2 and V_3
- Interpretation: Sinus tachycardia with acute anterior MI

PRACTICE 9-5
- Rhythm: Regular
- Rate: 136 beats/minute
- Axis: Normal
- T wave: Within normal limits
- ST segment: Elevation in leads aV_L, V_5, V_6; slight elevation in lead I
- Q wave: None
- Leads I, II, III: Slight ST-segment elevation in lead I
- Leads aV_R, aV_L, aV_F: ST-segment elevation in lead aV_L
- Leads V_1 to V_6: ST-segment elevation in leads V_5 and V_6
- Interpretation: Sinus tachycardia with lateral wall MI

PRACTICE 9-6
- Rhythm: Regular
- Rate: 136 beats/minute
- Axis: Normal
- T wave: Inverted in leads I, aV_L, V_5, and V_6
- ST segment: Within normal limits
- Q wave: None
- Leads I, II, III: Inverted T waves in lead I
- Leads aV_R, aV_L, aV_F: Inverted T waves in lead aV_L
- Leads V_1 to V_6: Inverted T waves in leads V_5 and V_6
- Interpretation: Sinus tachycardia with lateral wall ischemia

■ APPENDICES AND INDEX

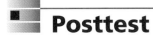

Posttest

This comprehensive posttest is designed to gauge what you've learned by presenting random rhythm strips for you to interpret. For each strip, record the rhythm, rates, and waveform characteristics in the blank spaces provided. Then compare your findings with the answers, beginning on page 358.

■ **STRIP 1**

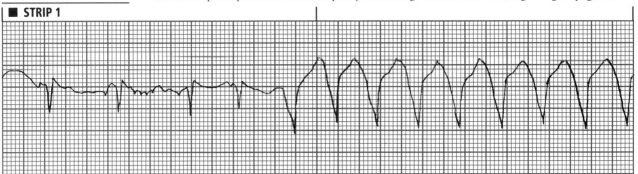

Rhythm:	PR interval:	QT interval:
Rate:	QRS complex:	Other:
P wave:	T wave:	Interpretation:

■ **STRIP 2**

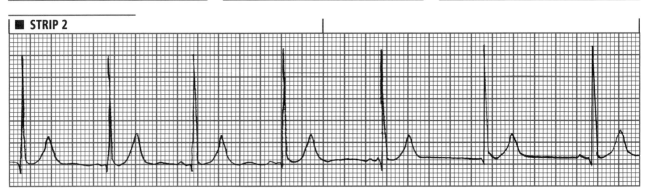

Rhythm:	PR interval:	QT interval:
Rate:	QRS complex:	Other:
P wave:	T wave:	Interpretation:

■ **STRIP 3**

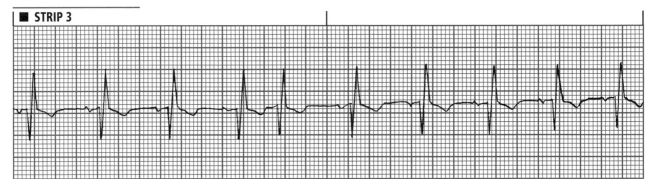

Rhythm:	PR interval:	QT interval:
Rate:	QRS complex:	Other:
P wave:	T wave:	Interpretation:

■ STRIP 4

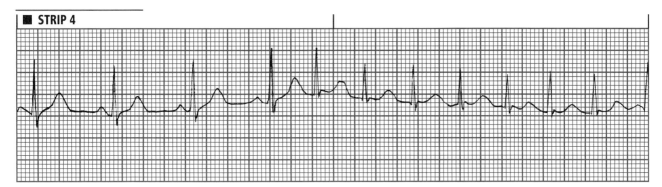

Rhythm: _____   PR interval: _____   QT interval: _____

Rate: _____   QRS complex: _____   Other: _____

P wave: _____   T wave: _____   Interpretation: _____

■ STRIP 5

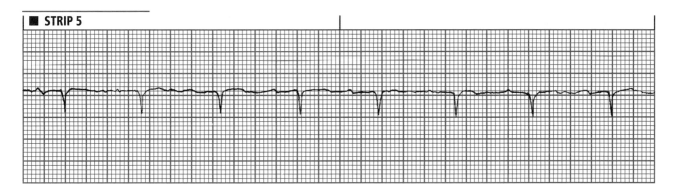

Rhythm: _____   PR interval: _____   QT interval: _____

Rate: _____   QRS complex: _____   Other: _____

P wave: _____   T wave: _____   Interpretation: _____

■ STRIP 6

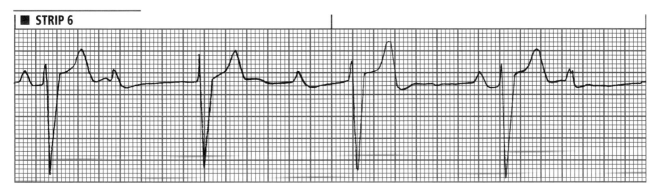

Rhythm: _____   PR interval: _____   QT interval: _____

Rate: _____   QRS complex: _____   Other: _____

P wave: _____   T wave: _____   Interpretation: _____

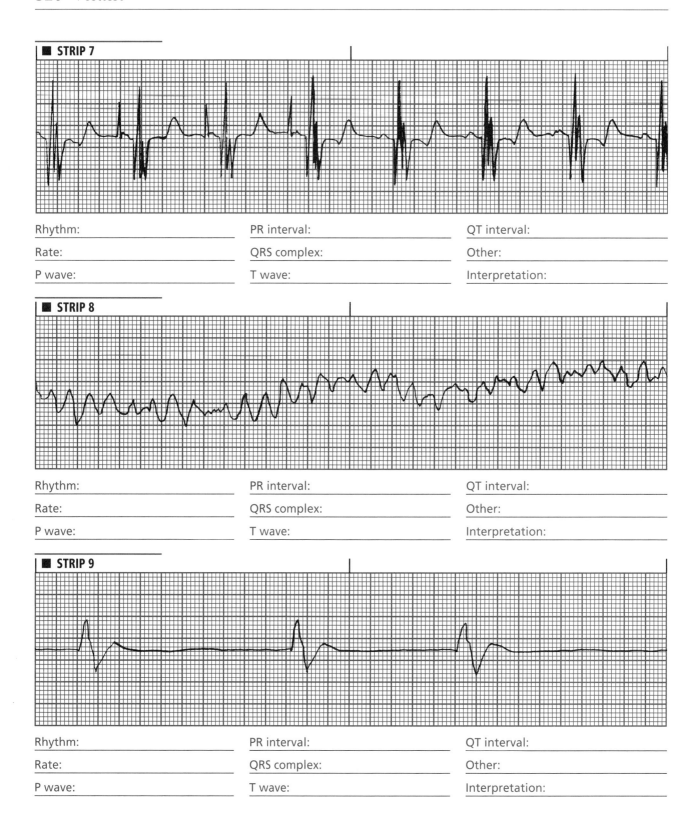

■ **STRIP 7**

Rhythm: _____   PR interval: _____   QT interval: _____

Rate: _____   QRS complex: _____   Other: _____

P wave: _____   T wave: _____   Interpretation: _____

■ **STRIP 8**

Rhythm: _____   PR interval: _____   QT interval: _____

Rate: _____   QRS complex: _____   Other: _____

P wave: _____   T wave: _____   Interpretation: _____

■ **STRIP 9**

Rhythm: _____   PR interval: _____   QT interval: _____

Rate: _____   QRS complex: _____   Other: _____

P wave: _____   T wave: _____   Interpretation: _____

■ **STRIP 10**

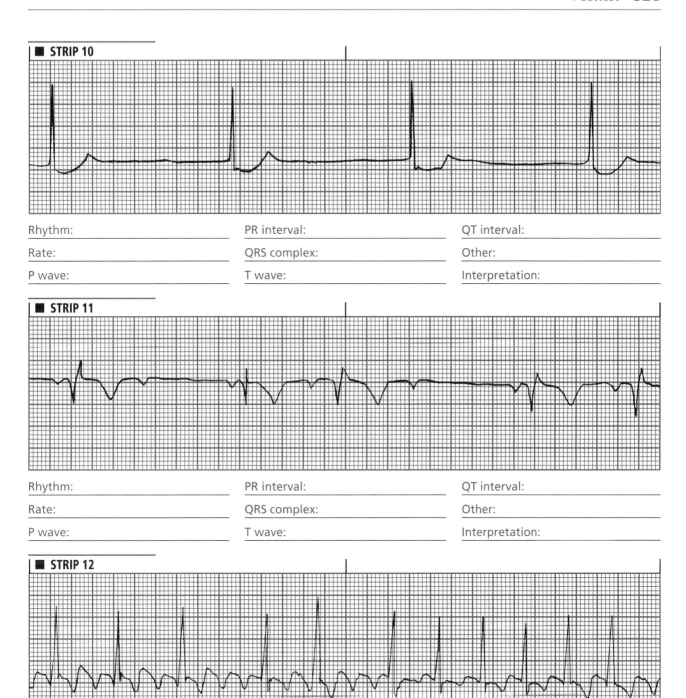

Rhythm: _____   PR interval: _____   QT interval: _____

Rate: _____   QRS complex: _____   Other: _____

P wave: _____   T wave: _____   Interpretation: _____

■ **STRIP 11**

Rhythm: _____   PR interval: _____   QT interval: _____

Rate: _____   QRS complex: _____   Other: _____

P wave: _____   T wave: _____   Interpretation: _____

■ **STRIP 12**

Rhythm: _____   PR interval: _____   QT interval: _____

Rate: _____   QRS complex: _____   Other: _____

P wave: _____   T wave: _____   Interpretation: _____

■ **STRIP 13**

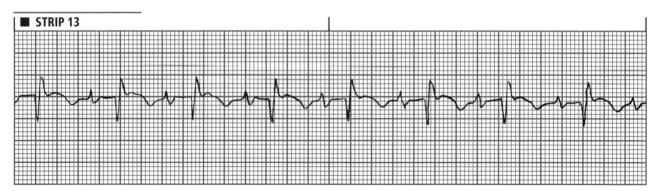

Rhythm: _____   PR interval: _____   QT interval: _____

Rate: _____   QRS complex: _____   Other: _____

P wave: _____   T wave: _____   Interpretation: _____

■ **STRIP 14**

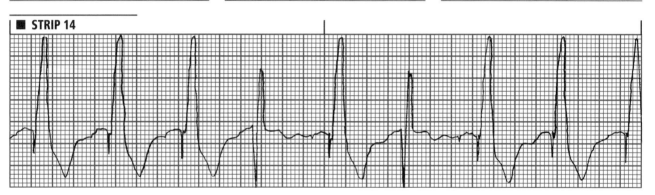

Rhythm: _____   PR interval: _____   QT interval: _____

Rate: _____   QRS complex: _____   Other: _____

P wave: _____   T wave: _____   Interpretation: _____

■ **STRIP 15**

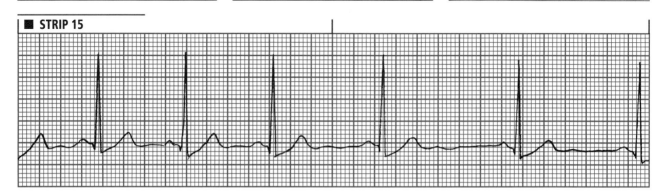

Rhythm: _____   PR interval: _____   QT interval: _____

Rate: _____   QRS complex: _____   Other: _____

P wave: _____   T wave: _____   Interpretation: _____

■ **STRIP 16**

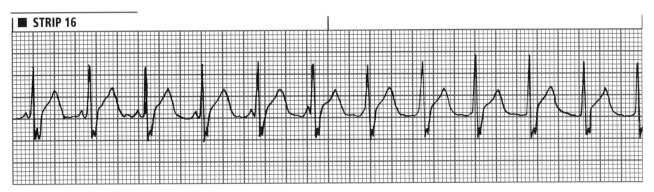

Rhythm: _____   PR interval: _____   QT interval: _____

Rate: _____   QRS complex: _____   Other: _____

P wave: _____   T wave: _____   Interpretation: _____

■ **STRIP 17**

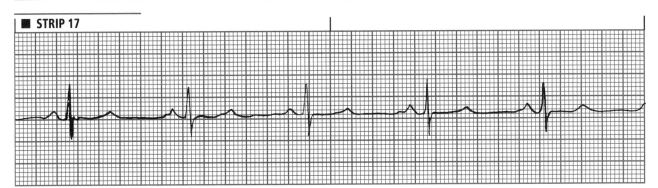

Rhythm: _____   PR interval: _____   QT interval: _____

Rate: _____   QRS complex: _____   Other: _____

P wave: _____   T wave: _____   Interpretation: _____

■ **STRIP 18**

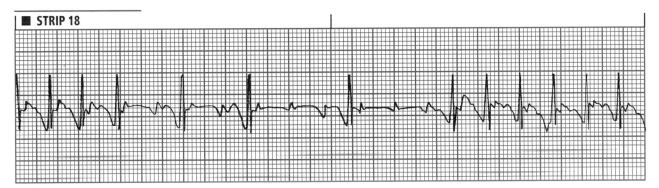

Rhythm: _____   PR interval: _____   QT interval: _____

Rate: _____   QRS complex: _____   Other: _____

P wave: _____   T wave: _____   Interpretation: _____

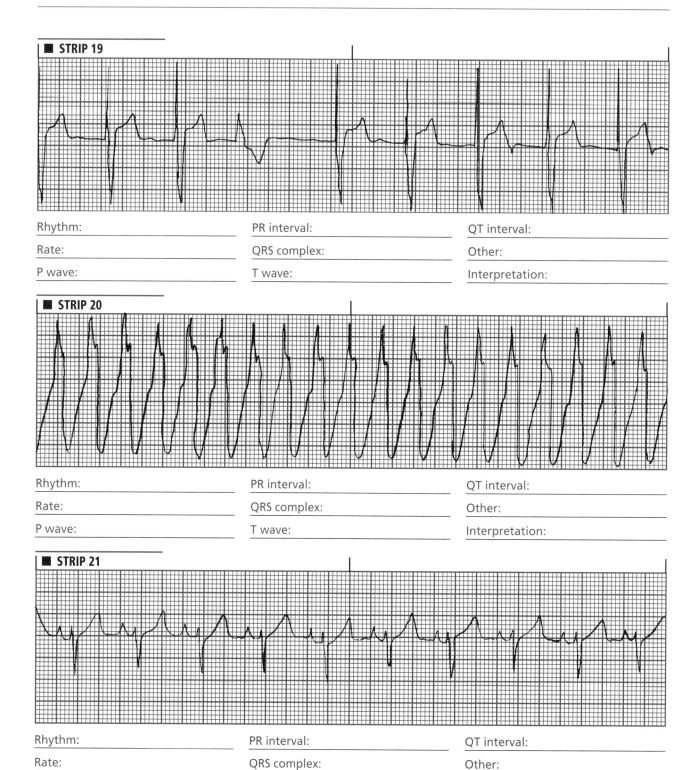

■ **STRIP 19**

Rhythm: _____   PR interval: _____   QT interval: _____

Rate: _____   QRS complex: _____   Other: _____

P wave: _____   T wave: _____   Interpretation: _____

■ **STRIP 20**

Rhythm: _____   PR interval: _____   QT interval: _____

Rate: _____   QRS complex: _____   Other: _____

P wave: _____   T wave: _____   Interpretation: _____

■ **STRIP 21**

Rhythm: _____   PR interval: _____   QT interval: _____

Rate: _____   QRS complex: _____   Other: _____

P wave: _____   T wave: _____   Interpretation: _____

■ **STRIP 22**

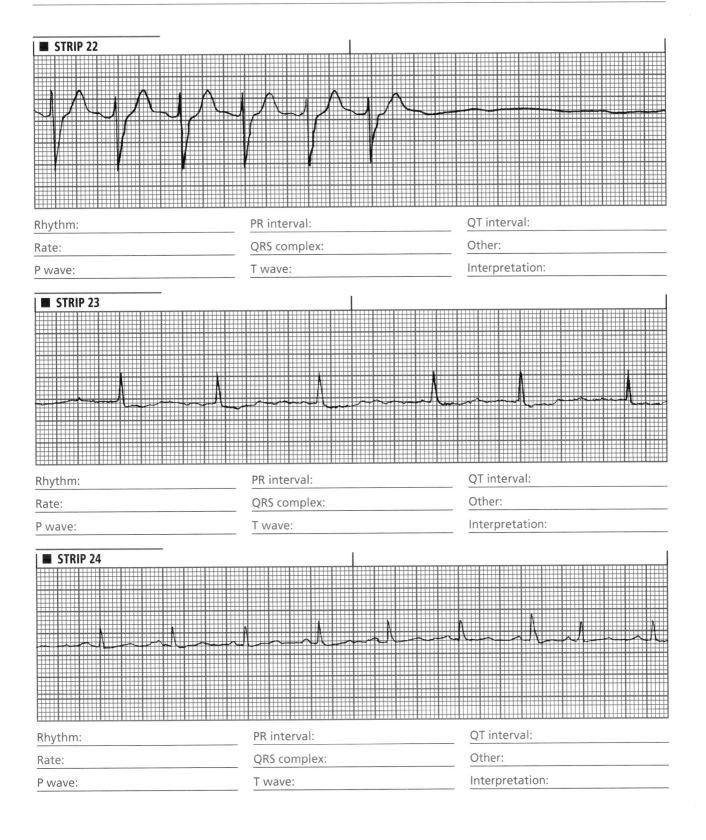

Rhythm: _____

Rate: _____

P wave: _____

PR interval: _____

QRS complex: _____

T wave: _____

QT interval: _____

Other: _____

Interpretation: _____

■ **STRIP 23**

Rhythm: _____

Rate: _____

P wave: _____

PR interval: _____

QRS complex: _____

T wave: _____

QT interval: _____

Other: _____

Interpretation: _____

■ **STRIP 24**

Rhythm: _____

Rate: _____

P wave: _____

PR interval: _____

QRS complex: _____

T wave: _____

QT interval: _____

Other: _____

Interpretation: _____

■ **STRIP 25**

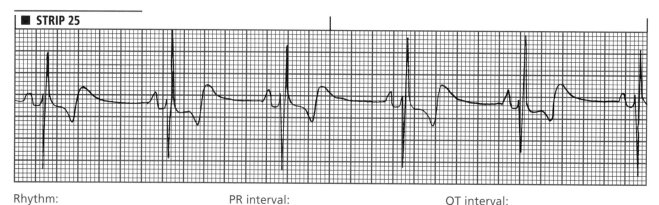

Rhythm: _____   PR interval: _____   QT interval: _____

Rate: _____   QRS complex: _____   Other: _____

P wave: _____   T wave: _____   Interpretation: _____

■ **STRIP 26**

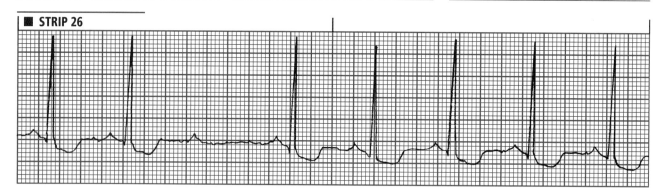

Rhythm: _____   PR interval: _____   QT interval: _____

Rate: _____   QRS complex: _____   Other: _____

P wave: _____   T wave: _____   Interpretation: _____

■ **STRIP 27**

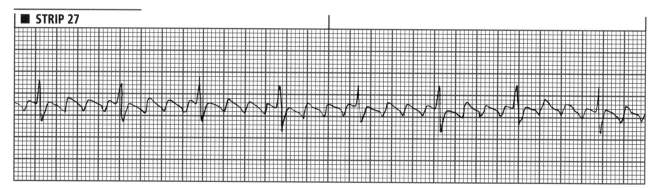

Rhythm: _____   PR interval: _____   QT interval: _____

Rate: _____   QRS complex: _____   Other: _____

P wave: _____   T wave: _____   Interpretation: _____

■ STRIP 28

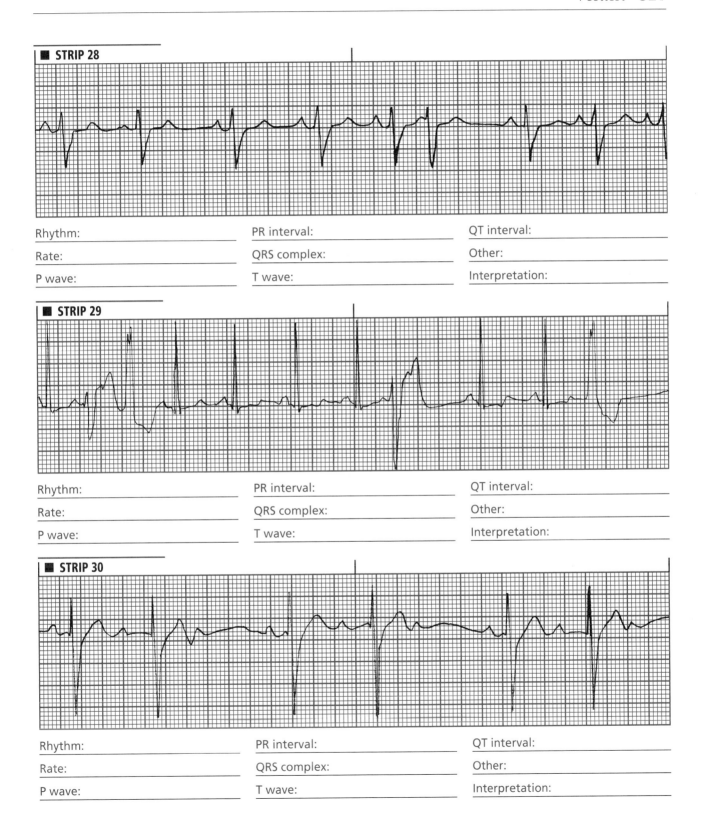

Rhythm: _____

Rate: _____

P wave: _____

PR interval: _____

QRS complex: _____

T wave: _____

QT interval: _____

Other: _____

Interpretation: _____

■ STRIP 29

Rhythm: _____

Rate: _____

P wave: _____

PR interval: _____

QRS complex: _____

T wave: _____

QT interval: _____

Other: _____

Interpretation: _____

■ STRIP 30

Rhythm: _____

Rate: _____

P wave: _____

PR interval: _____

QRS complex: _____

T wave: _____

QT interval: _____

Other: _____

Interpretation: _____

■ STRIP 31

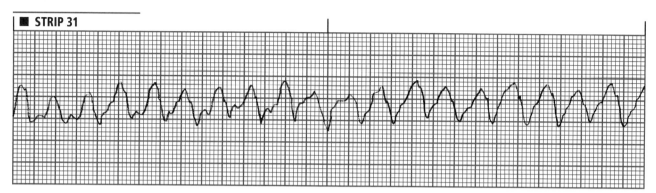

Rhythm: _____   PR interval: _____   QT interval: _____

Rate: _____   QRS complex: _____   Other: _____

P wave: _____   T wave: _____   Interpretation: _____

■ STRIP 32

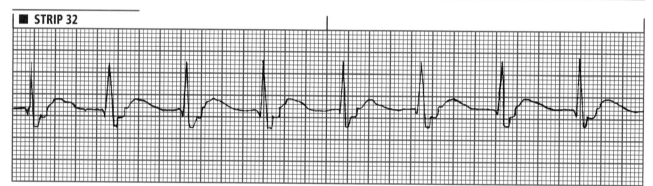

Rhythm: _____   PR interval: _____   QT interval: _____

Rate: _____   QRS complex: _____   Other: _____

P wave: _____   T wave: _____   Interpretation: _____

■ STRIP 33

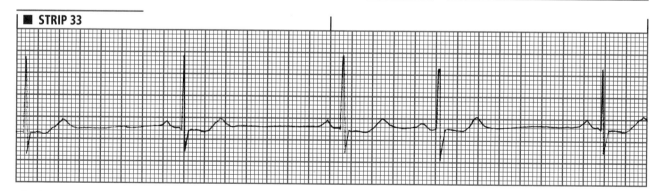

Rhythm: _____   PR interval: _____   QT interval: _____

Rate: _____   QRS complex: _____   Other: _____

P wave: _____   T wave: _____   Interpretation: _____

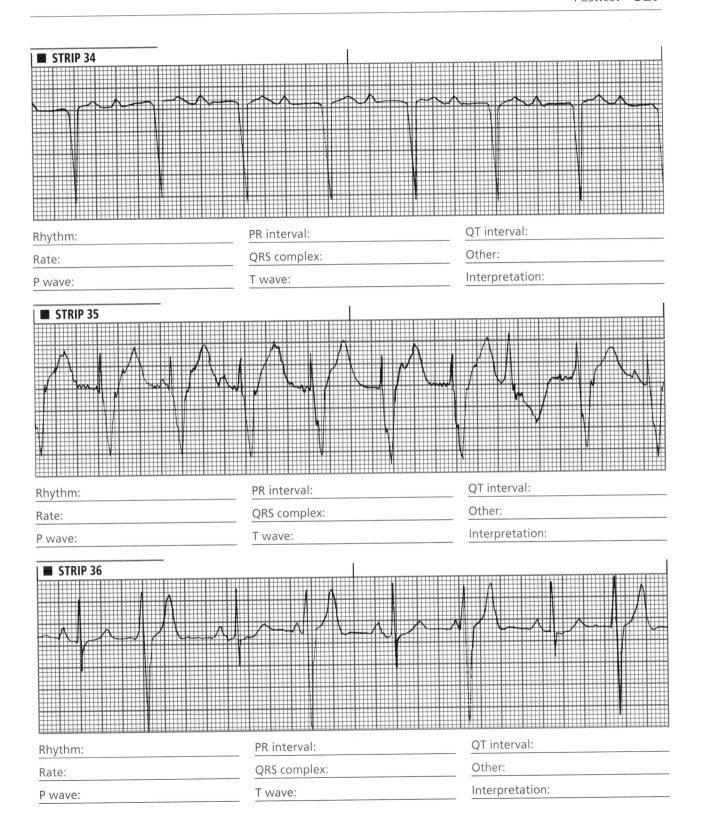

STRIP 34

Rhythm: _____

Rate: _____

P wave: _____

PR interval: _____

QRS complex: _____

T wave: _____

QT interval: _____

Other: _____

Interpretation: _____

STRIP 35

Rhythm: _____

Rate: _____

P wave: _____

PR interval: _____

QRS complex: _____

T wave: _____

QT interval: _____

Other: _____

Interpretation: _____

STRIP 36

Rhythm: _____

Rate: _____

P wave: _____

PR interval: _____

QRS complex: _____

T wave: _____

QT interval: _____

Other: _____

Interpretation: _____

■ STRIP 37

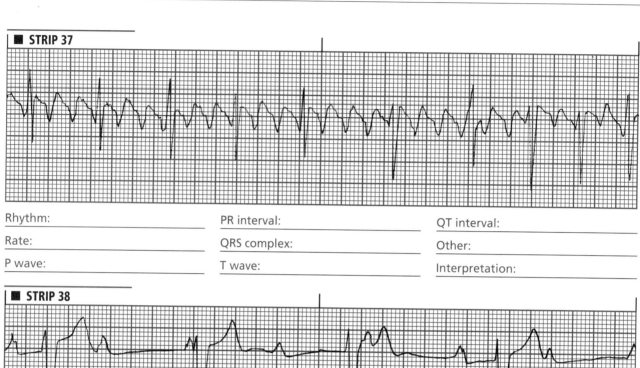

Rhythm: _____ PR interval: _____ QT interval: _____

Rate: _____ QRS complex: _____ Other: _____

P wave: _____ T wave: _____ Interpretation: _____

■ STRIP 38

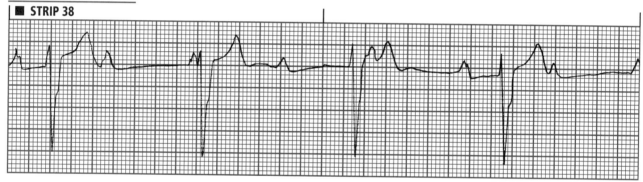

Rhythm: _____ PR interval: _____ QT interval: _____

Rate: _____ QRS complex: _____ Other: _____

P wave: _____ T wave: _____ Interpretation: _____

■ STRIP 39

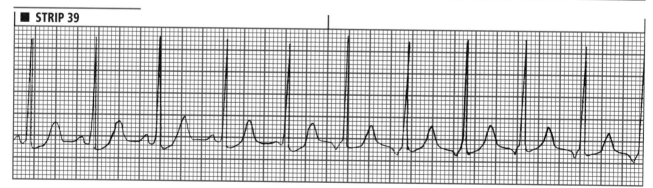

Rhythm: _____ PR interval: _____ QT interval: _____

Rate: _____ QRS complex: _____ Other: _____

P wave: _____ T wave: _____ Interpretation: _____

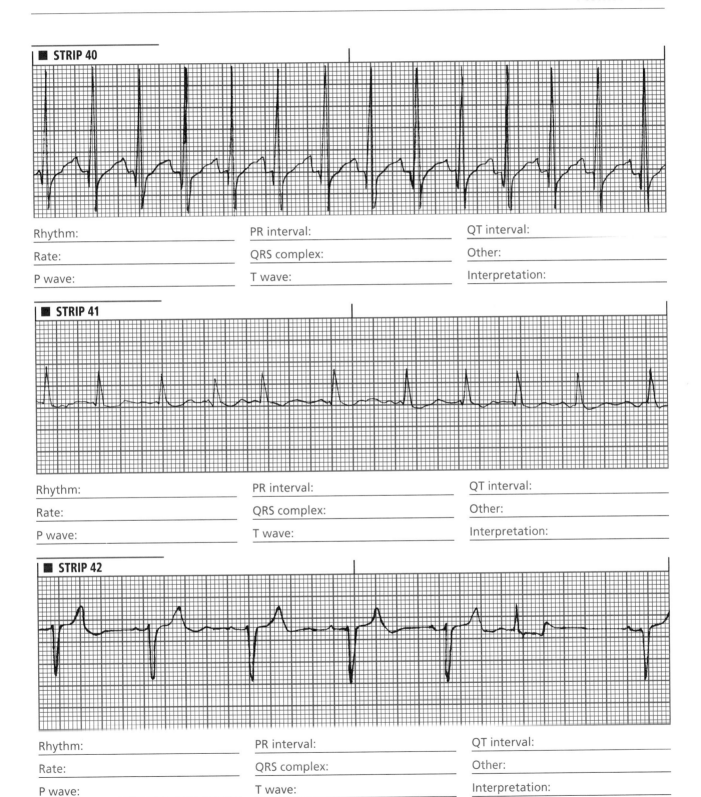

■ STRIP 40

Rhythm: _____

Rate: _____

P wave: _____

PR interval: _____

QRS complex: _____

T wave: _____

QT interval: _____

Other: _____

Interpretation: _____

■ STRIP 41

Rhythm: _____

Rate: _____

P wave: _____

PR interval: _____

QRS complex: _____

T wave: _____

QT interval: _____

Other: _____

Interpretation: _____

■ STRIP 42

Rhythm: _____

Rate: _____

P wave: _____

PR interval: _____

QRS complex: _____

T wave: _____

QT interval: _____

Other: _____

Interpretation: _____

■ **STRIP 43**

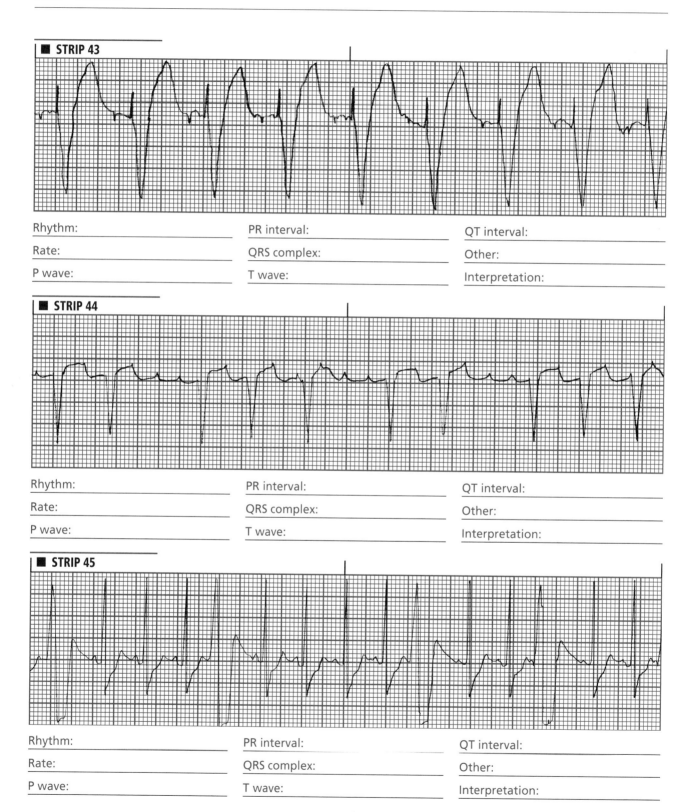

Rhythm: _____ PR interval: _____ QT interval: _____

Rate: _____ QRS complex: _____ Other: _____

P wave: _____ T wave: _____ Interpretation: _____

■ **STRIP 44**

Rhythm: _____ PR interval: _____ QT interval: _____

Rate: _____ QRS complex: _____ Other: _____

P wave: _____ T wave: _____ Interpretation: _____

■ **STRIP 45**

Rhythm: _____ PR interval: _____ QT interval: _____

Rate: _____ QRS complex: _____ Other: _____

P wave: _____ T wave: _____ Interpretation: _____

■ STRIP 46

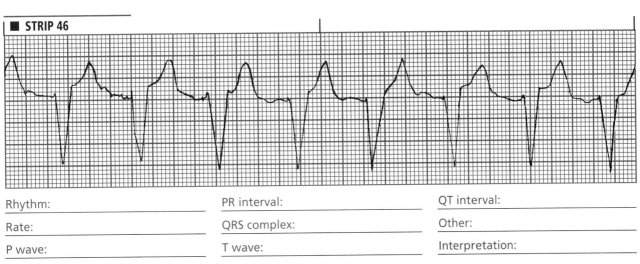

Rhythm: _____   PR interval: _____   QT interval: _____

Rate: _____   QRS complex: _____   Other: _____

P wave: _____   T wave: _____   Interpretation: _____

■ STRIP 47

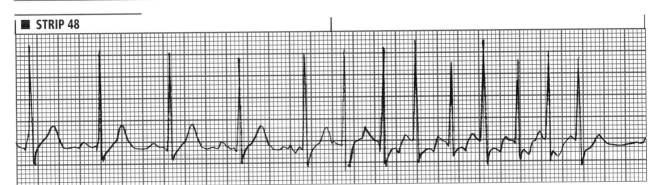

Rhythm: _____   PR interval: _____   QT interval: _____

Rate: _____   QRS complex: _____   Other: _____

P wave: _____   T wave: _____   Interpretation: _____

■ STRIP 48

Rhythm: _____   PR interval: _____   QT interval: _____

Rate: _____   QRS complex: _____   Other: _____

P wave: _____   T wave: _____   Interpretation: _____

■ **STRIP 49**

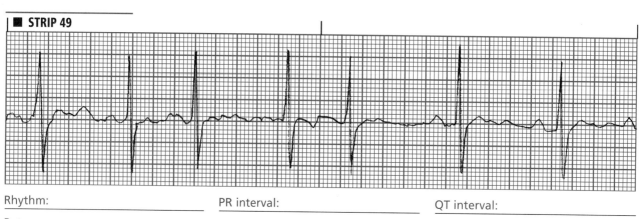

Rhythm: _____   PR interval: _____   QT interval: _____

Rate: _____   QRS complex: _____   Other: _____

P wave: _____   T wave: _____   Interpretation: _____

■ **STRIP 50**

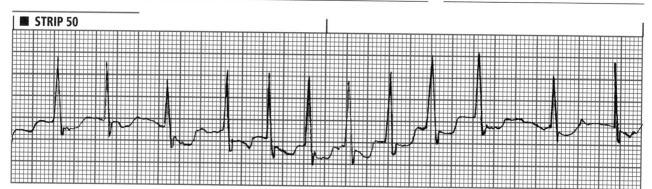

Rhythm: _____   PR interval: _____   QT interval: _____

Rate: _____   QRS complex: _____   Other: _____

P wave: _____   T wave: _____   Interpretation: _____

■ **STRIP 51**

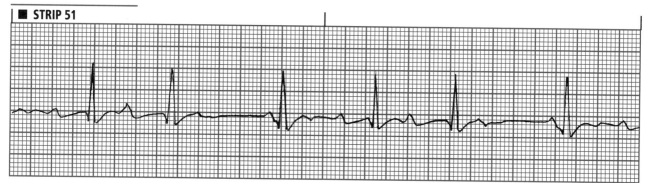

Rhythm: _____   PR interval: _____   QT interval: _____

Rate: _____   QRS complex: _____   Other: _____

P wave: _____   T wave: _____   Interpretation: _____

■ **STRIP 52**

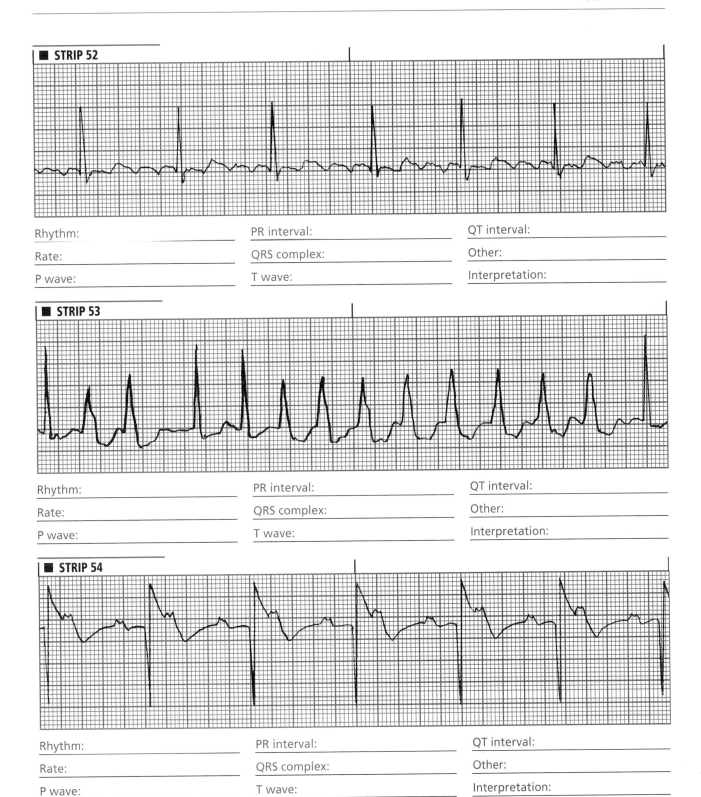

Rhythm: _____   PR interval: _____   QT interval: _____

Rate: _____   QRS complex: _____   Other: _____

P wave: _____   T wave: _____   Interpretation: _____

■ **STRIP 53**

Rhythm: _____   PR interval: _____   QT interval: _____

Rate: _____   QRS complex: _____   Other: _____

P wave: _____   T wave: _____   Interpretation: _____

■ **STRIP 54**

Rhythm: _____   PR interval: _____   QT interval: _____

Rate: _____   QRS complex: _____   Other: _____

P wave: _____   T wave: _____   Interpretation: _____

■ STRIP 55

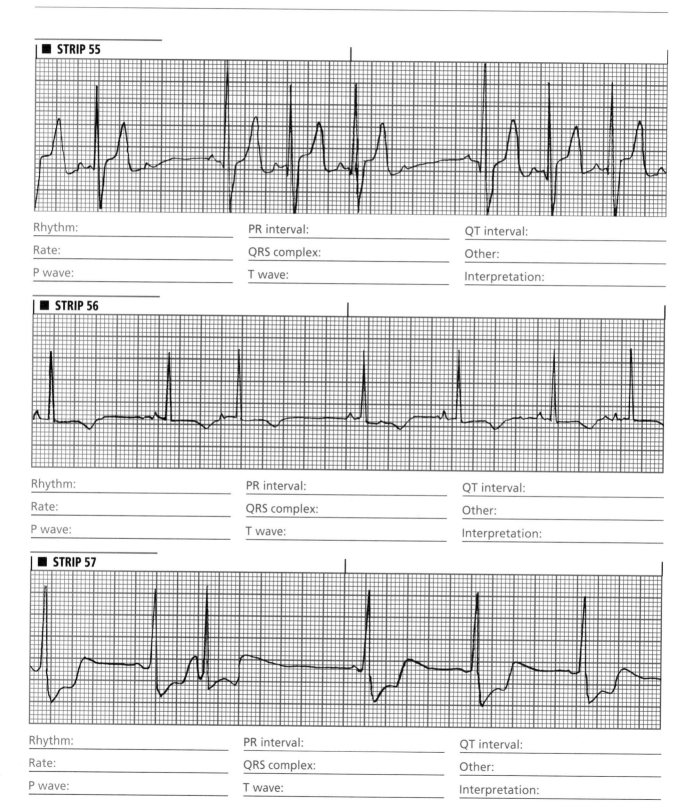

Rhythm: _____   PR interval: _____   QT interval: _____

Rate: _____   QRS complex: _____   Other: _____

P wave: _____   T wave: _____   Interpretation: _____

■ STRIP 56

Rhythm: _____   PR interval: _____   QT interval: _____

Rate: _____   QRS complex: _____   Other: _____

P wave: _____   T wave: _____   Interpretation: _____

■ STRIP 57

Rhythm: _____   PR interval: _____   QT interval: _____

Rate: _____   QRS complex: _____   Other: _____

P wave: _____   T wave: _____   Interpretation: _____

■ STRIP 58

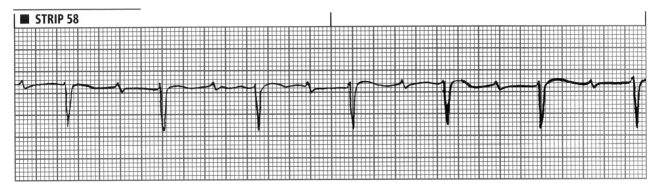

Rhythm: _____

Rate: _____

P wave: _____

PR interval: _____

QRS complex: _____

T wave: _____

QT interval: _____

Other: _____

Interpretation: _____

■ STRIP 59

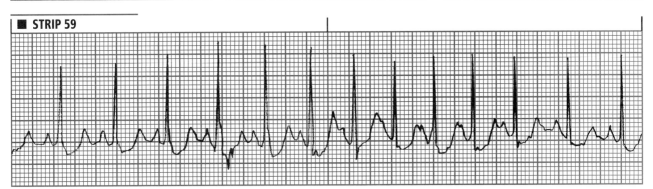

Rhythm: _____

Rate: _____

P wave: _____

PR interval: _____

QRS complex: _____

T wave: _____

QT interval: _____

Other: _____

Interpretation: _____

■ STRIP 60

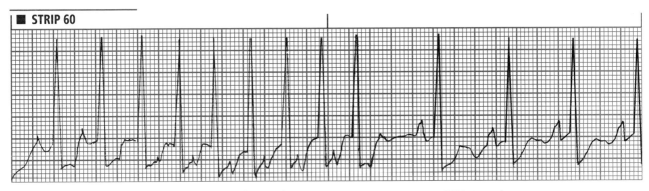

Rhythm: _____

Rate: _____

P wave: _____

PR interval: _____

QRS complex: _____

T wave: _____

QT interval: _____

Other: _____

Interpretation: _____

■ STRIP 61

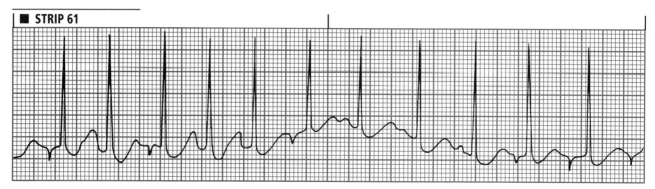

Rhythm: _____ PR interval: _____ QT interval: _____

Rate: _____ QRS complex: _____ Other: _____

P wave: _____ T wave: _____ Interpretation: _____

■ STRIP 62

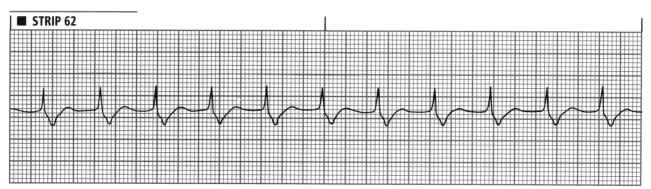

Rhythm: _____ PR interval: _____ QT interval: _____

Rate: _____ QRS complex: _____ Other: _____

P wave: _____ T wave: _____ Interpretation: _____

■ STRIP 63

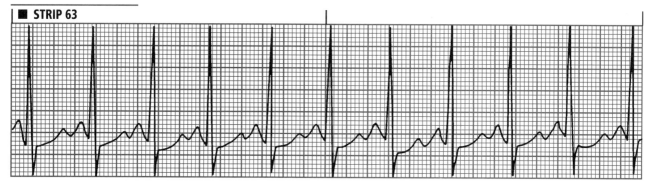

Rhythm: _____ PR interval: _____ QT interval: _____

Rate: _____ QRS complex: _____ Other: _____

P wave: _____ T wave: _____ Interpretation: _____

■ **STRIP 64**

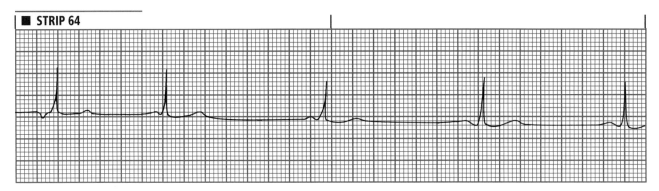

Rhythm: _____   PR interval: _____   QT interval: _____

Rate: _____   QRS complex: _____   Other: _____

P wave: _____   T wave: _____   Interpretation: _____

■ **STRIP 65**

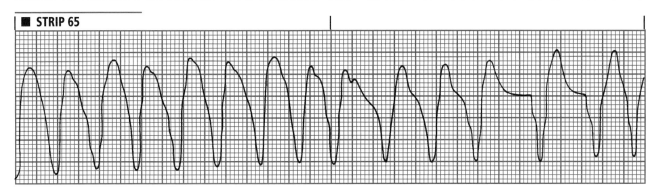

Rhythm: _____   PR interval: _____   QT interval: _____

Rate: _____   QRS complex: _____   Other: _____

P wave: _____   T wave: _____   Interpretation: _____

■ **STRIP 66**

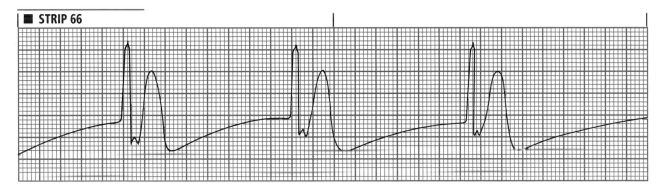

Rhythm: _____   PR interval: _____   QT interval: _____

Rate: _____   QRS complex: _____   Other: _____

P wave: _____   T wave: _____   Interpretation: _____

■ STRIP 67

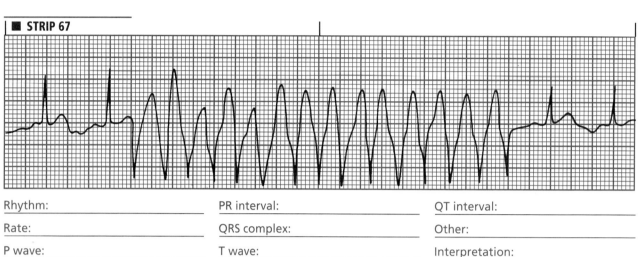

Rhythm: _____   PR interval: _____   QT interval: _____

Rate: _____   QRS complex: _____   Other: _____

P wave: _____   T wave: _____   Interpretation: _____

■ STRIP 68

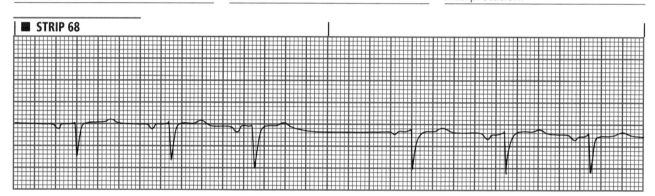

Rhythm: _____   PR interval: _____   QT interval: _____

Rate: _____   QRS complex: _____   Other: _____

P wave: _____   T wave: _____   Interpretation: _____

■ STRIP 69

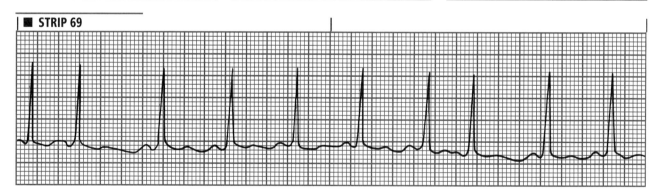

Rhythm: _____   PR interval: _____   QT interval: _____

Rate: _____   QRS complex: _____   Other: _____

P wave: _____   T wave: _____   Interpretation: _____

■ **STRIP 70**

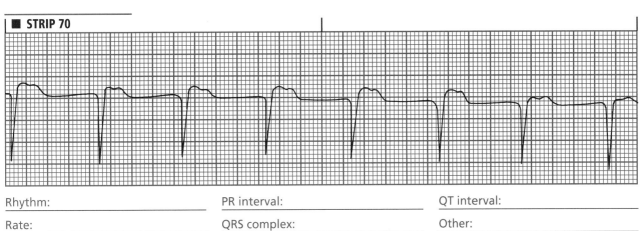

Rhythm: _____

Rate: _____

P wave: _____

PR interval: _____

QRS complex: _____

T wave: _____

QT interval: _____

Other: _____

Interpretation: _____

■ **STRIP 71**

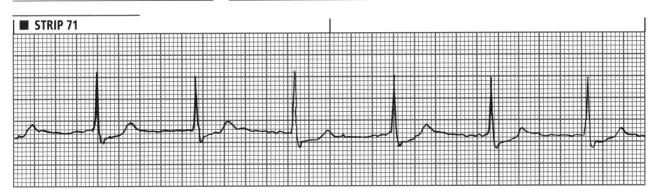

Rhythm: _____

Rate: _____

P wave: _____

PR interval: _____

QRS complex: _____

T wave: _____

QT interval: _____

Other: _____

Interpretation: _____

■ **STRIP 72**

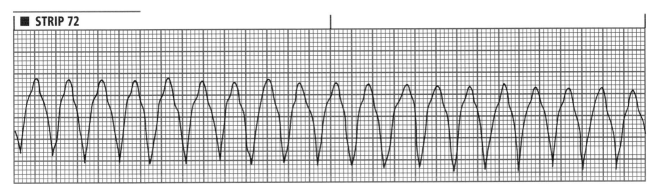

Rhythm: _____

Rate: _____

P wave: _____

PR interval: _____

QRS complex: _____

T wave: _____

QT interval: _____

Other: _____

Interpretation: _____

■ STRIP 73

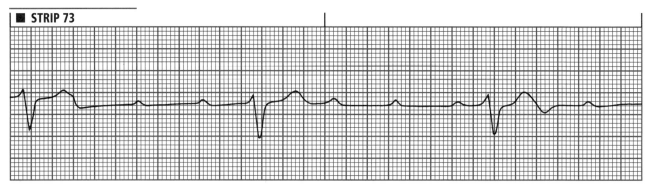

Rhythm: _____   PR interval: _____   QT interval: _____

Rate: _____   QRS complex: _____   Other: _____

P wave: _____   T wave: _____   Interpretation: _____

■ STRIP 74

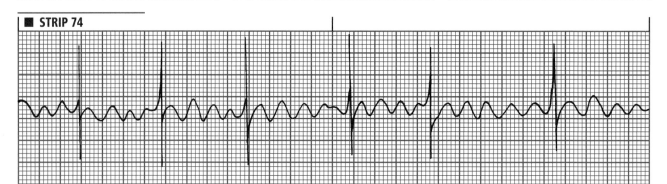

Rhythm: _____   PR interval: _____   QT interval: _____

Rate: _____   QRS complex: _____   Other: _____

P wave: _____   T wave: _____   Interpretation: _____

■ STRIP 75

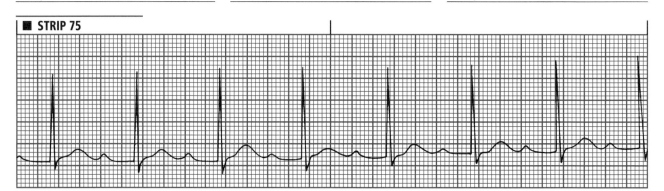

Rhythm: _____   PR interval: _____   QT interval: _____

Rate: _____   QRS complex: _____   Other: _____

P wave: _____   T wave: _____   Interpretation: _____

■ STRIP 76

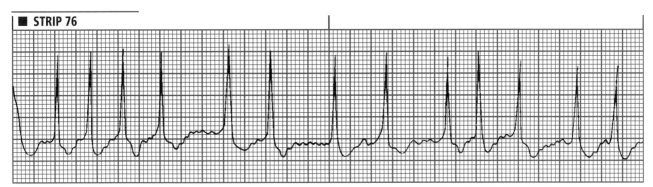

Rhythm: _____   PR interval: _____   QT interval: _____

Rate: _____   QRS complex: _____   Other: _____

P wave: _____   T wave: _____   Interpretation: _____

■ STRIP 77

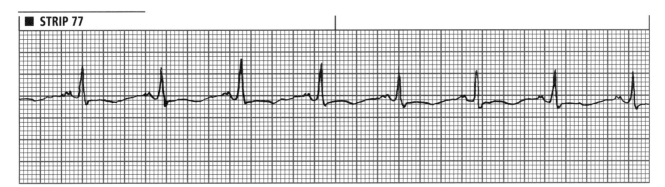

Rhythm: _____   PR interval: _____   QT interval: _____

Rate: _____   QRS complex: _____   Other: _____

P wave: _____   T wave: _____   Interpretation: _____

■ STRIP 78

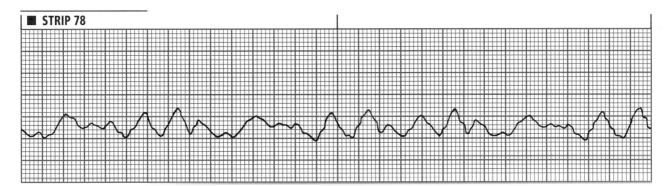

Rhythm: _____   PR interval: _____   QT interval: _____

Rate: _____   QRS complex: _____   Other: _____

P wave: _____   T wave: _____   Interpretation: _____

■ STRIP 79

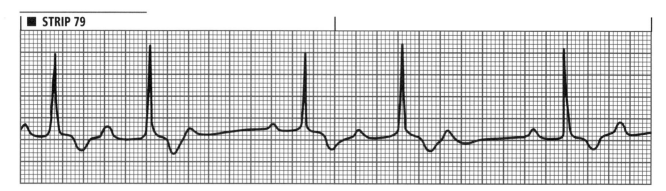

Rhythm: _____/ PR interval: _____ QT interval: _____

Rate: _____ QRS complex: _____ Other: _____

P wave: _____ T wave: _____ Interpretation: _____

■ STRIP 80

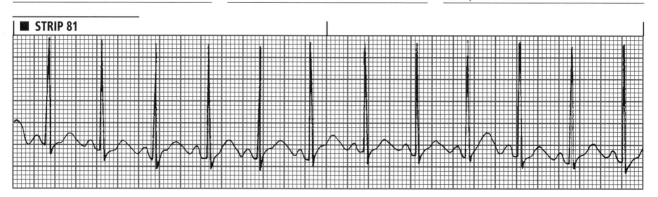

Rhythm: _____ PR interval: _____ QT interval: _____

Rate: _____ QRS complex: _____ Other: _____

P wave: _____ T wave: _____ Interpretation: _____

■ STRIP 81

Rhythm: _____ PR interval: _____ QT interval: _____

Rate: _____ QRS complex: _____ Other: _____

P wave: _____ T wave: _____ Interpretation: _____

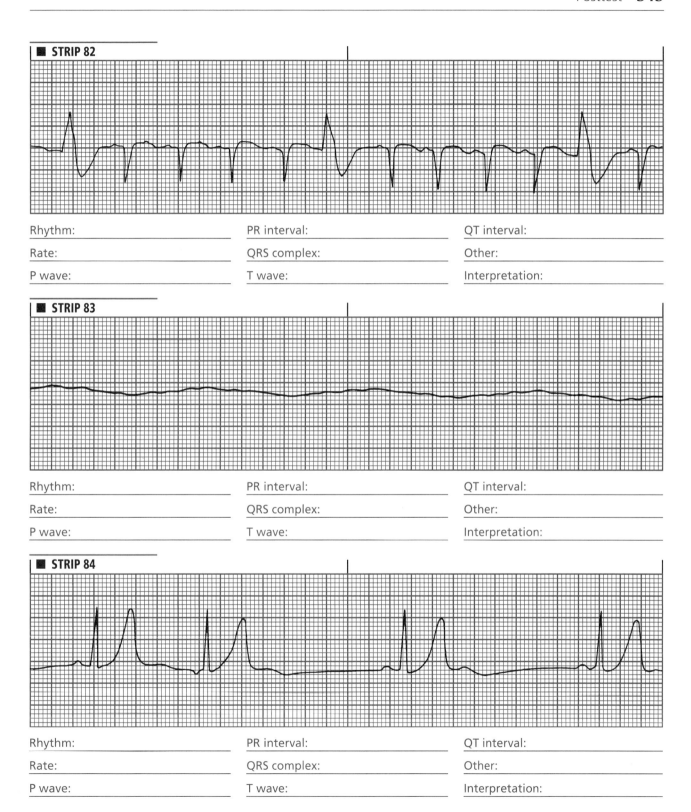

■ STRIP 82

Rhythm: _____   PR interval: _____   QT interval: _____

Rate: _____   QRS complex: _____   Other: _____

P wave: _____   T wave: _____   Interpretation: _____

■ STRIP 83

Rhythm: _____   PR interval: _____   QT interval: _____

Rate: _____   QRS complex: _____   Other: _____

P wave: _____   T wave: _____   Interpretation: _____

■ STRIP 84

Rhythm: _____   PR interval: _____   QT interval: _____

Rate: _____   QRS complex: _____   Other: _____

P wave: _____   T wave: _____   Interpretation: _____

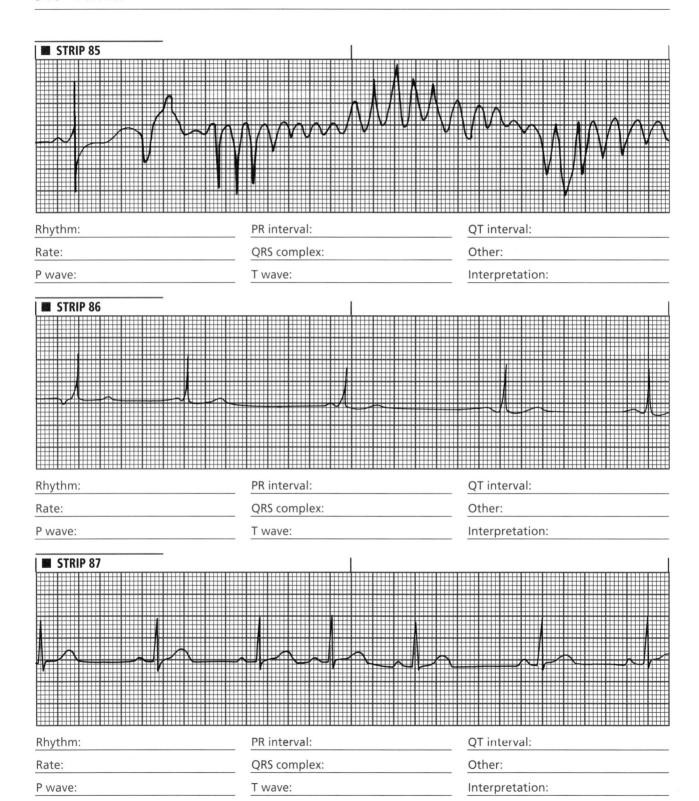

■ STRIP 85

Rhythm: _____ PR interval: _____ QT interval: _____

Rate: _____ QRS complex: _____ Other: _____

P wave: _____ T wave: _____ Interpretation: _____

■ STRIP 86

Rhythm: _____ PR interval: _____ QT interval: _____

Rate: _____ QRS complex: _____ Other: _____

P wave: _____ T wave: _____ Interpretation: _____

■ STRIP 87

Rhythm: _____ PR interval: _____ QT interval: _____

Rate: _____ QRS complex: _____ Other: _____

P wave: _____ T wave: _____ Interpretation: _____

■ STRIP 88

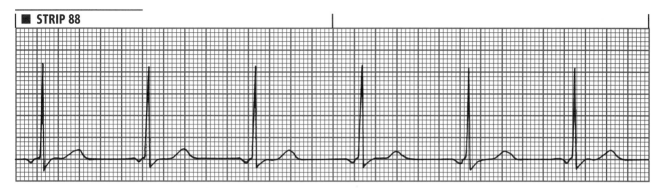

Rhythm: _____ PR interval: _____ QT interval: _____

Rate: _____ QRS complex: _____ Other: _____

P wave: _____ T wave: _____ Interpretation: _____

■ STRIP 89

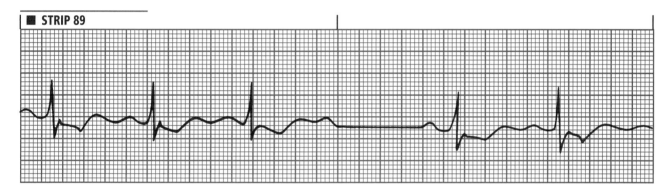

Rhythm: _____ PR interval: _____ QT interval: _____

Rate: _____ QRS complex: _____ Other: _____

P wave: _____ T wave: _____ Interpretation: _____

■ STRIP 90

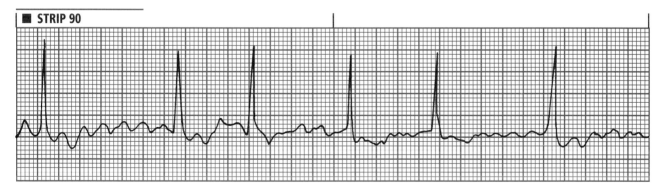

Rhythm: _____ PR interval: _____ QT interval: _____

Rate: _____ QRS complex: _____ Other: _____

P wave: _____ T wave: _____ Interpretation: _____

■ **STRIP 91**

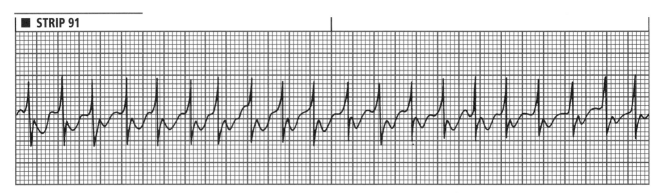

Rhythm: _____   PR interval: _____   QT interval: _____

Rate: _____   QRS complex: _____   Other: _____

P wave: _____   T wave: _____   Interpretation: _____

■ **STRIP 92**

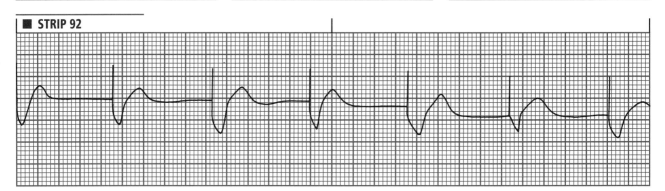

Rhythm: _____   PR interval: _____   QT interval: _____

Rate: _____   QRS complex: _____   Other: _____

P wave: _____   T wave: _____   Interpretation: _____

■ **STRIP 93**

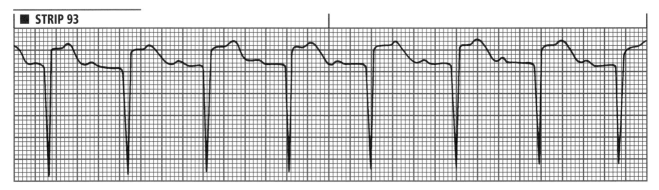

Rhythm: _____   PR interval: _____   QT interval: _____

Rate: _____   QRS complex: _____   Other: _____

P wave: _____   T wave: _____   Interpretation: _____

■ STRIP 94

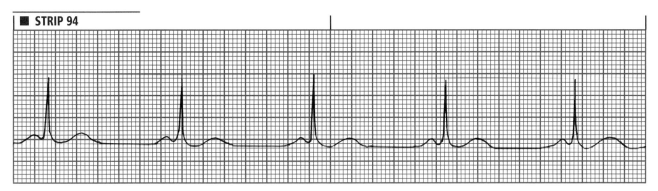

Rhythm: _____   PR interval: _____   QT interval: _____

Rate: _____   QRS complex: _____   Other: _____

P wave: _____   T wave: _____   Interpretation: _____

■ STRIP 95

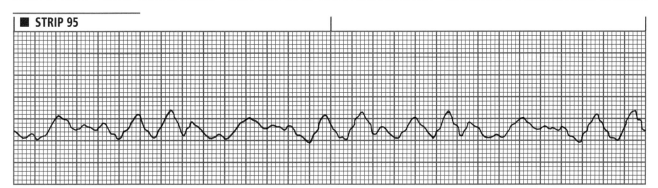

Rhythm: _____   PR interval: _____   QT interval: _____

Rate: _____   QRS complex: _____   Other: _____

P wave: _____   T wave: _____   Interpretation: _____

■ STRIP 96

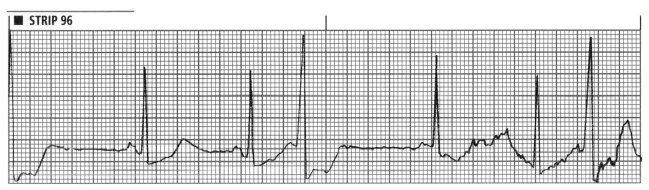

Rhythm: _____   PR interval: _____   QT interval: _____

Rate: _____   QRS complex: _____   Other: _____

P wave: _____   T wave: _____   Interpretation: _____

■ **STRIP 97**

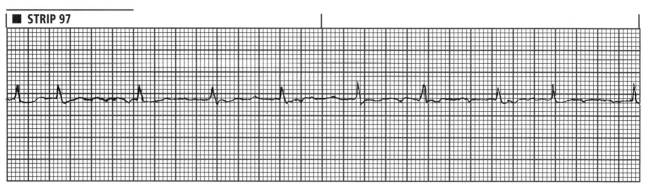

Rhythm: _____   PR interval: _____   QT interval: _____

Rate: _____   QRS complex: _____   Other: _____

P wave: _____   T wave: _____   Interpretation: _____

■ **STRIP 98**

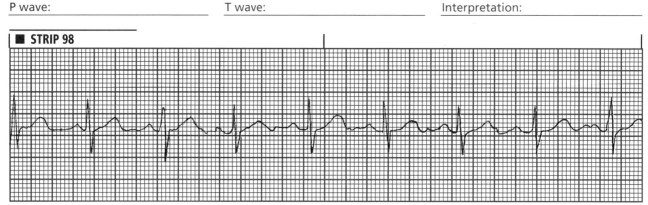

Rhythm: _____   PR interval: _____   QT interval: _____

Rate: _____   QRS complex: _____   Other: _____

P wave: _____   T wave: _____   Interpretation: _____

■ **STRIP 99**

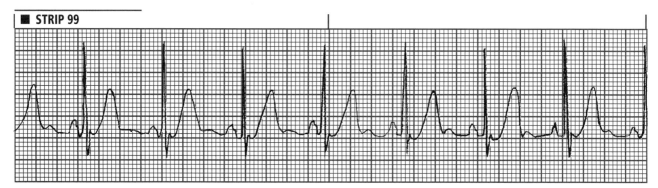

Rhythm: _____   PR interval: _____   QT interval: _____

Rate: _____   QRS complex: _____   Other: _____

P wave: _____   T wave: _____   Interpretation: _____

■ STRIP 100

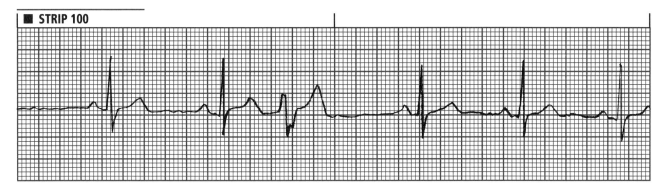

Rhythm: _____   PR interval: _____   QT interval: _____

Rate: _____   QRS complex: _____   Other: _____

P wave: _____   T wave: _____   Interpretation: _____

■ STRIP 101

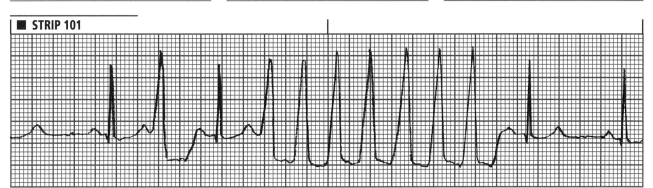

Rhythm: _____   PR interval: _____   QT interval: _____

Rate: _____   QRS complex: _____   Other: _____

P wave: _____   T wave: _____   Interpretation: _____

■ STRIP 102

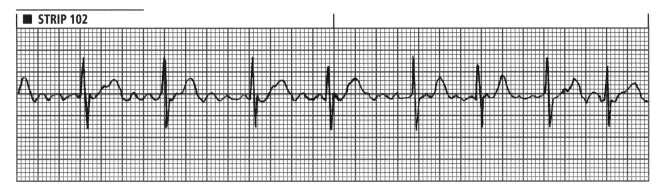

Rhythm: _____   PR interval: _____   QT interval: _____

Rate: _____   QRS complex: _____   Other: _____

P wave: _____   T wave: _____   Interpretation: _____

■ **STRIP 103**

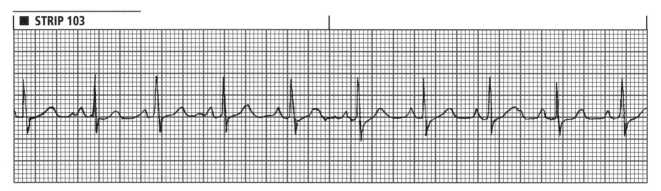

Rhythm: _____ PR interval: _____ QT interval: _____

Rate: _____ QRS complex: _____ Other: _____

P wave: _____ T wave: _____ Interpretation: _____

■ **STRIP 104**

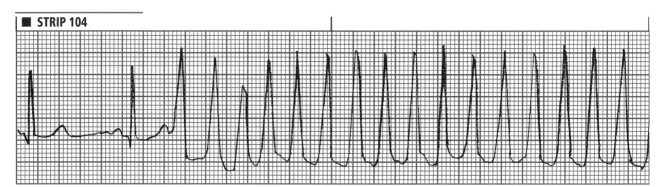

Rhythm: _____ PR interval: _____ QT interval: _____

Rate: _____ QRS complex: _____ Other: _____

P wave: _____ T wave: _____ Interpretation: _____

■ **STRIP 105**

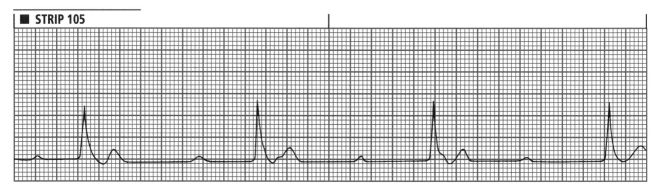

Rhythm: _____ PR interval: _____ QT interval: _____

Rate: _____ QRS complex: _____ Other: _____

P wave: _____ T wave: _____ Interpretation: _____

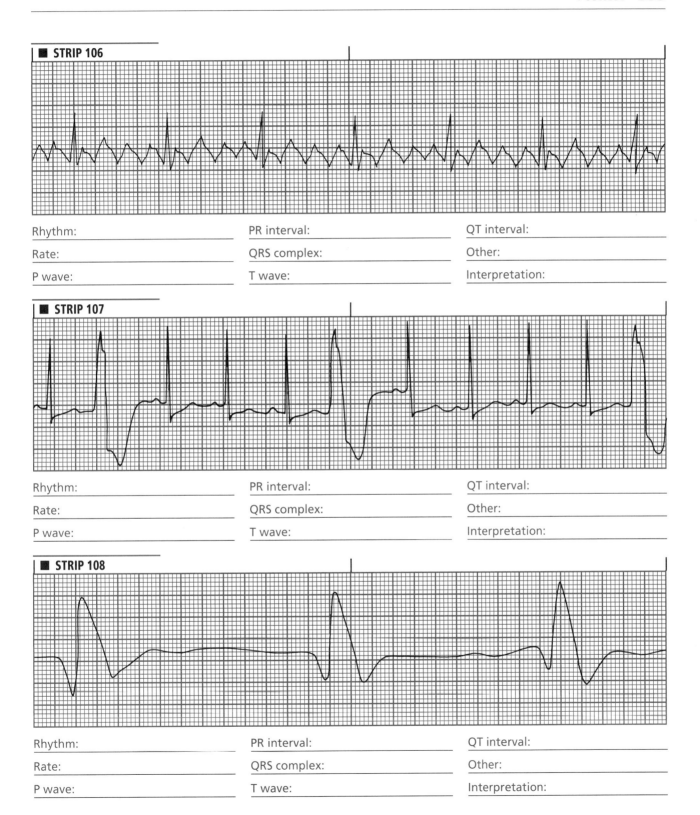

■ STRIP 106

Rhythm: _____   PR interval: _____   QT interval: _____

Rate: _____   QRS complex: _____   Other: _____

P wave: _____   T wave: _____   Interpretation: _____

■ STRIP 107

Rhythm: _____   PR interval: _____   QT interval: _____

Rate: _____   QRS complex: _____   Other: _____

P wave: _____   T wave: _____   Interpretation: _____

■ STRIP 108

Rhythm: _____   PR interval: _____   QT interval: _____

Rate: _____   QRS complex: _____   Other: _____

P wave: _____   T wave: _____   Interpretation: _____

■ **STRIP 109**

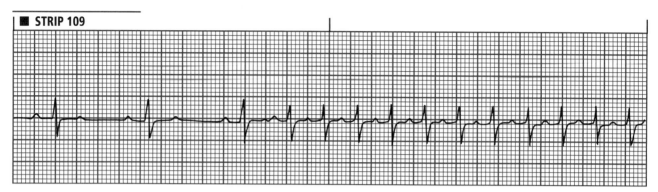

Rhythm: _____

Rate: _____

P wave: _____

PR interval: _____

QRS complex: _____

T wave: _____

QT interval: _____

Other: _____

Interpretation: _____

■ **STRIP 110**

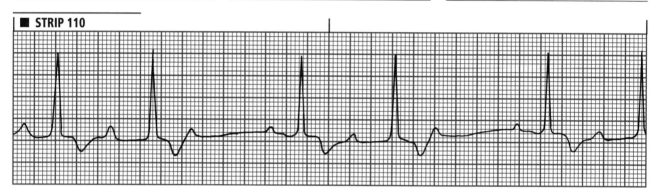

Rhythm: _____

Rate: _____

P wave: _____

PR interval: _____

QRS complex: _____

T wave: _____

QT interval: _____

Other: _____

Interpretation: _____

■ **STRIP 111**

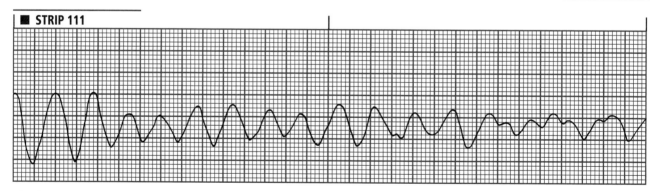

Rhythm: _____

Rate: _____

P wave: _____

PR interval: _____

QRS complex: _____

T wave: _____

QT interval: _____

Other: _____

Interpretation: _____

■ STRIP 112

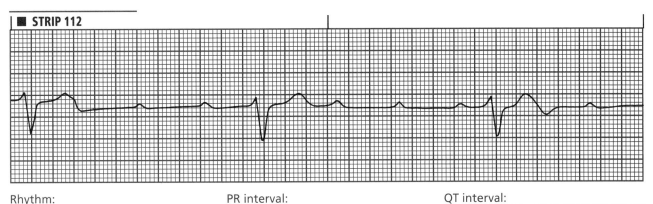

Rhythm: _____   PR interval: _____   QT interval: _____

Rate: _____   QRS complex: _____   Other: _____

P wave: _____   T wave: _____   Interpretation: _____

■ STRIP 113

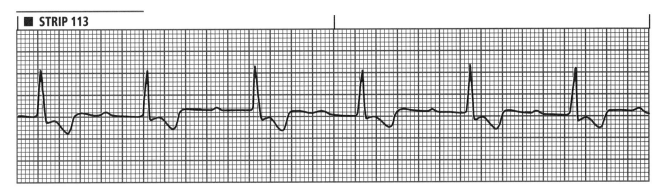

Rhythm: _____   PR interval: _____   QT interval: _____

Rate: _____   QRS complex: _____   Other: _____

P wave: _____   T wave: _____   Interpretation: _____

■ STRIP 114

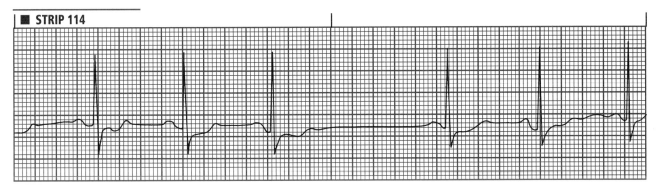

Rhythm: _____   PR interval: _____   QT interval: _____

Rate: _____   QRS complex: _____   Other: _____

P wave: _____   T wave: _____   Interpretation: _____

■ STRIP 115

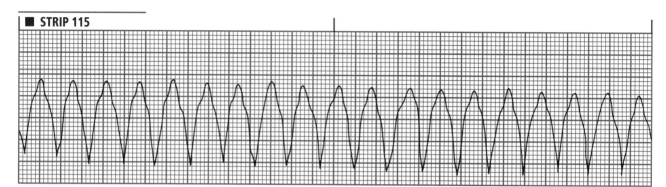

Rhythm: _____   PR interval: _____   QT interval: _____

Rate: _____   QRS complex: _____   Other: _____

P wave: _____   T wave: _____   Interpretation: _____

■ STRIP 116

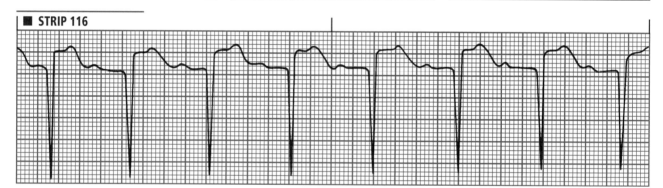

Rhythm: _____   PR interval: _____   QT interval: _____

Rate: _____   QRS complex: _____   Other: _____

P wave: _____   T wave: _____   Interpretation: _____

■ STRIP 117

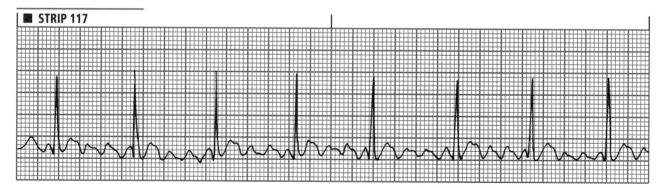

Rhythm: _____   PR interval: _____   QT interval: _____

Rate: _____   QRS complex: _____   Other: _____

P wave: _____   T wave: _____   Interpretation: _____

■ **STRIP 118**

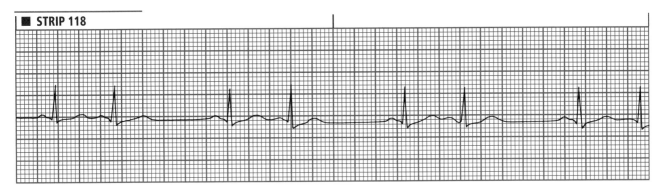

Rhythm: _____   PR interval: _____   QT interval: _____

Rate: _____   QRS complex: _____   Other: _____

P wave: _____   T wave: _____   Interpretation: _____

■ **STRIP 119**

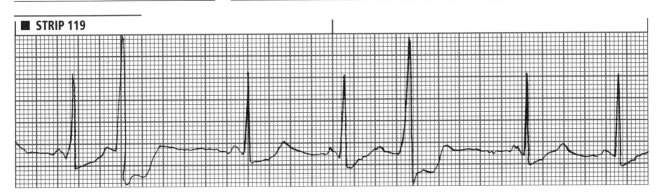

Rhythm: _____   PR interval: _____   QT interval: _____

Rate: _____   QRS complex: _____   Other: _____

P wave: _____   T wave: _____   Interpretation: _____

■ **STRIP 120**

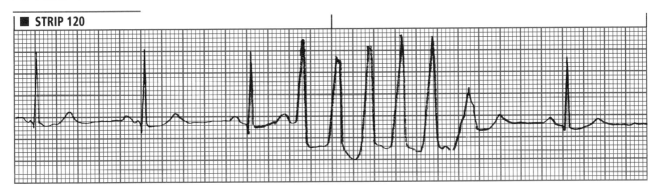

Rhythm: _____   PR interval: _____   QT interval: _____

Rate: _____   QRS complex: _____   Other: _____

P wave: _____   T wave: _____   Interpretation: _____

Posttest answers

STRIP 1
- Rhythm: Irregular
- Rate: 94 beats/minute for underlying rhythm; 150 beats/minute for run
- P wave: Indiscernible
- PR interval: Unmeasurable
- QRS complex: 0.08 second for underlying rhythm
- T wave: Indiscernible
- QT interval: Unmeasurable
- Other: Artifact present
- Interpretation: Normal sinus rhythm (NSR) with a run of ventricular tachycardia (VT)

STRIP 2
- Rhythm: Irregular
- Rate: 70 beats/minute
- P wave: Normal in most beats
- PR interval: 0.16 second
- QRS complex: 0.08 second
- T wave: Normal
- QT interval: 0.40 second
- Other: None
- Interpretation: NSR with junctional beat

STRIP 3
- Rhythm: Irregular
- Rate: 108 beats/minute
- P wave: Normal; absent with premature beats
- PR interval: 0.12 second
- QRS complex: 0.08 second
- T wave: Inverted
- QT interval: 0.28 second
- Other: None
- Interpretation: NSR with premature junctional contractions (PJCs)

STRIP 4
- Rhythm: Irregular
- Rate: 120 beats/minute
- P wave: Normal, then absent
- PR interval: 0.16 second
- QRS complex: 0.08 second
- T wave: Normal
- QT interval: 0.36 second
- Other: None
- Interpretation: NSR with premature atrial tachycardia (PAT)

STRIP 5
- Rhythm: Regular
- Rate: 80 beats/minute
- P wave: Flattened
- PR interval: 0.24 second
- QRS complex: 0.08 second
- T wave: Flattened
- QT interval: 0.32 second
- Other: None
- Interpretation: NSR with first-degree atrioventricular (AV) block

STRIP 6
- Rhythm: Regular
- Rate: 44 beats/minute
- P wave: Normal
- PR interval: Unmeasurable
- QRS complex: 0.12 second
- T wave: Normal
- QT interval: 0.44 second
- Other: P wave not related to QRS complex
- Interpretation: Third-degree AV block

STRIP 7
- Rhythm: Regular
- Rate: 72 beats/minute
- P wave: Some preceded by a pacemaker spike; intrinsic waves normal
- PR interval: 0.16 second in sinus beats
- QRS complex: Unmeasurable
- T wave: Normal
- QT interval: Unmeasurable
- Other: None
- Interpretation: AV pacing leading to sinus rhythm with tracking

STRIP 8
- Rhythm: Chaotic
- Rate: Unmeasurable
- P wave: Indiscernible
- PR interval: Unmeasurable
- QRS complex: Indiscernible
- T wave: Indiscernible
- QT interval: Unmeasurable
- Other: None
- Interpretation: Ventricular fibrillation (VF)

STRIP 9
- Rhythm: Slightly irregular
- Rate: 30 beats/minute
- P wave: Absent
- PR interval: Unmeasurable
- QRS complex: 0.24 second
- T wave: Abnormal
- QT interval: 0.44 second
- Other: None
- Interpretation: Idioventricular rhythm

STRIP 10
- Rhythm: Regular
- Rate: 38 beats/minute
- P wave: Absent
- PR interval: Unmeasurable
- QRS complex: 0.04 second
- T wave: Normal
- QT interval: 0.44 second
- Other: None
- Interpretation: Junctional rhythm

STRIP 11
- Rhythm: Irregular
- Rate: 60 beats/minute
- P wave: Inverted
- PR interval: Variable
- QRS complex: 0.10 second
- T wave: Inverted
- QT interval: 0.40 second
- Other: PR interval increases until dropped beat
- Interpretation: Second-degree AV block, type I

STRIP 12
- Rhythm: Irregular
- Rate: Approximately 110 beats/minute
- P wave: Flutter waves
- PR interval: Indiscernible
- QRS complex: 0.08 second
- T wave: Indiscernible
- QT interval: Indiscernible
- Other: None
- Interpretation: Atrial flutter

STRIP 13
- Rhythm: Regular
- Rate: 79 beats/minute
- P wave: Normal
- PR interval: 0.24 second
- QRS complex: 0.12 second
- T wave: Normal
- QT interval: 0.36 second
- Other: None
- Interpretation: NSR with first-degree AV block

STRIP 14
- Rhythm: Slightly irregular
- Rate: 88 beats/minute
- P wave: Pacemaker generated
- PR Interval: 0.16 second; pacemaker generated
- QRS complex: Follows ventricular spike; unmeasurable
- T wave: Normal
- QT interval: Unmeasurable
- Other: None
- Interpretation: AV pacing with two beats atrial pacing

STRIP 15
- Rhythm: Irregular
- Rate: 60 beats/minute
- P wave: Normal
- PR interval: 0.16 second
- QRS complex: 0.06 second
- T wave: Normal
- QT interval: 0.40 second
- Other: Phasic slowing and quickening
- Interpretation: Sinus arrhythmia

STRIP 16
- Rhythm: Regular
- Rate: 115 beats/minute
- P wave: Abnormal or absent
- PR interval: Unmeasurable
- QRS complex: 0.10 second
- T wave: Normal
- QT interval: 0.32 second
- Other: None
- Interpretation: Junctional tachycardia

STRIP 17
- Rhythm: Regular
- Rate: 52 beats/minute
- P wave: Normal
- PR interval: 0.20 second
- QRS complex: 0.10 second
- T wave: Normal
- QT interval: 0.48 second
- Other: None
- Interpretation: Sinus bradycardia

STRIP 18
- Rhythm: Irregular
- Rate: 130 beats/minute
- P wave: Normal
- PR interval: Unmeasurable
- QRS complex: 0.08 second
- T wave: Variable
- QT interval: Unmeasurable
- Other: None
- Interpretation: Atrial tachycardia with block

STRIP 19
- Rhythm: Irregular
- Rate: 90 beats/minute
- P wave: Absent
- PR interval: Unmeasurable
- QRS complex: Unmeasurable
- T wave: Normal
- QT interval: Unmeasurable
- Other: None
- Interpretation: VVI pacing with premature ventricular contraction (PVC)

STRIP 20
- Rhythm: Regular
- Rate: 88 beats/minute
- P wave: Absent
- PR interval: Absent
- QRS complex: Abnormal
- T wave: Indiscernible
- QT interval: Unmeasurable
- Other: None
- Interpretation: Monomorphic VT

STRIP 21
- Rhythm: Regular
- Rate: 100 beats/minute
- P wave: Normal
- PR interval: 0.16 second
- QRS complex: 0.12 second
- T wave: Normal
- QT interval: 0.32 second
- Other: None
- Interpretation: Sinus tachycardia

STRIP 22
- Rhythm: Regular initially, then absent
- Rate: 107 beats/minute initially, then absent
- P wave: Flattened with sinus beats
- PR interval: 0.20 second
- QRS complex: 0.12 second
- T wave: Normal
- QT interval: 0.36 second
- Other: None
- Interpretation: Sinus tachycardia leading to asystole

STRIP 23
- Rhythm: Irregular
- Rate: 60 beats/minute
- P wave: Fine fibrillation waves
- PR interval: Indiscernible
- QRS complex: 0.08 second
- T wave: Indiscernible
- QT interval: Indiscernible
- Other: None
- Interpretation: Atrial fibrillation

STRIP 24
- Rhythm: Irregular
- Rate: 90 beats/minute
- P wave: Normal
- PR interval: 0.20 second
- QRS complex: 0.12 second
- T wave: Normal
- QT interval: 0.40 second
- Other: None
- Interpretation: NSR with premature atrial contractions (PACs)

STRIP 25
- Rhythm: Regular
- Rate: 54 beats/minute
- P wave: Normal
- PR interval: 0.20 second
- QRS complex: 0.12 second
- T wave: Inverted
- QT interval: 0.36 second
- Other: None
- Interpretation: Sinus bradycardia

STRIP 26
- Rhythm: Irregular
- Rate: 88 beats/minute
- P wave: Normal
- PR interval: 0.20 second
- QRS complex: 0.08 second
- T wave: Normal
- QT interval: 0.28 second
- Other: P wave with missed QRS complex is regular
- Interpretation: Second-degree AV block, type II

STRIP 27
- Rhythm: Regular
- Rate: /9 beats/minute
- P wave: Flutter waves
- PR interval: Unmeasurable
- QRS complex: 0.12 second
- T wave: Indiscernible
- QT interval: Unmeasurable
- Other: None
- Interpretation: Atrial flutter (4:1 block)

STRIP 28

- Rhythm: Irregular
- Rate: 90 beats/minute
- P wave: Normal when present
- PR interval: 0.16 second
- QRS complex: 0.16 second
- T wave: Normal
- QT interval: 0.44 second
- Other: None
- Interpretation: Sinus rhythm with PJCs

STRIP 29

- Rhythm: Irregular
- Rate: 107 beats/minute for underlying rhythm
- P wave: Normal; absent with premature beats
- PR interval: 0.12 second
- QRS complex: 0.08 second for underlying rhythm
- T wave: Variable
- QT interval: Unmeasurable
- Other: None
- Interpretation: Sinus tachycardia with multifocal PVCs (one couplet)

STRIP 30

- Rhythm: Irregular
- Rate: 60 beats/minute
- P wave: Normal
- PR interval: Variable
- QRS complex: 0.16 second
- T wave: Normal
- QT interval: 0.40 second
- Other: PR interval increases until dropped beat
- Interpretation: Second-degree AV block, type I

STRIP 31

- Rhythm: Regular
- Rate: 188 beats/minute
- P wave: Absent
- PR interval: Unmeasurable
- QRS complex: Abnormal
- T wave: Indiscernible
- QT interval: Unmeasurable
- Other: None
- Interpretation: VT

STRIP 32

- Rhythm: Regular
- Rate: 79 beats/minute
- P wave: Retrograde
- PR interval: Unmeasurable
- QRS complex: 0.12 second
- T wave: Normal
- QT interval: 0.52 second
- Other: None
- Interpretation: Accelerated junctional rhythm

STRIP 33

- Rhythm: Irregular
- Rate: 50 beats/minute
- P wave: Normal
- PR interval: 0.20 second
- QRS complex: 0.08 second
- T wave: Normal
- QT interval: 0.44 second
- Other: None
- Interpretation: Sinus bradycardia with PACs

STRIP 34

- Rhythm: Regular
- Rate: 75 beats/minute
- P wave: Normal
- PR interval: 0.36 second
- QRS complex: 0.08 second
- T wave: Normal
- QT interval: 0.36 second
- Other: None
- Interpretation: NSR with first-degree AV block

STRIP 35

- Rhythm: Irregular
- Rate: 88 beats/minute
- P wave: Absent
- PR interval: Unmeasurable
- QRS complex: 0.24 second; pacemaker generated
- T wave: Normal
- QT interval: 0.44 second
- Other: None
- Interpretation: VVI pacing

STRIP 36

- Rhythm: Irregular
- Rate: 80 beats/minute
- P wave: Normal for underlying rhythm; absent for premature beats
- PR interval: 0.20 second
- QRS complex: 0.08 second for underlying rhythm; 0.16 second for premature beats
- T wave: Normal
- QT interval: 0.32 second
- Other: None
- Interpretation: NSR with PVCs (bigeminy)

STRIP 37

- Rhythm: Irregular
- Rate: Approximately 160 beats/minute
- P wave: Flutter waves
- PR interval: Unmeasurable
- QRS complex: 0.08 second
- T wave: Indiscernible
- QT interval: Unmeasurable
- Other: None
- Interpretation: Atrial flutter with varying conduction ratios

STRIP 38

- Rhythm: Regular
- Rate: 43 beats/minute
- P wave: Normal
- PR interval: Unmeasurable
- QRS complex: 0.12 second
- T wave: Normal
- QT interval: Unmeasurable
- Other: P wave not related to QRS complex
- Interpretation: Third-degree AV block

STRIP 39

- Rhythm: Regular
- Rate: 100 beats/minute
- P wave: Normal initially, then becomes inverted with shortened PR interval
- PR interval: 0.14 second initially, then unmeasurable
- QRS complex: 0.08 second
- T wave: Normal
- QT interval: 0.36 second
- Other: None
- Interpretation: Sinus tachycardia leading to junctional tachycardia

STRIP 40
- Rhythm: Regular
- Rate: 150 beats/minute
- P wave: Indiscernible
- PR interval: Unmeasurable
- QRS complex: 0.08 second
- T wave: Indiscernible
- QT interval: Unmeasurable
- Other: None
- Interpretation: Atrial tachycardia

STRIP 41
- Rhythm: Irregular
- Rate: 110 beats/minute
- P wave: Fine fibrillation waves
- PR interval: Indiscernible
- QRS complex: 0.08 second
- T wave: Indiscernible
- QT interval: Unmeasurable
- Other: None
- Interpretation: Atrial fibrillation

STRIP 42
- Rhythm: Irregular
- Rate: 70 beats/minute
- P wave: Normal; absent during premature beat
- PR interval: 0.16 second
- QRS complex: 0.08 second
- T wave: Normal
- QT interval: 0.40 second
- Other: None
- Interpretation: NSR with PJCs

STRIP 43
- Rhythm: Regular
- Rate: 88 beats/minute
- P wave: Pacemaker generated
- PR interval: 0.12 second; pacemaker generated
- QRS complex: 0.20 second; pacemaker generated
- T wave: Indiscernible
- QT interval: Unmeasurable
- Other: None
- Interpretation: AV pacing

STRIP 44
- Rhythm: Irregular
- Rate: 100 beats/minute
- P wave: Abnormal; slight sawtooth appearance
- PR interval: Unmeasurable
- QRS complex: 0.10 second
- T wave: Abnormal
- QT interval: Unmeasurable
- Other: None
- Interpretation: Atrial flutter with varying conduction ratios

STRIP 45
- Rhythm: Irregular
- Rate: 150 beats/minute
- P wave: Normal for underlying rhythm; absent for premature beats
- PR interval: 0.12 second
- QRS complex: 0.08 second for sinus beats
- T wave: Normal
- QT interval: 0.24 second
- Other: None
- Interpretation: Sinus tachycardia with unifocal PVCs

STRIP 46
- Rhythm: Slightly irregular
- Rate: 80 beats/minute
- P wave: Absent
- PR interval: Unmeasurable
- QRS complex: 0.16 second for underlying rhythm
- T wave: Normal
- QT interval: 0.44 second
- Other: None
- Interpretation: Accelerated idioventricular rhythm (AIVR)

STRIP 47
- Rhythm: Irregular
- Rate: 88 beats/minute
- P wave: Normal
- PR Interval: 0.16 second
- QRS complex: 0.08 second
- T wave: Normal
- QT interval: 0.40 second
- Other: ST-segment depression
- Interpretation: NSR with PACs

STRIP 48
- Rhythm: Irregular
- Rate: 94 beats/minute for underlying rhythm; 167 beats/minute for run
- P wave: Normal with sinus beats
- PR interval: 0.16 second
- QRS complex: 0.08 second
- T wave: Normal
- QT interval: 0.36 second
- Other: None
- Interpretation: NSR with PAT

STRIP 49
- Rhythm: Irregular
- Rate: 70 beats/minute
- P wave: Fine fibrillation waves initially, then normal
- PR interval: Unmeasurable initially, then 0.24 second
- QRS complex: 0.12 second
- T wave: Indiscernible initially, then normal
- QT interval: Unmeasurable initially, then 0.32 second
- Other: None
- Interpretation: Atrial fibrillation converting to NSR

STRIP 50
- Rhythm: Irregular
- Rate: 120 beats/minute
- P wave: Fine fibrillation waves
- PR interval: Unmeasurable
- QRS complex: 0.08 second
- T wave: Normal
- QT interval: Unmeasurable
- Other: None
- Interpretation: Atrial fibrillation

STRIP 51
- Rhythm: Irregular
- Rate: 60 beats/minute
- P wave: Normal
- PR interval: Variable
- QRS complex: 0.08 second
- T wave: Distorted by P waves
- QT interval: Unmeasurable
- Other: PR interval increases until dropped beat
- Interpretation: Second-degree AV block, type I

STRIP 52
- Rhythm: Slightly irregular
- Rate: 70 beats/minute
- P wave: Flutter waves
- PR interval: Unmeasurable
- QRS complex: 0.08 second
- T wave: Indiscernible
- QT interval: Indiscernible
- Other: None
- Interpretation: Atrial flutter (4:1 block)

STRIP 53
- Rhythm: Irregular
- Rate: 140 beats/minute
- P wave: Fine fibrillation waves present for underlying rhythm; absent for pair and run
- PR interval: Absent
- QRS complex: 0.04 second for underlying rhythm
- T wave: Indiscernible
- QT interval: Indiscernible
- Other: None
- Interpretation: Atrial fibrillation with a pair of PVCs and a run of VT

STRIP 54
- Rhythm: Regular
- Rate: 63 beats/minute
- P wave: Notched
- PR interval: 0.28 second
- QRS complex: 0.08 second
- T wave: Distorted by P wave
- QT interval: Unmeasurable
- Other: None
- Interpretation: Second-degree AV block, type II (2:1)

STRIP 55
- Rhythm: Irregular
- Rate: Underlying, 70 beats/minute
- P wave: Normal
- PR interval: 0.16 second
- QRS complex: 0.12 second
- T wave: Normal
- QT interval: 0.36 second
- Other: P wave on time with missing QRS complex
- Interpretation: Second-degree AV block, type II

STRIP 56
- Rhythm: Irregular
- Rate: 70 beats/minute
- P wave: Normal
- PR interval: 0.16 second
- QRS complex: 0.08 second
- T wave: Inverted
- QT interval: 0.48 second
- Other: None
- Interpretation: NSR with PACs

STRIP 57
- Rhythm: Irregular
- Rate: 60 beats/minute
- P wave: Variable
- PR interval: Variable
- QRS complex: 0.08 second
- T wave: Inverted
- QT interval: 0.36 second
- Other: None
- Interpretation: Wandering atrial pacemaker with PJCs

STRIP 58
- Rhythm: Regular
- Rate: 65 beats/minute
- P wave: Normal
- PR interval: 0.40 second
- QRS complex: 0.08 second
- T wave: Normal
- QT interval: 0.28 second
- Other: None
- Interpretation: NSR with first-degree AV block

STRIP 59
- Rhythm: Irregular
- Rate: 125 beats/minute for underlying rhythm; 150 to 167 beats/minute for run
- P wave: Normal with sinus beats
- PR interval: 0.12 second
- QRS complex: 0.04 second
- T wave: Normal
- QT interval: 0.32 second
- Other: None
- Interpretation: Sinus tachycardia with PAT

STRIP 60
- Rhythm: Irregular
- Rate: 94 beats/minute for underlying rhythm; 167 beats/minute for run
- P wave: Normal with sinus beats
- PR interval: 0.20 second
- QRS complex: 0.08 second
- T wave: Normal with sinus beats
- QT interval: 0.40 second
- Other: None
- Interpretation: PAT leading to NSR

STRIP 61
- Rhythm: Slightly irregular
- Rate: 110 beats/minute
- P wave: P wave shape different for multiple P waves
- PR interval: Unmeasurable
- QRS complex: 0.08 second
- T wave: Indiscernible
- QT interval: Unmeasurable
- Other: None
- Interpretation: Multifocal atrial tachycardia

STRIP 62
- Rhythm: Regular
- Rate: 115 beats/minute
- P wave: Absent
- PR interval: Unmeasurable
- QRS complex: 0.08 second
- T wave: Normal
- QT interval: 0.36 second
- Other: None
- Interpretation: Junctional tachycardia

STRIP 63
- Rhythm: Regular
- Rate: 107 beats/minute
- P wave: Normal
- PR interval: 0.16 second
- QRS complex: 0.12 second
- T wave: Normal
- QT interval: 0.36 second
- Other: None
- Interpretation: Sinus tachycardia

STRIP 64
- Rhythm: Slightly irregular
- Rate: 40 beats/minute
- P wave: Variable
- PR interval: 0.16 second
- QRS complex: 0.08 second
- T wave: Normal
- QT interval: 0.44 second
- Other: None
- Interpretation: Wandering atrial pacemaker

STRIP 65
- Rhythm: Irregular
- Rate: 140 beats/minute
- P wave: Absent
- PR interval: Absent
- QRS complex: Abnormal
- T wave: Indiscernible
- QT interval: Unmeasurable
- Other: None
- Interpretation: VT

STRIP 66
- Rhythm: Irregular
- Rate: 30 beats/minute
- P wave: Absent
- PR Interval: Absent
- QRS complex: 0.20 second
- T wave: Abnormal
- QT interval: Unmeasurable
- Other: None
- Interpretation: Idioventricular rhythm

STRIP 67
- Rhythm: Irregular
- Rate: 100 beats/minute for underlying rhythm; 214 to 300 beats/minute for run
- P wave: Variable
- PR interval: Variable
- QRS complex: 0.08 second for underlying rhythm
- T wave: Normal for underlying rhythm
- QT interval: 0.28 second
- Other: None
- Interpretation: Possible NSR with a run of VT

STRIP 68
- Rhythm: Irregular
- Rate: 60 beats/minute
- P wave: Inverted
- PR interval: 0.20 second
- QRS complex: 0.08 second
- T wave: Normal
- QT interval:0.44 second
- Other: Pause occurs at 1.48 second
- Interpretation: Accelerated junctional rhythm with pause

STRIP 69
- Rhythm: Irregular
- Rate: 100 beats/minute
- P wave: Normal
- PR interval: 0.16 second
- QRS complex: 0.08 second
- T wave: Normal
- QT interval: 0.40 second
- Other: None
- Interpretation: NSR with PACs

STRIP 70
- Rhythm: Regular
- Rate: 75 beats/minute
- P wave: Abnormal within T wave
- PR interval: Unmeasurable
- QRS complex: 0.08 second
- T wave: Distorted by P wave
- QT interval: Unmeasurable
- Other: None
- Interpretation: Accelerated junctional rhythm

STRIP 71
- Rhythm: Regular
- Rate: 63 beats/minute
- P wave: Absent
- PR interval: Unmeasurable
- QRS complex: 0.08 second
- T wave: Normal
- QT interval: 0.40 second
- Other: None
- Interpretation: Junctional rhythm

STRIP 72
- Rhythm: Regular
- Rate: 188 beats/minute
- P wave: Absent
- PR interval: Unmeasurable
- QRS complex: Abnormal
- T wave: Indiscernible
- QT interval: Unmeasurable
- Other: None
- Interpretation: VT

STRIP 73
- Rhythm: Regular
- Rate: 28 beats/minute
- P wave: Normal
- PR interval: Unmeasurable
- QRS complex: 0.16 second
- T wave: Distorted by P wave
- QT interval: Unmeasurable
- Other: P wave not related to QRS complex
- Interpretation: Third-degree AV block

STRIP 74
- Rhythm: Irregular
- Rate: 60 beats/minute
- P wave: Flutter waves
- PR interval: Unmeasurable
- QRS complex: 0.08 second
- T wave: Indiscernible
- QT interval: Unmeasurable
- Other: None
- Interpretation: Atrial flutter with varying conduction ratios

STRIP 75
- Rhythm: Regular
- Rate: 75 beats/minute
- P wave: Normal
- PR interval: 0.32 second
- QRS complex: 0.08 second
- T wave: Normal
- QT interval: 0.44 second
- Other: None
- Interpretation: NSR with first-degree AV block

STRIP 76
- Rhythm: Irregular
- Rate: 130 beats/minute
- P wave: Fine fibrillation waves
- PR interval: Unmeasurable
- QRS complex: 0.08 second
- T wave: Indiscernible
- QT interval: Unmeasurable
- Other: None
- Interpretation: Atrial fibrillation

STRIP 77
- Rhythm: Regular
- Rate: 84 beats/minute
- P wave: Normal
- PR interval: 0.16 second
- QRS complex: 0.08 second
- T wave: Normal
- QT interval: 0.40 second
- Other: None
- Interpretation: NSR

STRIP 78
- Rhythm: Chaotic
- Rate: Unmeasurable
- P wave: Absent
- PR interval: Unmeasurable
- QRS complex: Absent
- T wave: Absent
- QT interval: Unmeasurable
- Other: None
- Interpretation: VF

STRIP 79
- Rhythm: Irregular
- Rate: 50 beats/minute
- P wave: Normal
- PR interval: Variable
- QRS complex: 0.08 second
- T wave: Inverted
- QT interval: 0.44 second
- Other: PR interval increases until dropped beat
- Interpretation: Second-degree AV block, type I

STRIP 80
- Rhythm: Regular
- Rate: 84 beats/minute
- P wave: Absent
- PR interval: Unmeasurable
- QRS complex: 0.16 second
- T wave: Normal
- QT interval: 0.52 second
- Other: None
- Interpretation: AIVR

STRIP 81
- Rhythm: Regular
- Rate: 115 beats/minute
- P wave: Normal
- PR interval: 0.16 second
- QRS complex: 0.08 second
- T wave: Normal
- QT interval: 0.36 second
- Other: None
- Interpretation: Sinus tachycardia

STRIP 82
- Rhythm: Irregular
- Rate: 120 beats/minute
- P wave: Fine fibrillation waves
- PR interval: Unmeasurable
- QRS complex: 0.08 second
- T wave: Indiscernible
- QT interval: Unmeasurable
- Other: None
- Interpretation: Atrial fibrillation with unifocal PVCs

STRIP 83
- Rhythm: Absent
- Rate: Absent
- P wave: Absent
- PR interval: Unmeasurable
- QRS complex: Absent
- T wave: Absent
- QT interval: Unmeasurable
- Other: None
- Interpretation: Asystole

STRIP 84
- Rhythm: Irregular
- Rate: 40 beats/minute
- P wave: Normal for underlying rhythm; inverted with shortened PR interval for premature beat
- PR interval: 0.20 second; shortened with premature beat
- QRS complex: 0.08 second
- T wave: Peaked
- QT interval: 0.44 second
- Other: None
- Interpretation: Sinus bradycardia with PJCs

STRIP 85
- Rhythm: Irregular
- Rate: Unmeasurable
- P wave: Indiscernible
- PR interval: Unmeasurable
- QRS complex: Abnormal
- T wave: Indiscernible
- QT interval: Unmeasurable
- Other: Continuous switching of ventricular rhythm between positive and negative directions
- Interpretation: Torsades de pointes

STRIP 86
- Rhythm: Slightly irregular
- Rate: 50 beats/minute
- P wave: Variable
- PR interval: Variable
- QRS complex: 0.08 second
- T wave: Normal
- QT interval: 0.40 second
- Other: None
- Interpretation: Wandering atrial pacemaker

STRIP 87
- Rhythm: Slightly irregular
- Rate: 70 beats/minute
- P wave: Normal
- PR interval: 0.20 second
- QRS complex: 0.08 second
- T wave: Normal
- QT interval: 0.36 second
- Other: Phasic slowing and quickening
- Interpretation: Sinus arrhythmia

STRIP 88
- Rhythm: Regular
- Rate: 60 beats/minute
- P wave: Inverted
- PR interval: 0.10 second
- QRS complex: 0.12 second
- T wave: Normal
- QT interval: 0.44 second
- Other: None
- Interpretation: Junctional rhythm

STRIP 89
- Rhythm: Irregular
- Rate: 50 beats/minute
- P wave: Normal
- PR interval: 0.28 second
- QRS complex: 0.12 second
- T wave: Normal
- QT interval: 0.60 second
- Other: P wave on time with dropped QRS complex
- Interpretation: Second-degree AV block, type II

STRIP 90
- Rhythm: Irregular
- Rate: 60 beats/minute
- P wave: Fine fibrillation waves; some flutter waves
- PR interval: Unmeasurable
- QRS complex: 0.08 second
- T wave: Indiscernible
- QT interval: Unmeasurable
- Other: None
- Interpretation: Atrial fibrillation/atrial flutter

STRIP 91
- Rhythm: Regular
- Rate: 188 beats/minute
- P wave: Indiscernible
- PR interval: Unmeasurable
- QRS complex: 0.12 second
- T wave: Distorted by P wave
- QT interval: Unmeasurable
- Other: None
- Interpretation: Atrial tachycardia

STRIP 92
- Rhythm: Regular
- Rate: 65 beats/minute
- P wave: Absent
- PR interval: Absent
- QRS complex: 0.20 second; pacemaker generated
- T wave: Distorted by pacer beat
- QT interval: Unmeasurable
- Other: None
- Interpretation: Ventricular pacing

STRIP 93
- Rhythm: Regular
- Rate: 75 beats/minute
- P wave: Normal
- PR interval: 0.36 second
- QRS complex: 0.08 second
- T wave: Normal
- QT interval: 0.48 second
- Other: None
- Interpretation: NSR with first-degree AV block

STRIP 94
- Rhythm: Regular
- Rate: 47 beats/minute
- P wave: Normal
- PR interval: 0.20 second
- QRS complex: 0.08 second
- T wave: Normal
- QT interval: 0.52 second
- Other: None
- Interpretation: Sinus bradycardia

STRIP 95
- Rhythm: Chaotic
- Rate: Unmeasurable
- P wave: Absent
- PR interval: Unmeasurable
- QRS complex: Abnormal
- T wave: Absent
- QT interval: Unmeasurable
- Other: None
- Interpretation: VF

STRIP 96
- Rhythm: Irregular
- Rate: 60 beats/minute
- P wave: Normal
- PR interval: 0.16 second
- QRS complex: 0.08 second
- T wave: Normal
- QT interval: 0.60 second
- Other: None
- Interpretation: Sinus bradycardia with unifocal PVCs

STRIP 97
- Rhythm: Irregular
- Rate: 100 beats/minute
- P wave: Fine fibrillation waves
- PR interval: Unmeasurable
- QRS complex: 0.08 second
- T wave: Indiscernible
- QT interval: Unmeasurable
- Other: None
- Interpretation: Atrial fibrillation

STRIP 98
- Rhythm: Regular
- Rate: 84 beats/minute
- P wave: Normal
- PR interval: 0.20 second
- QRS complex: 0.08 second
- T wave: Normal
- QT interval: 0.36 second
- Other: None
- Interpretation: NSR

STRIP 99
- Rhythm: Regular
- Rate: 79 beats/minute
- P wave: Normal
- PR interval: 0.16 second
- QRS complex: 0.08 second
- T wave: Normal
- QT interval: 0.40 second
- Other: None
- Interpretation: NSR

STRIP 100
- Rhythm: Irregular
- Rate: 60 beats/minute
- P wave: Normal
- PR interval: 0.20 second
- QRS complex: 0.08 second
- T wave: Normal
- QT interval: 0.40 second
- Other: None
- Interpretation: Sinus bradycardia with PVC

STRIP 101
- Rhythm: Irregular
- Rate: 68 beats/minute for underlying rhythm; 188 beats/minute for run
- P wave: Normal
- PR interval: 0.20 second
- QRS complex: 0.08 second
- T wave: Normal
- QT interval: 0.40 second
- Other: None
- Interpretation: Sinus rhythm with a run of VT

STRIP 102
- Rhythm: Irregular
- Rate: 90 beats/minute
- P wave: Flutter waves
- PR interval: Unmeasurable
- QRS complex: 0.08 second
- T wave: Distorted by P waves
- QT interval: Unmeasurable
- Other: None
- Interpretation: Atrial flutter with varying conduction ratios

STRIP 103
- Rhythm: Regular
- Rate: 100 beats/minute
- P wave: Normal
- PR interval: 0.16 second
- QRS complex: 0.08 second
- T wave: Normal
- QT interval: 0.32 second
- Other: None
- Interpretation: Sinus tachycardia

STRIP 104
- Rhythm: Irregular
- Rate: 63 beats/minute initially, then 188 to 214 beats/minute
- P wave: Normal initially, then absent
- PR interval: 0.16 second initially, then absent and unmeasurable
- QRS complex: 0.08 second initially, then abnormal and variable
- T wave: Normal initially, then indiscernible
- QT interval: Unmeasurable
- Other: None
- Interpretation: NSR leading to sustained VT

STRIP 105
- Rhythm: Regular
- Rate: 36 beats/minute
- P wave: Normal
- PR interval: Unmeasurable
- QRS complex: 0.12 second
- T wave: Normal
- QT interval: 0.36 second
- Other: P wave not related to QRS complex
- Interpretation: Third-degree AV block

STRIP 106
- Rhythm: Regular
- Rate: 70 beats/minute
- P wave: Flutter waves
- PR interval: Unmeasurable
- QRS complex: 0.08 second
- T wave: Indiscernible
- QT interval: Unmeasurable
- Other: None
- Interpretation: Atrial flutter (4:1 block)

STRIP 107
- Rhythm: Irregular
- Rate: 110 beats/minute
- P wave: Normal
- PR interval: 0.16 second
- QRS complex: 0.08 second
- T wave: Normal
- QT interval: 0.32 second
- Other: None
- Interpretation: Sinus tachycardia with unifocal PVCs

STRIP 108
- Rhythm: Regular
- Rate: 30 beats/minute
- P wave: Absent
- PR interval: Unmeasurable
- QRS complex: Abnormal
- T wave: Abnormal
- QT interval: Unmeasurable
- Other: None
- Interpretation: Idioventricular rhythm

STRIP 109
- Rhythm: Irregular
- Rate: 75 beats/minute for underlying rhythm; 188 beats/minute for run
- P wave: Normal
- PR interval: 0.20 second initially, then unmeasurable
- QRS complex: 0.08 second for underlying rhythm and run
- T wave: Normal
- QT interval: 0.36 second
- Other: None
- Interpretation: NSR leading to PAT

STRIP 110
- Rhythm: Irregular
- Rate: 60 beats/minute
- P wave: Normal
- PR interval: Variable
- QRS complex: 0.08 second
- T wave: Distorted by P waves
- QT interval: Unmeasurable
- Other: PR interval increases until dropped beat
- Interpretation: Second-degree AV block, type I

STRIP 111
- Rhythm: Chaotic
- Rate: Unmeasurable
- P wave: Absent
- PR interval: Unmeasurable
- QRS complex: Unmeasurable
- T wave: Absent
- QT interval: Unmeasurable
- Other: None
- Interpretation: VF

STRIP 112
- Rhythm: Regular
- Rate: 30 beats/minute
- P wave: Normal
- PR interval: Unmeasurable
- QRS complex: 0.16 second
- T wave: Distorted by P waves
- QT interval: Unmeasurable
- Other: P wave not related to QRS complex
- Interpretation: Third-degree AV block

STRIP 113
- Rhythm: Regular
- Rate: 58 beats/minute
- P wave: Normal
- PR interval: 0.36 second
- QRS complex: 0.08 second
- T wave: Inverted
- QT interval: 0.44 second
- Other: None
- Interpretation: Sinus bradycardia with first-degree AV block

STRIP 114
- Rhythm: Irregular
- Rate: 60 beats/minute
- P wave: Normal
- PR interval: 0.16 second
- QRS complex: 0.08 second
- T wave: Normal
- QT interval: 0.40 second
- Other: None
- Interpretation: NSR with sinus arrest

STRIP 115
- Rhythm: Regular
- Rate: 214 beats/minute
- P wave: Absent
- PR interval: Unmeasurable
- QRS complex: Abnormal
- T wave: Indiscernible
- QT interval: Unmeasurable
- Other: None
- Interpretation: VT

STRIP 116
- Rhythm: Regular
- Rate: 75 beats/minute
- P wave: Normal
- PR interval: 0.32 second
- QRS complex: 0.08 second
- T wave: Normal
- QT interval: 0.44 second
- Other: None
- Interpretation: NSR with first-degree AV block

STRIP 117
- Rhythm: Regular
- Rate: 84 beats/minute
- P wave: Flutter waves
- PR interval: Unmeasurable
- QRS complex: 0.08 second
- T wave: Indiscernible
- QT interval: Indiscernible
- Other: None
- Interpretation: Atrial flutter (4:1 block)

STRIP 118
- Rhythm: Irregular
- Rate: 80 beats/minute
- P wave: Normal
- PR interval: 0.20 second
- QRS complex: 0.06 second
- T wave: Normal
- QT interval: 0.36 second
- Other: None
- Interpretation: NSR with PACs (atrial bigeminy)

STRIP 119
- Rhythm: Irregular
- Rate: 65 beats/minute
- P wave: Normal
- PR interval: 0.14 second
- QRS complex: 0.06 second
- T wave: Normal
- QT interval: 0.44 second
- Other: None
- Interpretation: NSR with unifocal PVCs

STRIP 120
- Rhythm: Irregular
- Rate: 63 beats/minute for underlying rhythm; 167 to 214 beats/minute for run
- P wave: Normal with sinus beats
- PR interval: 0.16 second
- QRS complex: 0.04 second
- T wave: Normal
- QT interval: 0.40 second
- Other: None
- Interpretation: NSR with a run of VT

Electrolyte and drug effects on ECGs

ECG effects of hyperkalemia

The classic and most striking electrocardiogram (ECG) feature of hyperkalemia is tall, peaked T waves. This rhythm strip below shows a typical peaked T wave (shaded area).

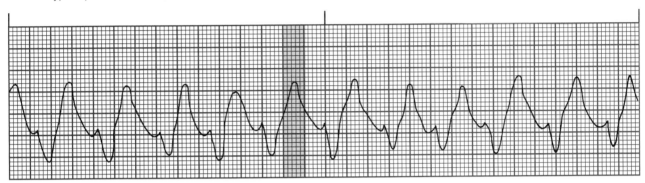

ECG effects of hypokalemia

As serum potassium concentration drops, T waves become flat and U waves appear (shaded area). This rhythm strip below shows the typical ECG effects of hypokalemia.

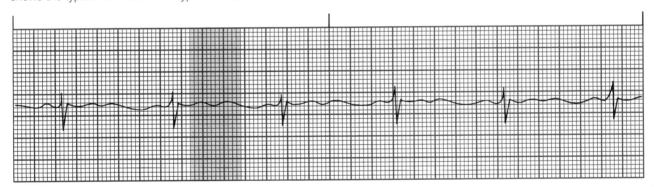

ECG effects of hypercalcemia

Increased serum concentrations of calcium cause shortening of the QT intervals, as shown in the ECG strip below (see shaded area).

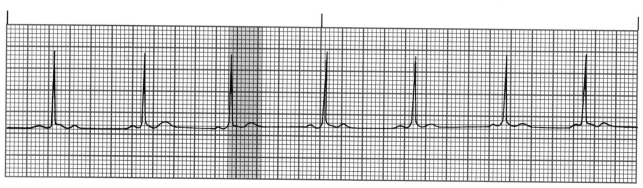

ECG effects of hypocalcemia

Decreased serum concentrations of calcium prolong the QT intervals, as shown in the ECG strip below (see shaded area).

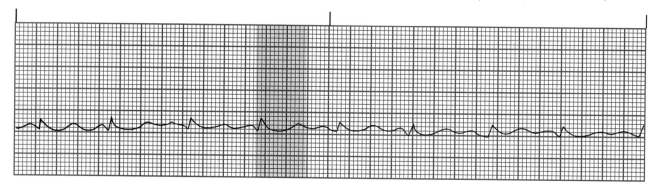

ECG effects of class IA antiarrhythmics

Class IA antiarrhythmics—such as procainamide and quinidine—affect the cardiac cycle in specific ways and lead to specific ECG changes, including slightly widened QRS complexes and prolonged QT intervals (see shaded area below). These drugs:

- block sodium influx during phase 0, which depresses the rate of depolarization
- prolong repolarization and the duration of the action potential
- lengthen the refractory period
- decrease contractility.

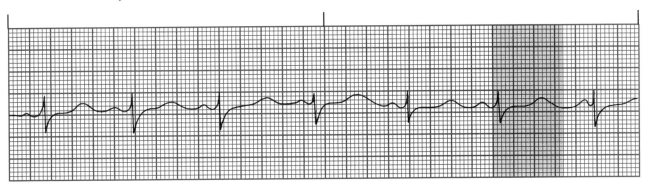

ECG effects of class IB antiarrhythmics

Class IB antiarrhythmics—such as lidocaine and tocainide—can cause QRS complexes to be slightly widened (see shaded area below). The PR intervals may also be prolonged. Class IB antiarrhythmics can also:

- block sodium influx during phase 0, which depresses the rate of depolarization
- shorten repolarization and the duration of the action potential
- suppress ventricular automaticity in ischemic tissue.

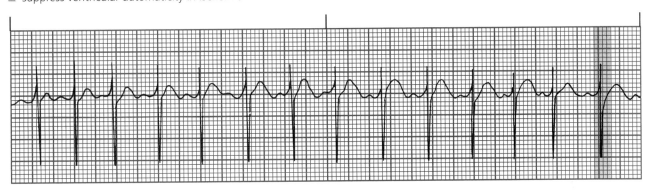

ECG effects of class IC antiarrhythmics

Class IC antiarrhythmics—such as flecainide, moricizine, and propafenone—exert particular actions on the cardiac cycle and lead to:

■ prolonged PR intervals (see shaded area, below left)
■ widened QRS complexes (see shaded area, below center)
■ prolonged QT intervals (see shaded area, below right).

These agents block sodium influx during phase 0, which depresses the rate of depolarization. Class IC antiarrhythmics exert no effect on repolarization or the duration of the action potential.

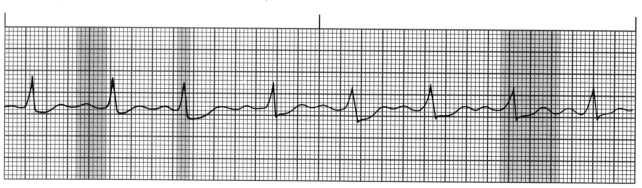

ECG effects of class II antiarrhythmics

Class II antiarrhythmics, including such beta-adrenergic blockers as acebutolol, esmolol, and propranolol:

■ depress sinoatrial node automaticity
■ shorten the duration of the action potential
■ increase the refractory period of atrial and atrioventricular (AV) junctional tissues, which slows conduction
■ inhibit sympathetic activity.
  ECG changes include:
■ slightly prolonged PR intervals (see shaded area, below left)
■ slightly shortened QT intervals (see shaded area, below right).

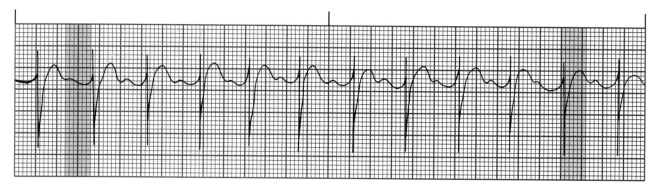

ECG effects of class III antiarrhythmics

Class III antiarrhythmics, such as amiodarone, ibutilide, and sotalol:
- block potassium movement during phase 3
- increase the duration of the action potential
- prolong the effective refractory period.
  ECG changes include:
- slightly prolonged PR intervals (see shaded area, below left)
- widened QRS complexes (see shaded area, below center)
- prolonged QT intervals (see shaded area, below right).

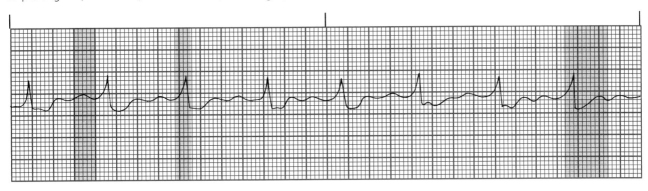

ECG effects of class IV antiarrhythmics

Class IV antiarrhythmics—including such calcium channel blockers as diltiazem and verapamil—can cause prolonged PR intervals (see shaded area below). These drugs:
- block calcium movement during phase 2
- prolong the conduction time and increase the refractory period in the AV node
- decrease contractility.

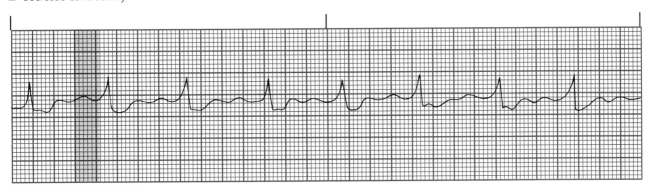

ECG effects of digoxin

Digoxin affects the cardiac cycle in various ways and may lead to:

■ gradual sloping of ST segments, causing ST-segment depression in the opposite direction of the QRS deflection (see shaded area below)

■ possible notched P waves.

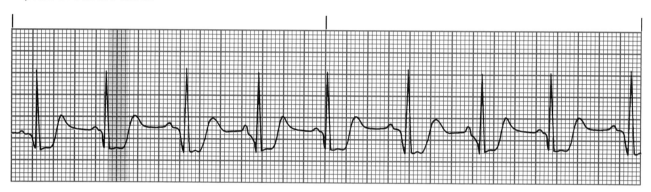

Selected references

ACLS Review Made Incredibly Easy. Philadelphia: Lippincott Williams & Wilkins, 2006.

Chiu, C., et al. "Diagnosis and Treatment of Idiopathic Ventricular Tachycardia," *AACN Advanced Critical Care* 15(3):449-461, July-September 2004.

Ebert, H. *Easy ECG: Interpretation—Differential Diagnosis.* New York: Thieme New York, 2004.

ECG Interpretation: An Incredibly Easy Pocket Guide. Philadelphia: Lippincott Williams & Wilkins, 2006.

Hesselson, A. *Simplified Interpretations of Pacemaker ECGs.* Oxford: Blackwell Publishing, 2003.

Interpreting Difficult ECGs. Philadelphia: Lippincott Williams & Wilkins, 2006.

Jones, S. *ECG Notes: Interpretation and Management Guide.* Philadelphia: F.A. Davis Co., 2005.

Page, B. *12-lead ECG for the Acute Care Provider.* New Jersey: Prentice Hall Health, 2005.

Poon, K., et al. "Diagnostic Performance of a Computer-Based ECG Rhythm Algorithm," *Journal of Electrocardiology* 38(4):235-38, October 2005.

Phalen, T., and Aehlert, B. *The 12-lead ECG in Acute Coronary Syndrome,* 2nd ed. Philadelphia: Mosby–Year Book, Inc., 2006.

Schiavone, W. *Clinically Relevant Electrocardiology.* Ontario: B.C. Decker, Inc., 2006.

Wellens, H., and Conover, M.B. *The ECG in Emergency Decision Making,* 2nd ed. Philadelphia: W.B. Saunders Co., 2006.

Zimmerman, F. *Clinical Electrocardiography: Review and Study Guide,* 2nd ed. New York: McGraw-Hill Professional, 2004.

Index

i refers to an illustration; t refers to a table.

i refers to an illustration; t refers to a table.

i refers to an illustration; t refers to a table.